"Phelan and Lloyd have assembled a highly informative and readable text that focuses first on what the concept of equitable, person-centered care can actually mean and then on how to operationalise that in practice. They provide living examples from community action researchers in several countries and across the life course, but are particularly focused on the care of older people. I expect this to be a go-to publication that will be widely used by health professionals across many caring disciplines".

Cecily Kelleher, *Professor of Public Health Medicine & Epidemiology, School of Public Health, Physiotherapy and Sports Science, University College Dublin*

"The authors offer a comprehensive and integrative overview of the diverse perspectives and contexts that together form a compelling vision of person-centered care as a collective endeavour. [...] This is an invaluable contribution to the field, providing a nuanced understanding of 'community' as a dynamic network of shared identity, mutuality and evolving relationships, rather than a fixed geographical space".

Axel Wolf, *Professor, senior consultant anesthesia (CRNA) and affiliated researcher at the University of Gothenburg, Director, Centre for Person-Centred Care (GPCC).*

COMMUNITY CENTRED HEALTH AND WELL-BEING

This insightful volume examines how the principles and practice of person-centred care can be extended to operate at the level of community health and well-being.

Split into three parts, this book articulates the conditions under which community-centred health and well-being can be made possible, discussing issues such as capacity building, community participation, determinants of health (social, economic and cultural) and the political landscape around governmental and non-governmental organizations. The first part sets the context, highlighting the reorientation of care from a bio-medical model to a psychosocial one. The second part outlines a number of different approaches through which community-centred health and well-being can be fostered, while the final part features some of these approaches in action, from social prescribing and adult education to early childhood visiting and integrated care technology for older people.

Thought-provoking and cohesive, this important collection will interest students, scholars, policymakers and voluntary organizations working across public health, social care and community development.

Amanda Phelan is Full Professor in General Nursing, School of Nursing, Psychotherapy and Community Health, Dublin City University, Ireland.

Helen Lloyd is Full Professor in Applied Social and Cultural Psychology, School of Psychology, Faculty of Health, University of Plymouth, UK.

COMMUNITY CENTRED HEALTH AND WELL-BEING

Approaches and Cases

Edited by
Amanda Phelan and Helen Lloyd

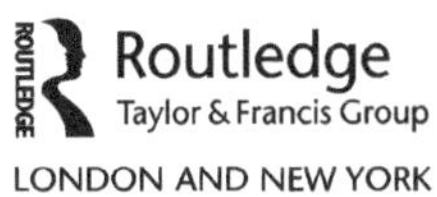

LONDON AND NEW YORK

Designed cover image: Getty Images

First published 2026
by Routledge
4 Park Square, Milton Park, Abingdon, Oxon OX14 4RN

and by Routledge
605 Third Avenue, New York, NY 10158

Routledge is an imprint of the Taylor & Francis Group, an informa business

British Library Cataloguing-in-Publication Data
A catalogue record for this book is available from the British Library

ISBN: 978-1-032-66279-4 (hbk)
ISBN: 978-1-032-66262-6 (pbk)
ISBN: 978-1-032-66265-7 (ebk)

DOI: 10.4324/9781032662657

Typeset in Times New Roman
by codeMantra

CONTENTS

DEDICATION AND ACKNOWLEDGEMENTS

This book is dedicated to all the communities of people who suffer the effects of marginalisation and poverty, and in particular, to all those communities that are currently being destroyed by acts of political violence and war.

This book would not be possible without numerous collaborations with the co-authors, who have brought such expertise to the project. Bringing together such a diverse conceptual, practice-based based and research exemplars would not be possible without the generosity of their contribution. We thank you.

Many colleagues have also offered engaging conversations and alternative insights into the development of the book, and we are grateful for their insights and debate.

Helen Lloyd owes a debt of thanks to Alex Vessis, Suvi Rehell and all the staff at Devon and Cornwall Refugee Support. The work you do to support displaced people is inspiring and heartwarming. I am also immensely grateful to you for being generous research collaborators in the research presented in Chapter 5. Research of which would not have been possible without an amazingly sensitive and intelligent team of researchers committed to social justice. Special thanks are therefore due to Dr Wen-Yu Wu, Dr Hoayda Darkal, Yasmin Ansbro, Dr Megan Stuart Richards, Jet Newcomb, Dr Zahraa Abdulreda and Dr Louise Morgan.

A particular debt of thanks goes to Lucy Howling who supported the creation of this book during the editing stage and the School of Psychology at the University of Plymouth who also supported this work.

Finally, thanks to our families who were always at our shoulders. For Amanda Phelan, thanks go to Gary for your friendship, love and encouragement, and our children, Amy, Aoife and Jack who have always been such a support. A special thanks to our grandchildren Oliver, Annabel and Theo for providing so many fun interludes.

Helen Lloyd owes a special thank you to Gregg for his love and support, and for providing a little haven in which to write and escape the distractions of a busy house and office. To my children Eli and Mia, your love and encouragement are always a source of motivation for me. My love for you is immeasurable and I owe you a big thank you for tolerating the busyness of an academic mother!

ABOUT THE EDITORS

Amanda Phelan is a Full Professor in General Nursing at the School of Nursing, Psychotherapy & Community Health, Dublin City University. She previously held positions at the School of Nursing, Midwifery & Health Systems, University College Dublin, where she also served as Deputy Director of the National Centre for the Protection of Older People, and at the School of Nursing & Midwifery, Trinity College Dublin. Amanda has edited four books on the topics of gerontology, elder abuse and person-centered care in community contexts. She also has numerous peer-reviewed publications and has been involved in multiple studies, reports and collaborations totaling over 4.5 million euros. Her work has been cited by the Irish Law Reform Commission and the World Health Organization and contributed to policy and practice in healthcare related to adult safeguarding and older person care. Amanda has held visiting professorships at Belmont University, Nashville, and Leiden University, the Netherlands, as well as holding a visiting researcher post at the Norwegian University of Science and Technology. She has also held research advisory roles at the University of Toronto, Canada, and the University of Turku, Finland.

Helen Lloyd is Professor in Applied Social and Cultural Psychology at the University of Plymouth. Helen holds a master's degree in Medical Anthropology and a doctorate in Social Psychiatry and Anthropology from the University of Oxford. Her research aims to create real-world change for society's most vulnerablised populations by examining how social structures, epistemic injustice and issues of race, ethnicity and identity shape health experiences and outcomes. Her innovative multidisciplinary approach integrates psychology, anthropology, sociology of medicine and creative arts to deliver powerful interventions that transform lives and reduce health and social inequalities. Helen is currently leading NIHR-funded research to develop peer-led mental health support for refugees. Her previous research work on digital harm explored the intersection between online gaming and gambling to explore emerging digital health threats. Helen's interest in person-centered care began when she created and led the person-centered coordinated care (P3C) collaborative to improve healthcare delivery for people with long-term conditions. With 40 years of applied health services experience, her aim has been to translate research into practical solutions that strengthen healthcare systems. Helen has published numerous peer-reviewed publications, and has attracted research income totalling 4.5 million pounds. She is visiting professor at the Universities of Syndey and has active collaborations with international researchers across the globe. Her current teaching includes research methods and modules in critical psychology.

CONTRIBUTOR BIOGRAPHIES

Rengin Aslanoğlu is Assistant Professor in the Department of Systems Research at the Wrocław University of Environmental and Life Sciences, Poland. Her works focus on the domains of socio-environmental systems, including adaptation of urban space to climate change, nature-based solutions, aging society and visual perception of the built environment. She has a wide scientific cooperation in projects at the international level.

Tina Bedenik is a senior postdoctoral fellow at the Royal College of Surgeons Ireland University of Medicine and Health Sciences, School of Population Health, where she leads a qualitative study that explores the application of artificial intelligence in clinical decision-making in neurological healthcare. Prior to that, Tina led research projects on secondary use of health data and the role of gender in technology entrepreneurship, and she held research posts in the healthcare sector in Ireland. Tina taught at both undergraduate and postgraduate levels, and she currently supervises postgraduate students and advises on health data regulation and implementation. Her earlier research focused on women's body image and reproductive health. Tina has an interdisciplinary background with a PhD in Social Justice from University College Dublin (Ireland), a joint MA in Human Rights from the University of Tromsø (Norway), the University of Gothenburg (Sweden), and the University of Roehampton (UK) and an MA in Political Science and a BA (Hons) from the University of Zagreb (Croatia). She has received multiple international awards for academic excellence.

Josephine Bleach has been the Director of the Early Learning Initiative at the National College of Ireland since 2008. Dr Josephine Bleach holds a PhD in Education from the University of Dublin, Trinity College, 2004–2008. She began her career as a primary school teacher before getting involved in various national initiatives by the Department of Education and Skills, including the Home School Community Liaison, Early Start Pre-School Intervention Programme and School Development Planning Support Service. She is a published academic who contributes to national and international journals, publications and conferences. Her research interests include community action research; parenting, early learning; literacy, numeracy; and professional development, community development, policy development and implementation.

Sarah Bowman is the Vice President of Operations and Development at Blue Zones, LLC, where she leads policy reform and large-scale engagement initiatives to create healthier, more livable communities. With more than 20 years of experience in strategic planning, public engagement and policy development, she has guided transformation efforts in over 1,400 communities across the United States, Canada and Ireland. She blends local priorities with national best practices to design context-sensitive, culturally responsive strategies and has helped teams secure more than $400M for initiatives that measurably improve well-being. Specializing in community engagement for the built environment and food systems transformation, Sarah integrates health and sustainability goals into public policy and community planning. A former Planning Commissioner in Port Townsend, Washington, she brings deep knowledge of government processes. She has held senior national policy, research and engagement roles in both the United States and Ireland, including as Director of Strategic Engagement and Impact Assessment at Trinity College Dublin, Ireland. Sarah is the author and co-author of several widely used frameworks and guides, including the *Engaged Research Framework*, *Researcher Impact Framework* and *Planning for Impact Framework*, which help universities and partners strengthen community engagement, assess impact and embed public involvement in research. Her publications span walkability, livability, active transportation and well-being, developed with government agencies, universities and nonprofits. Committed to lasting change, Sarah works with residents, community leaders, policymakers and partner organizations to ensure that strategies are evidence-based and outcomes-focused, creating environments where the healthy choice is the easy choice and well-being is a shared, sustained priority.

Gobnait Byrne is Assistant Professor at the School of Nursing & Midwifery, Trinity College Dublin, University of Dublin, Ireland. She is the current Director of Trinity Centre for Practice Health Care Innovation in the School. Gobnait's research interests include health promotion, cardiology nursing, critical care, community nursing, public health, health education and migration. She has published in several peer-reviewed journals and serves as a journal reviewer for the *Journal of Clinical Nursing* and the *Journal of Nursing & Healthcare of Chronic Illness*. Gobnait has also completed the Johanna Briggs Training Program on Systematic Reviews.

Marion Byrne holds a diploma in Nursery Nursing and Montessori Teaching. She has recently completed an Honours BA in Early Childhood Education & Care at the National College of Ireland. Currently, she is pursuing a Master of Arts in Educational Practice. Marion has over 20 years of experience in early years services and Montessori teaching. In 2015, she used this wealth of experience to join the Early Learning Initiative, focusing on marginalized families in the inner city of Dublin. She started as the coordinator for the 0–2 home visiting program when it launched; it is now known as the Community Families Programme. In 2018, she created the My Place to Play Programme designed for parents and infants aged 0–12 months and centered on a baby play mat with age-appropriate toys and resources to support baby development. In the following year, it received an Irish Health Care Award. Through recommendations, this project has been developed and enhanced with the design of a Toddler Pack and is now rolled out nationally. In 2023, Marion became a senior specialist with the Community Families Programme and the My Place to Play Programme. Marion has a keen interest in supporting all parents to give their children the best start from the beginning, and she has a passion for sharing her knowledge with other professionals through chairing the local infant mental health network and presenting at conferences to share the work of Community Families.

Áine Carroll is Professor of Integrated Care and Improvement at University College Dublin. Prior to this role, she was National Director of the Clinical Strategy and Programmes Division at the Health Services Executive, a division encompassing the National Clinical Programmes, Integrated Care Programmes and the Office of the Nursing & Midwifery Services (ONMSD). During her tenure, Professor Carroll established the Integrated Care Programmes for older persons, chronic disease, children and patient flow to promote coordinated care and teamwork across services and specialities, ensuring that care is provided effectively and seamlessly to patients as they move through the system. Áine is acknowledged internationally for her expertise in large-scale change and implementation. As an experienced improvement advisor, she has provided advice, guidance and training on quality improvement and change to leaders of healthcare systems across the world. She is passionate about person-centered coordinated care, complexity and implementation science.

Grzegorz Chrobak is Assistant Professor at the Wrocław University of Environmental and Life Sciences, Poland, specializing in Urban Ecoacoustics and Complex Systems. His research combines acoustic measurements, graph theory and satellite data to analyze urban soundscapes, biodiversity and environmental connectivity. He is particularly focused on developing innovative methods for soundscape mapping, intelligent environmental databases and the use of complex networks in urban sustainability research and planning.

Catherine Comiskey is Professor of Healthcare Modeling, Global Addiction and Transformation in the School of Nursing and Midwifery at Trinity College Dublin, University of Dublin, Ireland. She is the former Head of School from 2014 to 2017 and again from 2019 to 2020. She holds a PhD in Biomathematics, Biostatistics and Epidemiology. She held Chair of the Scientific Committee of the EMCDDA, Lisbon (European Monitoring Centre for Drugs and Drug Addiction) from 2020 to 2024 and is the ministerial appointed academic expert to the Irish National Drug Strategy Implementation Committee. She is a member of the current Scientific Committee of the European Union Drugs Agency. She is the sole author of the book *Addiction Debates*, published by Sage UK in 2020, and the author of *Addiction Research and Evaluation: Addressing Key Challenges for Policy and Practice*, published by Springer New York in 2024. She is also the author of over 150 research papers in addiction, leadership and education.

Elizabeth A. Curtis is Assistant Professor and a member of the academic team at the School of Nursing and Midwifery, Trinity College Dublin (TCD), University of Dublin, Republic of Ireland. She received her PhD and MEd degrees from the School of Education, TCD. Elizabeth qualified as a general nurse in London and specialized in orthopedics and neurosciences while working in the National Health Service (NHS). During her time in clinical practice, she always had an interest in education, and this ultimately led to postgraduate study in this field when she relocated to Dublin. Completing her MEd degree provided her with a comprehensive background in the disciplines relating to the study of education and contributed to her move from clinical practice to a full-time position in academia. Elizabeth has taught leadership, management, change and research methods to both undergraduate and postgraduate students and supervised many research projects over the years. Her research interests include leadership, job satisfaction and organizational management, and she has collaborated with colleagues within and outside Trinity College on several research initiatives. Her published books include *Leadership for Intellectual Disability Service: Motivating Change and Improvement* (2019), among others.

Andrew Darley is Assistant Professor/Ad Astra Fellow in the School of Nursing, Midwifery and Health Systems at University College Dublin. Dr Darley is a lived experience researcher, and their interests include an interdisciplinary range of topics, including psychosocial well-being, patient and public involvement, arts and health, digital health, family caregiving and evidence synthesis. Dr Darley has ten years of experience as a research lead and project manager of European-funded research projects, focusing on designing, implementing and evaluating supportive digital health technology in healthcare settings, both nationally and internationally.

Anne Dempsey is a journalist, writer, trainer and counselor. She has worked mainly in print journalism, contributing to a broad range of Irish newspapers and magazines, primarily in the health/social affairs areas. She has taught journalism on the Vocational Education Committee programs and at a number of third-level colleges. She was commissioned to write the history of Women's Aid, has written a number of books on retirement and served on the Board of the Retirement Planning Council of Ireland and The Coombe Hospital. Anne gained her trainer experience with the Health Education Board and the Health Promotion Unit and ran a series of personal development courses for the Health Service Executive. She obtained her diploma in Counselling from the Creative Counselling Centre, ran a private practice and served on the editorial committee of *Eisteach*, the quarterly journal published by the Irish Association for Counselling and Psychotherapy. Anne joined Third Age in 2006 and is employed as communication manager and training facilitator.

Jeroen Dikken is a senior researcher with the Research Group of Urban Ageing in the Faculty of Social Work & Education at The Hague University of Applied Sciences in The Hague, the Netherlands. He also works for the Department of Nursing. He has a background in nursing, nursing sciences and gerontology. His research interests intersect between education and clinical practice, in particular, continuing education after graduation (life-long learning). He is involved in various projects related to clinimetrics, as well as life-long learning, educating and examining in (clinical) practice.

Michael Foley is the Civic Engagement for Societal Impact (CESI) Manager at Trinity College Dublin in Ireland, with a focus on fostering connections and relationships between academia and external communities. These communities include geographical communities, as well as civil and public service agencies, civil society organizations and non-governmental organizations. He is implementing the CESI Action Plan while also developing the unit for the university with the Associate Dean. Michael formerly managed Trinity's PPI Ignite Office, promoting public and patient involvement (PPI) in health-related research. Taking co-design and partnership as a principal tenet, his work included the co-development of a national values and principles framework for PPI and a Quality Improvement Framework for Ireland's PPI sector with a team of 40 patients and researchers. His portfolio includes co-designing and delivering training on engaged research to more than 60 university staff across Ireland; leading the inaugural IPPOSI Citizen Jury and creating, together with the health research charities sector, a toolkit to support early-stage PPI involvement. Prior to that, he served as Research and Development Officer at the Trinity Centre for Ageing and Intellectual Disability during its formative period, while also coordinating master's research modules at Maynooth University. Michael worked for ten years in the charity sector, most notably with Age & Opportunity, an organization running national programs for older people in the areas of arts, sport and personal development. Before that, he spent many years at the National Disability Authority, the state's research, policy and standards agency on disability issues.

Kate Harrison-Brennan is Director of the Sydney Policy Lab and Professor of Practice and Honorary Associate at the Sydney Law School. The primary questions driving her research are "How do we make policy for the common good?" and "How might universities, understood as a community of communities, actively conciliate estranged interests and knowledges?" As a result, her work and that of the Sydney Policy Lab are investigating the practice of politics through action research in policymaking. Her work explores the significance of person-centeredness, dignity, relationships, trust, communities and institutions. Prior to joining the University of Sydney in 2022, Kate was the Head of Policy and Design at the Paul Ramsay Foundation, working with communities in Australia to secure thriving futures. From 2015 to 2020, Kate was CEO of Anglican Deaconess Ministries, a 130-year-old Christian women's foundation, where she worked to reimagine the vision of the organization and re-establish their work in public and practical engagement. In government, Kate was an adviser to former Prime Minister Julia Gillard. Kate is a graduate of the University of Sydney and a NSW Rhodes scholar. She holds a DPhil in Politics and an MPhil in Development Studies (International Development, with Distinction) from the University of Oxford.

Loredana Ivan is Professor at the National University of Political Studies and Public Administration, Communication Department, Bucharest, Romania. She holds a PhD in Sociology and a post-doctorate in Social Psychology. During 2019–2022, she served as Chair of the European Network of Aging Studies (ENAS). Her areas of interest include interpersonal communication mediated by technology, fake news and generations and family communication. She has led some special issues in the area of aging and communication technology. She is the author and co-author of several book chapters that draw on ageism and digital communication later in life.

Jo-Hanna Ivers is Associate Professor of Addiction (Public Health & Primary Care) at Trinity College Dublin, where she holds Ireland's only academic post dedicated to addiction. She was the first to serve as Trinity's Associate Dean of Civic Engagement for Societal Impact, leading initiatives that connect world-class research to meaningful change in communities. As an internationally recognized researcher, Professor Ivers directs the MSc in Addiction Recovery and leads the Neurobehavioural Addiction Research Group, advancing understanding of addiction through neurobiological, behavioral and social science. Her work addresses critical issues including opioid use disorder, stigma reduction, non-fatal overdose prevention and equitable access to treatment. Professor Ivers plays a prominent role in shaping policy at national and European levels. She was a member of the Scientific Committee for the European Monitoring Centre for Drugs and Drug Addiction, the European Council Pompidou Group on Human Rights and Drugs Policy, and has served on governmental task forces and expert review groups. She was appointed to the Advisory Support Group for the Citizens' Assembly on Drug

Use. Her research drives innovation across prevention, treatment and recovery, influencing clinical practice, public health strategy and legislative reform. Through partnerships with frontline services, international networks and multidisciplinary teams, she translates evidence into action, strengthening systems of care and improving outcomes for people affected by addiction.

Jan K. Kazak is Associate Professor at the Wrocław University of Environmental and Life Sciences (Poland) and Visiting Professor at The Hague University of Applied Sciences (the Netherlands). He chairs the Leading Research Group: Sustainable Cities and Regions, which serves as a cross-cutting hub gathering experts from various domains, including geography, environmental and social sciences, real estate management and governance. He is a member of the Main Board of the Polish Real Estate Scientific Society. He was listed in Stanford's list of world's top 2% scientists, confirming his contribution to the development of science.

Hannah R. Marston is a senior research fellow in the School of Health, Wellbeing and Social Care at The Open University, UK. Her research focuses on digital health, digital literacy and digital practices of older and younger populations living in rural and urban environments. Her research and submitted evidence have been cited in policy documents, including the House of Lords "Beyond Digital: Planning for a Hybrid World" (2021), The Future of Ageing: Ethical Considerations for Research and Innovation (Nuffield Council on Bioethics, 2023) and the Smarter Homes for Independent Living: Putting People in Control of Their Lives report by Policy Connect (2022). She serves as an editorial board member for the *Cogent Gerontology* journal, and she is Visiting Professor in the Research Group of Urban Ageing part of the Centre for Expertise of Governance of Urban Transitions at The Hague University of Applied Sciences in The Hague, the Netherlands.

Brendan McCormack is Head of School and Dean at The Susan Wakil School of Nursing and Midwifery (including Sydney Nursing School), the Faculty of Medicine and Health at The University of Sydney. He is also the Academic Chair of "The CARE Program" at Sydney Policy Lab, University of Sydney. Brendan's research focuses on person-centered healthcare with a particular focus on the development of person-centered cultures, practices and processes. He has specialized as a clinical nurse in gerontology and dementia care. Brendan is a fellow of the American Academy of Nursing. He has been awarded the Sigma "International Nurse Researcher Hall of Fame". He is also a member of the Academia Europaea. He has >700 publications reflecting these research areas, including 310 peer-reviewed publications in international journals and 14 books. His h-index is 54. He has been featured in the Wiley Publishers' "Inspiring Minds" short films series https://www.youtube.com/watch?v=13c5C-tbcT4 in recognition of his extensive contributions to person-centered healthcare. In 2023, he was awarded an Honorary Doctorate from the University of Maribor, Slovenia, in recognition of his services to nursing and healthcare. In September 2024, Professor McCormack was selected to join the Lancet Global Commission on People-Centred Healthcare for Universal Health Coverage hosted by Harvard University and made an affiliate academic at Harvard Medical School Centre for Primary Care. In 2025, he was awarded the Paul Tournier Prize for Person-Centred Healthcare by the International College of Person-Centred Medicine.

Éidín Ní Shé is a senior lecturer in the Royal College of Surgeons Ireland Graduate School of Healthcare Management (GSM) at RCSI University of Medicine and Health Sciences. She is the Program Director of the MSc in Healthcare Management. Éidín's teaching experience in higher education spans over 20 years, with experience in both Ireland and Australia. She has a disciplinary research focus in co-design and applied health systems research. Her projects in Ireland have included work on developing interprofessional competencies in the care of older people with the national clinical program, assisted decision-making, frailty pathway co-design and supporting staff in speaking up about safety.

Michael John Norton is an early-career researcher currently studying for a PhD in Recovery at the Royal College of Surgeons, Ireland. He previously worked for the Health Service Executive as an Engagement and Recovery Programme Lead where he had responsibility for the development of peer support, family recovery and the co-production of the next iteration of "A National Framework for Recovery in Mental Health". Additionally, within his role, he led the implementation of a number of "Sharing the Vision" recommendations. Michael is an established author with 44 publications relating to peer support, co-production, mental health and recovery. He is also the author of *Co-Production in Mental Health: Implementing Policy into Practice*. Michael has recently authored another book *Peer Support Work in Mental Health Services: Theory, Research, Policy and Practice* which is due for publication in September 2025.

Deirdre O'Donnell is a registered nurse and a Full Professor of Nursing at Ulster University. She is also the Strategic Lead for the Nursing and Midwifery Council (NMC) Competence Test Centre in Northern Ireland. Deirdre is a senior fellow of the UK Higher Education Academy (HEA). Deirdre's doctoral research focused on the role of higher education (HE) in preparing the future healthcare workforce for person-centered practice. In recognition of her sustained contribution to the development of person-centeredness through HE, in 2023, Deirdre was awarded a prestigious Advance HE Collaborative Award for Teaching Excellence. She has since been an Advance HE reviewer for this award category. For 11 years, Deirdre held a Ministerial Public Appointment as a Non-Executive Director of the Northern Ireland Practice and Education Council (NIPEC) for Nurses and Midwives. During this time, she was the Chair of NIPEC's Audit and Risk Committee. She also served for two terms as an NMC fitness to practice registrant panelist.

Cormac Russell is a social explorer, an author and a much sought-after speaker. He is the Founding Director of Nurture Development and a member of the Asset-Based Community Development (ABCD) Institute at DePaul University, Chicago. Over the last 29 years, Cormac's work has demonstrated an enduring impact in 38 countries around the world. He has trained communities, agencies, NGOs and governments in ABCD and other community-based approaches in Africa, Asia, Australia/Oceania, Europe and North America. His most recent books are *The Connected Community: Discovering the Health, Wealth, and Power of Neighborhoods* (co-author John McKnight, 2022) and *Rekindling Democracy: A Professional's Guide to Working in Citizen Space* (2020).

Małgorzata Świąder is Assistant Professor in the Department of Systems Research at the Wrocław University of Environmental and Life Sciences, Poland. Her research focuses on spatial analysis using geographic information systems, socio-environmental assessments, human impact and environmental impact evaluations through metrics such as carbon and land footprints. She is particularly interested in the integration of geospatial data and sustainability indicators to support evidence-based environmental planning and policymaking.

Zsuzsu Tavy is a researcher with the Research Group of Urban Ageing in the Faculty of Social Work & Education at The Hague University of Applied Sciences in The Hague, the Netherlands. She also works for the Department of Nursing. She has a background in nursing and social and cultural anthropology. She specializes in the use of (audio) visual methodologies in participatory research. Her research focuses on the participation of older people. She is a curriculum leader of the course on participatory healthcare.

Lucia Thielman holds a bachelor's degree in Bio-medical Sciences from the University of Leiden and a master's in Management, Policy Analysis and Entrepreneurship in Health and Life Sciences from the Vrije Universiteit Amsterdam. She has worked as a researcher at VU Amsterdam and as an action researcher at the Leyden Academy on Vitality and Ageing. In recent years, her focus has shifted to fostering European collaboration on themes such as age-friendly environments, culture and well-being, working with organizations including the Age-Friendly Environments Academy, SHAFE Foundation and TrueMotion.

Stephanie Tierney is Associate Professor at the Nuffield Department of Primary Care Health Sciences, University of Oxford. Her research centers on social prescribing, which she has explored using realist research and mixed methods. In particular, she has studied the link worker role in England and the role of the cultural sector in social prescribing. She is also interested in skills mix in healthcare and the introduction of new roles into primary care (like social prescribing link workers). Stephanie leads a network of academics, clinicians, providers, policymakers and members of the public – the Oxford Social Prescribing Research Network (https://socialprescribing.phc.ox.ac.uk/).

Joost van Hoof works as a Full Professor of Urban Ageing in the Faculty of Social Work & Education at The Hague University of Applied Sciences in The Hague, the Netherlands. His research interests lie in the domain of age-friendly cities and the design of housing and gerontechnology for older people. He serves as the chairperson of the Knowledge Platform Age-Friendly The Hague and coordinates the national network of age-friendly municipalities. Since December 2017, he has also been affiliated with the Department of Systems Research, Faculty of Spatial Management and Landscape Architecture, Wrocław University of Environmental and Life Sciences, Wrocław, Poland. In Poland, he works as Professor in the field of social sciences in the discipline of socio-economic geography and spatial management. He was listed in Stanford's list of world's top 2% scientists, confirming his contribution to the development of science.

Wilhelmina H. van Staalduinen is the CEO of AFEdemy, an academy on age-friendly environments in Europe founder, and a co-director of the SHAFE Foundation (Smart Healthy Age-Friendly Environments). She graduated as a political scientist and was a nurse in practice in mental healthcare. Since 2013, Wilhelmina worked with the WHO concept of age-friendly cities and communities. She is actively involved in Age-Friendly City The Hague and co-developed with The Hague University of Applied Sciences the Age-Friendly Cities and Communities Questionnaire with which older adults themselves can express their opinions on the age-friendliness of their community. She was the Vice-Chair and Grant Holder of COST Action NET4Age-Friendly and is currently active as a co-coordinator of Stakeholders and Management Committee and a member of COST Action PAAR-net on participatory approaches with older adults (2023–2027).

Debra Westlake is a qualitative researcher in Applied Health Services Research, with expertise in realist approaches at the Nuffield Department for Primary Health Care Sciences, University of Oxford. She is passionate about embedded research that involves people in co-design, analysis and implementation of findings. Debra's specialist areas are person-centered care and social prescribing, and she has worked on a number of studies in these areas at the Universities of Liverpool, Plymouth and Oxford, as well as conducting embedded research in voluntary sector and NHS organizations. Debra is currently working on the TOUS study, which is examining how cultural and creative sector organizations can tailor their offers to older people from global majority backgrounds, and is a co-applicant on the Routes to Wellness, NIHR-funded study of a peer support intervention for refugee mental health. Debra originally qualified as a speech and language therapist and has practiced in education, health and social care settings. She was the founder and trustee for a charity in Lima, Peru, which for 35 years has provided preschool education in vulnerable communities. Debra also acts as a trustee for a local voluntary sector care organization in Devon.

PART 1

Laying the Foundations for Person-Centered Approaches in Community Well-being

1

INTRODUCTION

Amanda Phelan and Helen Lloyd

Introduction

Many countries have moved to a health and social care model of primary care, targeting community-level supports. In this book, we take a wide perspective on the term "community". Equally, we support a multidimensional understanding of health and social care, which proposes a social determinant of health foundation with the application of person-centered principles to the community. Accordingly, we commence with a brief consideration of what constitutes a community. The World Health Organization (2025:web) states that community is:

> ...a specific group of people who share a common culture, values and norms, identity, interest, action, place, practice, or circumstance, and are arranged in social connection according to relationships which have developed over a period of time and may be modified in the future.

Likewise, the United Nations (2020:1) observe that communities are often considered as a geographic entity; however, understandings transcend this narrow focus:

> Often a geographical subset of society at the local level, a "community" can be defined by commonalities such as, but not limited to, norms, religion, shared interests, customs, values and needs of civilians. A community is not static or closed, but constantly evolving subject to internal and external construction and reconstruction.

Within this broader framework, "community" has multiple meanings, but it generally reflects a network of people where relationships can be emotional, structural

DOI: 10.4324/9781032662657-2

or functional. While it can be perceived as an ambiguous term (Mannarini & Fedi, 2009), community suggests a network that is connected through some form of commonality or identity, which can be related to the place or environment people live or work in, ethnicity, the type of work or study people undertake or institution they are affiliated to, or illnesses shared. Community can also reflect the values or beliefs people identify with, such as religion or culture, nationality or people who share a common interest (i.e., a book club or sports club followers). In recent years, the meaning of community has expanded as social media and digital formats have evolved, for example, groups on Facebook, gaming sites or other online forums. Indeed, this has added a layer of complexity; many people now belong to multiple communities that can take various formats, such as in-person or virtual. Moreover, community can be manifested within a physical identity (neighborhood, church, school and club) or within a relational way of being (religion, culture and club). In working with communities, approaches may pivot on interacting with multiple system levels and focusing on structure (social, environment, organization, governance, educational and transport), demographics (population trends) and process (how things are done). A historical understanding is also important as issues such as expansion, changing populations, employment or politics may provide context to current community realities.

While belonging to a community is founded on mutuality and promotes social connectedness, it has also been used to marginalize people both historically and within contemporary times. For example, belonging to a particular community has been used to justify oppression based on aspects such as color, religion, ethnicity, gender, socio-economic group, age and disability (see David & Derthick, 2018; Brancho & Hayes, 2020; Liedauer, 2021). Additionally, individuals' intersectionality with multiple communities can increase vulnerability (Siller & Aydin, 2022) while such marginalization erodes their decision-making and influence (Robert Wood Johnson Foundation, 2019). This is typified by segregating practices, which can be legitimized, where "othering" is common, and justifies inequality in how community members experience their daily lives through prejudicial perspectives (Rohlelder, 2014). Moreover, even when belonging to a community, if individuals no longer share the group's values and beliefs, the community itself may resort to isolating members or worse. Not complying with such community norms can sometimes result in fatalities, for example, in the case of honor killings (Aksoy & Szekely, 2025). Recognizing these issues is important as they can define both inclusionary and exclusionary practices experienced by and within communities (Akbulut & Razum, 2022). Consequently, addressing community health often translates to systems change underpinned by a long-term commitment to collaboration and engagement.

This book is a result of many conversations about person-centered care (PCC) applied to the community. While developments within the space of PCC have expanded, its contextualization within the community level has lagged. Consequently, we aim to provide a framework to consider communities within the principles of

PCC. In this way, we can work with communities to co-create "a society in which everyone has a fair and just opportunity to live the healthiest life possible" (Robert Wood Johnson Foundation, 2019:1). This demands a re-orientation in health to address inequities (Higginson et al., 2024). This book offers several chapters that explore the foundations of working in partnership with communities emphasizing the uniqueness of each one, while appreciating the rich diversity of people who live and work within the neighborhoods or entities constituting the community. Following the foundational chapters that present the principles and concepts of PCC and other useful frameworks as applied to communities, we provide further discussions enabling an exploration of how this works in multiple environments such as education, environmental, population groups and community engagement with underserved populations. Our perspective supports the WHO (2020:3) definition of community engagement as:

...a process of developing relationships that enable stakeholders to work together to address health-related issues and promote well-being to achieve positive health impact and outcomes.

Our approach also underpins person-centered principles reflected by the United Nations' (2020) definition of community engagement as being strategic, with communities involved in all dimensions of decision-making and ownership through the establishment of sustained partnerships. This book presents 16 chapters divided into 3 sections. Part 1 focuses on laying the conceptual and operational foundations for person-centered approaches to facilitate community well-being. Part 2 provides examples of community engagement activities with various communities that demonstrate the principles of PCC. In Part 3, a number of research projects are presented that apply person-centered approaches in the context of working with communities to improve well-being.

Chapter 2 introduces the development of current understandings of PCC. Phelan observes PCC as reflecting the move from a biomedical, hierarchical relationship with people in care environments to a more humanistic, psychosocial orientation. Within many countries, the philosophical impetus of care pivots on a recognition of the uniqueness of human beings and their right to be involved in their care and decisions about their lives. Moreover, it encompasses the appreciation and validation of the lived experience of each individual in supporting people to have mastery over their own lives and, in this sense, having a deep and authentic drive to work in partnership to address what matters to them within their community. This chapter also provides an understanding of community health and how collaborations can be framed to address issues such as social deprivation. This chapter concludes by providing a lens to assess communities within Bronfenbrenner's (1977; 1979; 1995), Bronfenbrenner and Morris's (1998) ecological approach and Donabedian's (1966; 2005) quality model, a theme which is continued in Chapter 4.

Working with communities requires competencies that are founded on mutual trust and authentic collaboration. Chapter 3 considers the building blocks of working with communities. Phelan commences by articulating how the concept of need can be constituted in relation to community-level collaborations. Following on from this, drawing on Bronfenbrenner (1977; 1979), Bronfenbrenner and Morris (1998) and Donabedian (1966; 2005), Chapter 3 presents practical aspects pertaining to engaging with communities and how building up relationships of trust requires meaningful involvement of people within the targeted geographical, social, ethnic or other configurations of community. Engaging authentically should not be under-estimated; it is a complex activity that takes time and skilled communication, and the ability to synthesize information and context from multiple perspectives. It is imbued with mutual respect and truly valuing communities, their diversity and their unique characteristics. As McCance and McCormack (2025) discuss in the context of PCC, being authentic involves being committed and competent, shared decision-making, transparency and creating and sustaining relationships which foster healthful, equitable cultures within communities. Working with communities to identify need (profiling) means collecting relevant information that emanates from community-level characteristics and generating multiple, inclusive and diverse insights into the realities of people's lives. This differs from PCC in the sense that there is a need to authentically listen to multiple perspectives and represent all groups in order to frame their experiences, perspectives, beliefs and values. At all stages of working with communities, from preparing to engage to evaluating the collaborative activities, ensuring representation, voice and promoting equity requires careful negotiation and leadership skills, which are navigated in this chapter.

Communities are immersed in environments that impact health, opportunities, happiness and quality of life. A review of the community's social determinants of health is key in terms of inequities in social and economic benefits people experience throughout life (CDC, 2024). In Chapter 4, Lloyd examines health inequalities through a comprehensive ecological framework, exploring both the problems and potential solutions. Key concepts of health, health inequalities and the social determinants of health are defined along with an exploration of the Social Gradient of Health. This is followed by a presentation of the evidence on global health inequities. By advocating for a systems approach using Bronfenbrenner's ecological model (1977), this chapter outlines the value of stakeholder engagement, proportionate universalism and the importance of health creation through a framework of salutogenesis. Examples of promising community interventions are provided. This chapter concludes that successful interventions are those that are co-designed with communities, provide safe spaces for connection and meaning-making and address multiple social determinants simultaneously through a strengths-based, salutogenic approach.

In Chapter 5, Lloyd provides a depth overview of social capital and its relationship to community well-being. She begins by outlining the historical development of the concept of social capital, tracing its origins back to Karl Marx's "gesellschaftliche", through to contemporary and multidisciplinary definitions. Exploring the dimensional structure of social capital, this chapter also demonstrates how it impacts and relates to community well-being through interventions that often vary by context and population. Case studies are provided from the Southwest of England to illustrate the value of social capital for health promotion and community well-being. This chapter concludes by highlighting the complex nature of social capital and the context-dependent impact of interventions seeking to create it. The discussion emphasizes the importance of trust, reciprocity and shared understanding as essential mechanisms for social capital. Importantly, it is acknowledged that social capital can have both positive and negative effects, potentially reinforcing exclusion.

Asset-Based Community Development (ABCD) is discussed in Chapter 6 as a mechanism for transforming community health rather than traditional deficit-based approaches. Russell proposes that "generative communities" – neighborhoods where residents collaborate to cultivate growth and change – should become the primary actors in health creation, with external resources supplementing rather than replacing community capabilities. This chapter distinguishes between two operating systems: institutions that deliver services at scale through command-and-control mechanisms and associations that provide care and mutuality through trust-based relationships. Russell argues that many social problems arise from applying institutional solutions to issues better addressed through associational approaches – what the authors call "Maslow's hammer". Evidence supporting community-centered approaches in this chapter reveals that social connection reduces mortality risk by 50% and that neighborhood belonging and community control are key health determinants. The Milwaukee Blueprint for Peace is provided to exemplify this approach. This chapter concludes with the emphasis that ABCD cannot substitute for addressing structural inequalities or improving essential services, arguing, like many other chapters in this edition, that marginalized communities require ongoing equity investment, where community organizing combines with basic income support and comprehensive services to address environmental racism and institutional neglect. This chapter envisions a fundamental transformation where communities become the primary actors in well-being creation, with clinicians and services playing supplementary roles. This requires transferring authority and resources from acute healthcare systems to generative neighborhoods while maintaining proportionate universalism to ensure equity. The ultimate goal is creating societies where empowered communities co-create wellness, supported by enabling states with progressive policies that prioritize health as a common good.

Chapter 7 explores the evolution and current state of patient and public involvement (PPI) in health and social care systems. Ní Shé, Norton and Bedenik trace the historical development of PPI, providing an overview from the 1960s when patients were passive recipients of care, through Sherry Arnstein's influential "ladder of participation" (1969), to today's emphasis on co-design, co-production and co-creation approaches where patients become active partners in healthcare decisions and research. Key terms are defined, and current challenges are identified in creating barriers to effective PPI implementation. These include change fatigue following COVID-19, power imbalances between researchers and patients, tokenistic practices that limit meaningful participation, a lack of representation from diverse groups (men, ethnic minorities and socioeconomically disadvantaged) and resource constraints and training gaps. The key characteristics of effective leadership in PPI are discussed. This chapter concludes that while PPI is becoming increasingly complex and expected in healthcare, leaders must create the necessary conditions for it to flourish, with the overall emphasis on the critical message that effective PPI requires a fundamental shift from traditional hierarchical healthcare models to collaborative partnerships that value patients' experiential expertise alongside professional knowledge.

In Chapter 8, Westlake and Tierney introduce social prescribing as a non-clinical method of addressing health inequalities and promoting people's health in communities (HSE, 2021). The authors outline how social prescribing, the process of referring people to non-clinical, community-based activities rather than purely medical treatments in the English NHS, provides opportunities to enhance well-being. Social prescribing attempts to address the general practitioner visits in England, currently around 20%, which are a result of non-medical issues like loneliness, housing problems or financial difficulties. In the context of National Health Service policy, which positions social prescribing as serving both individual needs and community well-being, this chapter asks the question of whether this person-centered approach can also benefit communities beyond individual patients. The mechanism to enable this is through the expectation that social prescribers should spend up to one day per week on community development activities to strengthen community assets, in addition to providing personalized care. This chapter summarizes the evidence-based benefits of these activities at individual, community and primary care levels and describes the documented challenges to these schemes and notable resource constraints. Of particular note is the acknowledgment that these schemes operate less in deprived areas, with lower uptake among certain sectors of the community. The authors acknowledge the potential in these schemes to create community well-being but argue that without addressing important challenges, social prescribing risks reproducing existing inequalities rather than creating genuinely healthier, more resilient communities.

In Chapter 9, Curtis and Comiskey explore the potential for combining distributed leadership (DL) and community recovery models (CRM) to support the implementation of PCC in community mental health settings. The two primary aims of this chapter are to summarize the key tenets of PCC, DL and CRM and identify similarities between these concepts to suggest their combined use for implementing PCC in community settings. A practical research example is used to demonstrate how these constructs intersect in the Healthy Addiction Treatment (HAT) Recovery Model. The authors tentatively suggest that combining DL and CRM could effectively support PCC implementation, particularly given the WHO's (2015) call for "distributed leadership that involves multiple actors working together collaboratively." However, they emphasize that this suggestion is provisional and requires empirical research to establish compatibility and long-term utility. This chapter concludes that despite definitional and implementation challenges, these three approaches share fundamental strengths in promoting inclusivity, interaction and community-focused care – qualities deemed essential for addressing contemporary global healthcare challenges.

Chapter 10 articulates how an early childhood home visiting program applies a collaborative person-centered community approach. Byrne and Bleach detail the origins of Irish-based support programs, which are traced from the establishment of the Community Mothers' initiative in 1983, followed by the Area-Based Childhood program and, more recently, the establishment of the Community Families program. The current program pivots on the development of partnerships with parents to create flourishing environments for early childhood. These programs were launched to address poor health outcomes and lack of access to health information in Dublin's inner city. The programs described were designed to focus on maternal and child health, diet, sleep, attachment, parenting and infant development. They were built on three core principles: PCC, parents as first educators and wraparound interagency support. Parents are seen as key educators of their children and the program enables linkages to support systems if the child and family require additional support. The impact and success of the programs are described with demonstrable evidence of how community-based, relationship-focused home visiting can effectively support vulnerable families while adapting to local needs and changing circumstances.

In Chapter 11, Dempsey describes how a charitable organization evolved to meet a need for socialization for older people living in the community. Third Age, based in Summerhill, Co Meath, Ireland, developed from a local organization to provide a range of national supports both for older people (SeniorHelpline, AgeWell) and for communities (Fáilte Isteach) where language is a barrier to participation in Irish society. These programs are underpinned by person-centered principles of involvement, ownership and participation and were developed in partnership with communities to address gaps in quality of life issues and through empowerment strategies, to address real-life challenges in underserved communities.

Drawing on work with communities within third-level education institutions, Chapter 12 details the key role of universities in promoting civic engagement with communities. Ivers, Bowman and Foley detail the development and work within one Irish University, Trinity College Dublin (TCD), to initiate and sustain partnerships with diverse communities for research, community engagement, teaching and learning to address societal challenges. The authors emphasize that higher-level institutions have a responsibility to engage and collaborate with civil society to create mutually beneficial relationships that have a dual impact on addressing community needs and providing real-world learning for students, which has tangible impacts. Reflecting person-centered principles, this is underpinned by staff and students working with people in communities to focus on everyday realities, what matters to them and collaboratively consider how to create meaningful responses. In recognition of the need to be proactive, this chapter navigates TCD's Civic

Engagement for Societal Impact Action Plan (CESI) based on fostering meaningful community-based partnerships and initiatives and provides guidance for a blueprint for engaged research and activities.

In recent years, there have been calls to reimagine healthcare, particularly in the context of changing demographics and multi-morbidity, with calls for more focus on people's involvement in care that meets their needs (Phelan et al., 2021; Higginson et al., 2024). Chapter 13 presents findings from the Australia Cares Project, which aimed to reimagine care policy through community-led approaches rather than traditional top-down policymaking. McCormack and Harrison-Brennan describe the necessity and value of this approach, driven by the recognition that healthcare has become overly medical, fragmented and target-driven, losing focus on fundamental caring relationships. An innovative methodology which combined care labs (online workshops using Theory U methodology with 38 diverse participants), People's Assemblies (community deliberations in Westmead (South Asian families) and Stories of Care (personal narratives to complement other findings) is presented. Key findings are shared, identifying gaps in understanding, systemic problems and social and cultural barriers to care. The authors provide an outline of the principles of care upon which policy solutions were generated by the community. This chapter argues that current care systems, rooted in 1950s thinking, have fundamentally failed even by past standards and that community-led policy development offers a pathway to more effective, humane care systems.

Co-designing integrated care technology with older people and their support network in the community is the focus of Chapter 14. Acknowledging the changing needs of older people and the impetus to support aging in place, this chapter reflects on the Irish phase of a European project that aims to develop a person-centered, value-based digital health technology. Most importantly, Darley and Carroll note that working in partnership with older people translates to recognizing when plans need to be flexible and adapt to challenges in engagement and project scope. This underpins the autonomy of older people and promotes meaningful collaboration to enhance community living and quality of life. This chapter provides another dimension to how person-centered principles can be applied within communities.

Chapter 15 presents a thoughtful consideration of how both indoor and outdoor spaces can be facilitative or limiting for older people. van Hoof and colleagues note the growing demographic aging shift and the need to be innovative in creating places and spaces that support older people's quality of life. Key to environmental and settings' design is the collaboration of older people in what is important in planning, facilities and processes to co-create meaningful intergenerational spaces which foster inclusion and belonging. It is well recognized that the environment is a key feature that can enhance people's lives (National Research Council, 2013; Collins et al., 2024) and promote intergenerational solidarity (Nelischer & Loukaitou-Sideris, 2022). To illustrate how person-centeredness was applied in developing age-friendly environments, the authors present three case studies based on working with older people. The first describes older people involement in the development of a geopotal design using photoproduction research in Poland, Romania and the Netherlands; the second explores a European Age-friendly Environments Activists project and a third study from Delft in the Netherlands which focused on assessment of age-friendliness of cities.

To conclude, Chapter 16 provides an overview of a European project that applied PCC and the 7S (McKinsey Company, 2008) framework to develop a Person-centered Curriculum Framework (PcCF). Supported by European funding, six countries worked together to identify how each of the 7Ss applies within a PcCF. This involved a collaborative approach with higher education institutions' staff and students, healthcare professionals and regulators to distill components, thematic actions, mapping statements and activities which align with strategy, structure, systems, staff, style, skills and shared values. The project demonstrates an iterative process of working in partnership with stakeholders to represent core principles to support a PcCF to support healthcare professions' education.

Conclusion

This book provides both a foundation for understanding the complexity and dynamics of translating PCC to the community context. Part 1 provides the conceptual basis for understanding community and person-centered frameworks and approaches to collaboration are considered. Part 2 allows readers the opportunity to reflect on how person-centered principles are practically applied to communities within specific settings, environments, populations or geographical areas. Within Part 3, various illustrations of community engagement are discussed, demonstrating collaborative foundations for well-being enhancement. As health care systems advance, the involvement and participation of communities is a core impetus in navigating what is important and what matters to their health and well-being. Communities are dynamic and multidimensional entities that have demonstrable complex internal systems of being. Thus, working authentically translates to ensuring the establishment of inclusive and diverse trusting relationships, meaningful collaboration, participation, co-decision-making and implementation and evaluation of plans. As a system with interconnecting networks, the key is ensuring equitable representation, which fosters individual voices and perspectives to generate positive directions in addressing inequities and to improve community well-being. Such work requires skilled and thoughtful, authentic engagement and leadership, negotiation and communication abilities to forge plans while equally supporting the psychological safety of community members.

References

Akbulut, N., & Razum, O. (2022). Why othering should be considered in research on health in equalities: Theoretical perspectives and research needs. *SSM – Population Health*, *20*, 101286. https://doi.org/10.1016/j.ssmph.2022.101286

Aksoy, O., & Szekely, A. (2025). Making sense of honor killings. *American Sociological Review, 90*(3), 427–454.

Bracho, C., & Hayes, C. (2020). Gay voices without intersectionality is White supremacy: Narratives of gay and lesbian teachers of color on teaching and learning. *International Journal of Qualitative Studies in Education, 33*, 1–10. https://doi.org/10.1080/09518398.2020.1751897.

Bronfenbrenner, U. (1977). Toward an experimental ecology of human development. *American Psychologist, 32*(7), 513–531. https://doi.org/10.1037/0003-066X.32.7.513.

Bronfenbrenner, U. (1979). *The ecology of human development: Experiments by nature and design.* Harvard University Press, Massachusetts.

Bronfenbrenner, U. (1995). Developmental ecology through space and time: A future perspective. In *Examining lives in context: Perspectives on the ecology of human development* (P. Moen, Elder, G.H. Jr., & Lüscher, K., eds). American Psychological Association, Washington, pp. 619–647.

Bronfenbrenner, U., & Morris, P.A. (1998). The ecology of developmental processes. In *Handbook of child psychology: Vol. 1. Theoretical models of human development* (Damon, W. (Series Ed.) & Lerner R. M. (Vol. Ed.)), (5th ed.). Wiley, New York, pp. 993–1028.

Centre for Disease Control (2024). Social Determinants of Health (SDOH). Retrieved from https://www.cdc.gov/about/priorities/why-is-addressing-sdoh-important.html#:~:text=The%20impact%20is%20pervasive%20and,higher%20risk%20of%20poor%20health.

Collins, P.Y., Sinha, M., Concepcion, T., Patton, G., Way, T., McCay, L., Mensa-Kwao, A., Herrman, H., de Leeuw, E., Anand, N., Atwoli, L., Bardikoff, N., Booysen, C., Bustamante, I., Chen, Y., Davis, K., Dua, T., Foote, N., Hughsam, M., Juma, D., Khanal, S., Kumar, M., Lefkowitz, B., McDermott, P., Moitra, M., Ochieng, Y., Omigbodun, O., Queen, E., Unützer, J., Uribe-Restrepo, J.M., Wolpert, M., & Zeitz, L. (2024). Making cities mental health friendly for adolescents and young adults. *Nature, 627*(8002), 137–148. https://doi.org/10.1038/s41586-023-07005-4

David, E.J.R., & Derthick, A.O. (2018). *The psychology of oppression.* Springer Publishing Company, New York.

Donabedian, A. (1966; 2005) Evaluating the quality of medical care. *Milbank Memorial Fund Q, 44*(3), (suppl), 166–206. (Reprinted in *Milbank Quarterly, 83*(4), 691–729.

Health Service Executive (HSE) (2021). *HSE Social prescribing framework.* HSE, Dublin.

Higginson, I.J., Shand, J., Robert, G., Boaz, A., French, C., Carvalho N'Djai, A., Malone, M., Wolfe, I., Normand, C., & Hotopf, M. (2024). Reimagining health and care to tackle the rising tide of inequity, multimorbidity, and complex conditions. *NEJM Catalyst, 5*(5), Article 5. https://doi.org/10.1056/CAT.24.0266

Liedauer, S. (2021). Dimensions and causes of systemic oppression. In *Reduced inequalities. Encyclopedia of the UN sustainable development goals* (Leal Filho, W., Azul, A.M., Brandli, L., Lange Salvia, A., Özuyar, P.G., & Wall, T., eds). Springer, Cham. https://doi.org/10.1007/978-3-319-71060-0_91-1

Mannarini, T., & Fedi, A. (2009). Multiple senses of community: The experience and meaning of community. *Journal of Community Psychology, 37*(2), 211–227. https://doi.org/10.1002/jcop.20289

McCance, T., & McCormack, B. (2025). The person-centred nursing framework: A mid-range theory for nursing practice. *Journal of Research in Nursing: JRN*, 17449871241281428. Advance online publication. https://doi.org/10.1177/17449871241281428

McKinsey & Company (2008). *Enduring ideas: The 7-S framework.* Retrieved from https://www.mckinsey.com/capabilities/strategy-and-corporate-finance/our-insights/enduring-ideas-the-7-s-framework

National Research Council (2013). Physical and social environmental factors. In *U.S. health in international perspective: Shorter lives, poorer health.* (Woolf, S.H. & Aron, L., eds). National Academies, Washington, D.C.

Nelischer, C., & Loukaitou-Sideris, A. (2022). Intergenerational public space design and policy: A review of the literature. *Journal of Planning Literature, 38*(1),19–32. https://doi.org/10.1177/08854122221092175

Phelan, A., Rohde, D., Casey, M., Fealy, G., Felle, P., O'Kelly, G., Lloyd, H., & Carroll, A. (2021). Co-creating descriptors and a definition for person-centred coordinated health care: An action research study. *International Journal of Integrated Care, 21*(1), 11. https://doi.org/10.5334/ijic.5575

Robert Wood Johnson Foundation (2019). *Culture of health, sentinel community insights: Health equity.* Princeton, New Jersey.

Rohleder, P. (2014). Othering. In *Encyclopaedia of critical psychology* (Teo, T. ed.). Springer, New York, pp 1306–1308.

Siller, H., & Aydin, N. (2022). Using an intersectional lens on vulnerability and resilience in minority and/or marginalized groups during the COVID-19 pandemic: A narrative review. *Frontiers in Psychology, 13*, 894103. https://doi.org/10.3389/fpsyg.2022.894103

United Nations (2020). Community engagement guidelines on peacebuilding and sustaining peace. Retrieved from https://www.un.org/peacebuilding/sites/www.un.org.peacebuilding/files/documents/un_community-engagement_guidelines.august_2020.pdf

World Health Organization (2015). *WHO global strategy on people-centred and integrated health services: Interim report.* WHO, Geneva.

World Health Organisation (2020). *Community engagement: A health promotion guide for universal health coverage in the hands of the people.* WHO, Geneva.

World Health Organization (2025). Considerations at the community level. Retrieved from https://qualityhealthservices.who.int/quality-toolkit/new-to-health-system-quality-thinking/quality-considerations-at-the-community-level

2

TRANSLATING PERSON-CENTERED CARE TO THE COMMUNITY

Amanda Phelan

Introduction

Person-centeredness has emerged in the 20th century as a philosophical and practice-based foundation for healthcare. In particular, person-centered care represents an increasing resistance to the standardized rigidity of healthcare within the context of biomedical principles which focus on a disease-oriented model. Such approaches construct power differentials in the relationship between the person receiving care support and the professional/institution (Sobolewska et al., 2020; Phelan et al., 2020). The transformation to a psychosocial foundation acknowledges the unique needs of individuals, specifically recognizing personhood, autonomy, partnership, collaboration and the rights of people within their care journeys. While the majority of academic and practice-based focus is healthcare (Phelan et al., 2020), work has been undertaken to use person-centered principles in other areas such as education (Gray & Woods, 2022; McCormack, 2024), workplace (Caesens et al, 2020; Blackmon et al., 2023), policy articulation (WHO, 2025; Ndu, 2022; Buchanan & Sharma, 2024) and housing (Brown, 2025). Concurrently, many health systems have adapted the triple aim (Berwick et al., 2008), which promotes better care for individuals, better health for populations and lower per capita costs. In 2022, this was expanded to a quadruple aim, which includes the well-being of the healthcare workforce and advancing health equity (Nundy et al., 2022). A population health agenda seeks to address health disparities by examining the multiple influences related to ill health (Thomas, 2021). Community-centered care represents a collaborative commitment and empowerment-based contribution to addressing health disparities through leveraging local assets (people, history, physical environment, resources, social competence, partnerships with external agents), thus impacting

DOI: 10.4324/9781032662657-3

broader population health outcomes (Public Health England, 2018). While person-centered care has been applied at a community level (Public Health England & NHS, England, 2015; McCauley et al., 2021; Office for Health Improvement and Disparities, 2022), further application of its principles in this context is required. In this chapter, person-centered care's development and principles are presented together with its application to the community context, which enables a foundation for subsequent chapters.

Person-Centered Care

Person-centered care can be defined as:

> …an approach to practice established through the formation and fostering of healthful relationships between all care providers, service users and others significant to them in their lives. It is underpinned by values of respect for persons, individual right to self-determination, mutual respect and understanding. It is enabled by cultures of empowerment that foster continuous approaches to practice development.
>
> (McCormack et al., 2013: 193)

The origins of person-centered care have been traced to the work of philosopher Martin Buber, whose book I and Thou (1923) provides key insights into human relationships and dialogue. Buber argues that individuals' relationships in everyday life are framed as I-Thou and I-It. The I-Thou relationship is experienced with meaning, without judgment, and embraces deep engagement, intersubjectivity and genuine mutuality. I-It relationships represent reductionism; the "It" becomes an object. Buber (1923) does not deny the common role of I-it relationships, which are supported through the five senses, enabling us to categorize other people and the world. However, the I-Thou is the transformational experience of transcendence. Essentially, I-Thou is the connection that prizes personhood. White (2013) considers personhood as an essence of the human species with two key components. Firstly, personhood is existential, thus intrinsically bound to the status of human beings and, secondly, it is relational, that is, its value is inherently prescribed by others (individuals/society). Another proponent of the principles of person-centered care was Carl Rogers, a humanist psychologist who, from the 1940s, argued that client-centered care in psychotherapy demands that the therapist is non-directive and demonstrates unconditional positive regard, empathy, genuineness and congruence (Rogers, 1946). While there are criticisms of both proponents, Burber (neglect of the impact of oppression and tolerance of evil (Fackenheim, 1982; Saguy, 2018)) and Rogers (being vague or over-optimistic and unrealistic (May, 1990; Brodley & Bradburn, 2015)), each perspective provides key foundations of person-centered care.

While the work of such authors resonates with our current understandings, Tom Kitwood, a psychologist, is generally attributed to developing the initial theory of person-centered care. Kitwood (1997) observed care of older adults living with dementia and argued that the standard medical model created an environment that supported malignant social psychology, which negatively impacted the individual being cared for. Kitwood pointed to the necessity of individualized care which supports relationships and personhood within a positive social environment. Supporting the arguments of Buber and Rogers, personhood is described as "a standing or status that is bestowed upon one human being, by others, it implies recognition, respect and trust" (Kitwood, 1997: 8). In dementia care, creating the conditions for person-centered care is supported by attending to individuals' comfort, attachment, occupation, identity, supporting their inclusion and ensuring they experience feeling loved and valued (Kitwood, 1997). Building on the work of Kitwood (1997) and Brooker and Latham (2016) developed the Values, Individual Perspectives and Social (VIPS) framework to guide care environments' delivery of person-centered care. The four domains are presented in Table 2.1, and each one contains up to seven sub-domains.

TABLE 2.1 The Values, Individual Perspectives and Social (VIPS) framework (Brooker & Latham, 2016)

Values	*Individuals*	*Perspectives*	*Social*
V1: Vision	I1: Individual support and care	P1: Communication	S1: Inclusion
V2: Human resources	I2: Recognizing and responding to change	P2: Empathy and acceptable risk	S2: Respect
V3: Management ethos	I3: Personal possessions	P3: Physical environment	S3: Warmth
V4: Training and practice development	I4: Individual preferences	P4: Physical health needs	S4: Validation
V5: The service environment	I5: Life histories	P5: Challenging behavior as communication	S5: Enabling
V6: Quality assurance	I6: Activity and occupation	P6: Advocacy	S6: Part of the community S7: Partners, families, friends and relatives

Other frameworks have represented the inherent elements of person-centered care.

a. Nolan et al. (2006) developed the Senses' Framework, which encompasses six domains: (1) sense of security, (2) sense of belonging, (3) sense of continuity, (4) sense of purpose, (5) sense of achievement and (6) sense of significance.
b. Another impactful approach to person-centered care has been developed by the University of Gothenburg (2020) with three domains: (1) partnership, (2) patient narrative/story and (3) documentation. Further work by Lloyd et al. (2019) has expanded to a fourth domain (4) an agreement to act in conjunction with the person and other professionals to coordinate care.
c. Santana et al. (2017) developed a framework using Donabedian's (1988) quality of care framework, which navigates care as: *structure*-healthcare systems/organizational level, *process*: healthcare provider levels and *outcome:* patient-healthcare provider-healthcare system/organizational level.
d. McCormack and McCance's (2017) framework places the person at the center of care and is comprised of five domains: (1) macro-context, (2) pre-requisites, (3) care environment, (4) person-centered processes and (5) person-centered outcomes.

Within recent reviews of person-centered care, particular core qualities have been identified. These include the development and fostering of partnerships, self-management, collaboration and shared decision-making, which support personhood (Harding et al., 2015; Sharma et al., 2015; Hennelly et al., 2018). Ekman et al. (2021) argue that person-centered care translates to routines which involve initiating the partnership, implementing the partnership and safeguarding the partnership. Supporting personhood requires an authentic motivation that supports an ethical orientation (Ekman, 2022) and a human rights-based approach supporting the person's values and preferences (Safeguarding Ireland & HIQA, 2019). Accordingly, "doing the thing right" does not always equate to "doing the right thing". For example, in a case within the English Courts of Protection, Lord Justice Munby notes that protocols may be followed to keep people safe (overplaying risk), but that the lack of intersubjectivity and absent voice of the person can mean the outcomes meet criteria but not the intrinsic happiness of the person:

> The emphasis must be on sensible risk appraisal, not striving to avoid all risk, whatever the price, but instead seeking a proper balance and being willing to tolerate manageable or acceptable risks as the price appropriately to be paid, in order to achieve some other good-in particular to achieve the vital good of the elderly or vulnerable person's happiness. What good is it making someone safer if it merely makes them miserable.
>
> *(Munby, 2007)*

Thus, person-centered care involves a humanistic approach of equitable connection and vindication of rights, regardless of physical or cognitive ability. As person-centered care has become a key priority in many countries, an assessment of the people's subjective experience within healthcare has become increasingly valued within systems of care that recognize their accountability in quality service provision (Larson et al., 2019). Many institutions and healthcare regulators now include patient experience and patient satisfaction surveys as important measures of care quality (see the Irish Health Information and Quality Authority: https://www.hiqa.ie/areas-we-work/national-care-experience-programme). Equally, assessing person/patient-centeredness has resulted in several measurement scales (Jones et al., 2018), including various patient-reported outcomes measures and patient-reported experience measures, as well as gauging related key performance indicators (i.e. McCance et al., 2012).

Person-centered principles are important in community approaches. McCallum et al. (2024) illustrated how the community impacts health; in their study on multi-morbidity in a socially deprived community, the use of person-centered approaches was found to improve engagement and support responses. Furthermore, using a person-centered strengths approach when working with communities enables the visibility and leveraging of what communities can do rather than their deficits. This increases communities' self-determination and control over what is important to improve their well-being (Office for Health Improvement & Disparities, 2022). However, as discussed in Chapter 4, engagement must balance ambition with scope to influence or change circumstances using an asset-based community approach (NICE, 2016).

Further work has been undertaken in person-centered coordinated care (P3C), which recognizes that people rarely experience health in one setting but have multiple encounters with various healthcare professionals and non-statutory organizations in various settings (home, community, acute care, residential care). Moreover, healthcare systems are often structured within siloed specializations as they can be delivered around single issues (i.e. cardiac, respiratory), which can neglect the intricacy of an individual's health status, particularly related to chronic illness care (Lloyd et al., 2017a; Djukanovic et al., 2024). Consequently, navigating a complex health system has often resulted in fragmented and uncoordinated care which can lead to gaps in continuity of such care and adverse events (Akinyelure et al., 2022; WHO, 2023a). Person-centered coordinated care can be defined as:

"Care and support that is guided by and organized effectively around the needs and preferences of individuals" (Lloyd et al., 2019: 506).

Culture change is fundamental to transforming systems of care to reflect a joined-up coordinated health experience for people, yet this demands commitment from individual professionals, to organizations, to overall healthcare governance (Lloyd et al., 2017b). Moving to think, plan and transform services to P3C is underpinned by a trusting collaboration with key stakeholders to provide care that is both person-centered and coordinated within the complexity of the broader health system. Furthermore, Lloyd and colleagues (2019) propose P3C as encompassing five domains: (1) information and communication, (2) care planning, (3) transitions, (4) patient-defined goals or outcomes and (5) shared decision-making. Research on measuring these domains has demonstrated positive results with both patients and staff (Horrell et al., 2018; Lloyd et al., 2018, 2019; Sugavanam et al., 2018). Other examples of work undertaken to guide P3C are evident in separate patient narrative studies in the United Kingdom and Ireland, focusing on subjective "I" statements that reflect what people want from their healthcare system. In the United Kingdom, National Voices, a coalition of charities that advocates for person-centered care, developed six domains reflecting how care should be experienced related to my goals/outcomes; care planning; communication; information; decision-making (including budgets); and transitions, containing 38 narrative statements (Redding, 2013). Similarly, in Ireland, a multi-phase project developed 19 "I" statements under three domains – my healthcare experience, care that I am confident in and my journey through healthcare to remind healthcare professionals of what people expect from their care experience (Phelan et al., 2017).

Why Community Health?

As noted above, in delivering healthcare, there have been many calls to address issues of fragmentation, lack of continuity, improve people's experience of health care and maximize health outcomes leveraging interdisciplinary and service users' collaborations (WHO, 2007; Timmins et al., 2022; Prior et al., 2023; Kern et al., 2024). A concept akin to care coordination is integrated care, where care is coordinated across professionals, facilities and support systems. It meets people's individual needs over time and facilitates timely health professional contact (Singer et al., 2011). Valentijn et al. (2013) describe this as having multiple levels of integration; these are vertical, horizontal, system, organizational, professional, clinical and normative, with population-based and person-centered care as foundational. Integrated care encompasses care continuity which maps to the interconnection of health contacts over time, incorporating the person's needs and preferences (WHO, 2018). As such, although integrated care is a systems focus, its objective mirrors a person-centered coordinated approach with aspects related to interconnections of care for the person across settings and professionals and with care built around the individual's needs and preferences.

In 2015, the World Health Organization (WHO) advocated that people have access to an equitable and acceptable healthcare system that enables co-production of timely responses to their needs across both the life course and the continuum of care. This should be supported by five targeted strategies:

- Engaging and empowering people and communities.
- Strengthening governance and accountability.
- Reorienting the model of care.

- Coordinating services within and across sectors.
- Creating an enabling environment.

Using the term people-centered healthcare services, the WHO describes a supportive approach to fostering communities' well-being:

> ...an approach to care that consciously adopts the perspectives of individuals, families and communities, and sees them as participants as well as beneficiaries of trusted health systems that respond to their needs and preferences in humane and holistic ways. People-centred care requires that people have the education and support they need to make decisions and participate in their own care. It is organised around the health needs and expectations of people rather than diseases.
>
> *(WHO 2016a: 2)*

While this broad framework is founded on people-centered integrated care, there are key aspects within the approach that apply when working with communities (WHO 2016b). Engaging and empowering communities reflects a reorientation in how health is negotiated and how actions are implemented. Rather than a "one-size-fits-all" approach, the uniqueness and diversity of communities can provide a bottom-up approach to generating tailored and meaningful collaborations and partnerships. Through authentic and enabling engagement, the power dynamics shift and the model of care maps to need rather than the application of inflexible, universal, standardized approaches. Notably, this does not reduce the responsibility for governance and accountability; it is strengthened through the equitable participation and voice of the community stakeholders. This process refocuses on the relational aspects of collaboration and mirrors frameworks of person-centered care where personhood is equated to neighborhood, valuing individuality, identity and equity but also celebrating diversity and inclusion. It is in diversity that the community differs, and the key is to identify common issues that represent the community rather than privileging some of its members. This takes careful negotiation, as discussed in Chapter 3, to prioritize and compromise toward the goal of community flourishing. Furthermore, health disparities are experienced globally, particularly by underserved and at-risk populations (Tangcharoensathien et al., 2024). Yet, it is crucial to consider communities and neighborhoods individually, as examining wider regions or states' health can obscure health disparities that present "average" outcomes.

In the United Kingdom, the Marmot reports (2010; 2019) point to the importance of community capital and fostering social networks to support positive life experiences (see Chapter 3). Communities are considered an important pillar in responding to health disparities, and these reports argue the imperative of creating and developing healthy and sustainable spaces, places and communities to limit preventable social inequalities and inequities in people's health. A key point made in the 2019 Marmot report is the need for proportionate universalism. This means investment according to need. From this perspective, fostering community-centered approaches and working in partnership with communities translates to both identifying and addressing local issues, particularly related to the social determinants of health, with funding aimed at initiatives that provide equity in health opportunities. For example, Radley et al. (2024) point to the continuing racial and ethnic health disparities in the United States and argue that better access to services is required, but this depends on factors such as political will, investment, addressing health insurance administrative burden and universal, equitable health coverage for people.

Community-centered care is important, particularly in the context of addressing deprivation (Public Health England, 2018). Recognizing health disparities and working with communities means sharing power through a joint commitment to well-being. However, despite this, reports which can be traced to Chadwick (1842), Black (1980) and Marmot (2010; 2019) detail widening health inequalities related to the social determinants of health. Issues such as access and equity in healthcare, as well as socio-economic inequalities, gender, race and ethnicity, can lead to marginalized underserved communities, and this can be magnified through the intersectionality of community characteristics (WHO, 2023b; Tangcharoensathien et al., 2024). While arguments have demonstrated the need for social justice and empowering community solidarity, cohesion and self-determination, political (funding and structural supports), follow-through can be elusive. Therefore, the reorientation to community-centered care is crucial, but importantly, community, political and statutory stakeholders need to be committed to collaboration, partnership, compromise and negotiation to authentically meet needs.

Recent projects by the Robert Wood Johnson Foundation (RWJF) demonstrate the use of partnerships and initiatives to co-create healthy communities. Drawing on the discussion by Lloyd in Chapter 4, addressing health inequities is key to supporting communities to enhance their collective well-being. In the Culture of Health Action Framework, four action areas are core to supporting communities. These are:

1 Making Health a Shared Value.
2 Fostering Cross-Sector Collaboration to Improve Well-Being.
3 Creating Healthier, More Equitable Communities.
4 Strengthening Integration of Health Services and Systems (RWJF, 2019:1).

Within this approach, a triple perspective is needed which focuses on increasing economic and educational opportunities, reducing health disparities and addressing historical and system-level barriers. Moreover, while meeting the needs of underserved populations often demands immediate actions, the RWJF (2019) argues that sustainability of change is also a prerequisite to long-term success.

One method of civic engagement and collaboration is via deliberative democracy. Deliberative democracy has multiple understandings, but there are central common tenets (Ercan & Dryzek, 2015). Based on normative theory, deliberative democracy provides normative standards against which democracies can be examined, assessed and improved. As such, it provides a way of scrutinizing political practices within the real world, seeking to continually improve and refine the democratic process through a transformative and emancipatory approach. Layman (2016) argues that this involves a political liberty wherein citizens are instrumental in decision-making and become co-authors of legislation. However, such political liberty encompasses active citizen involvement in all stages of decision-making, from reflection, critique and debate on possible options by citizens and the selection and recommendation of the best proposals, which are subject to voting (Goodwin, 2017). While deliberative democracy is more recognizable in activities such as Citizens' Assemblies, its process and ethos are based on citizen decision-making, which, from this chapter's perspective, translates to people who live in the community. The application of this approach within a community context can be reviewed in McCormack et al.'s chapter (Chapter 7). A key aspect of deliberative democracy is engagement in dialogue that respects all perspectives, even those contrary or oppositional within the group membership (Verhasselt, 2025). Thus, deliberative democracy acknowledges the potential for conflict and diversity but provides a foundation of positive discussion. The key to change is the mobilization of collective action to effect sustainable change.

A Framework to Understand Communities

As we argue in this book, individuals, families and neighborhoods comprise communities and communities are complex entities. As such, communities are influenced by both internal and external factors. Understanding community means taking a multifaceted approach. In this regard, as Lloyd also recognizes in Chapter 4, taking an ecological approach is useful to appreciate the confluence of system levels that can impact a community. Bronfenbrenner (1977; 1979; 1995) originally developed the ecological framework to understand human development within multiple nested system levels. It is recognized that Bronfenbrenner's framework neglects issues such as resilience (Christensen, 2016), oversimplifying the complexity of interactions without due consideration to issues of power dynamics, intersectionality, issues related to inequities, casual relationships and other factors such as incorporating subjectivities of individuals (Kaushik et al., 2023). Moreover, Bronfenbrenner (1995) and Bronfenbrenner and Morris's (1998)'s application relate to the individual's development, whereas we are using the framework to explore community development. In other words, Bronfenbrenner's work focused on the individual as the unit of analysis, while we are using the ecological model to prioritize the community as the unit of analysis. To understand community and

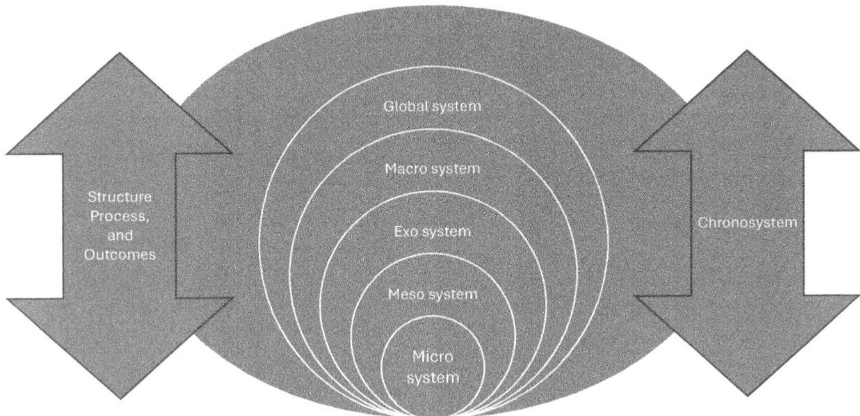

FIGURE 2.1 Combining Bronfenbrenner's Ecological model and Donabedian's model for community

address potential limitations in using the ecological approach, Donabedian's (1988) model is also incorporated, which accounts for structures, processes and outcomes. Figure 2.1 depicts an adapted representation of Bronfenbrenner's socio-ecological model (Phelan & Kirwan, 2020) combined with the adapted Donabedian model (1966; 2005).

Bronfenbrenner's (1977; 1979) ecological framework was developed to understand child development and was later extended to an ecological systems theory (Bronfenbrenner 1995; Bronfenbrenner & Morris, 1998). Bronfenbrenner's work has been used widely to understand individual and contextual issues within bidirectional nested systems as applied to health behaviors (Sallis et al., 2008), healthy living (Kim et al., 2021), mental health (Slimmens et al., 2024; Ghasemi, 2025), violence prevention (CDC, 2024), policy analysis (Ndu et al., 2022; Amorocho-Daza et al., 2025) and agriculture (Kilanowski, 2017). The ecological model has also been used to examine community engagement (Caperon et al., 2022) and underserved populations (Salihu et al., 2015). The framework provides a lens to examine how people are embedded in context (community) and successively adapt to their environment over time and are both influenced by and influence their environment (Phelan & Kirwan, 2020). For our focus, we are using the framework to understand the cultural, social, economic and political confluences that impact a community's development. Table 2.2 provides the context of each system level where Phelan and Kirwan (2020) have adapted the model to incorporate global influences, which are increasingly relevant in a globalized world where information and influence are advanced through technology.

The ecological model is used to consider the complex inter-relationships that produce communities. From the global system to the exo-system, there is a

TABLE 2.2 Modified Bronfenbrenner's socio-ecological model (Phelan & Kirwan, 2020) as applied to community

System level	*Representation*	*Examples*
Global system	Global	Global economics, political context, WHO, UN, pandemics, global alliances, membership (i.e. EU, NATO)
Macrosystem	National	Legislation, policy, ideologies, culture, regulations, systems of welfare, housing policy, education supports, politics, national economy, open or closed system.
Exo-system	Regional level	Relationships within regions and communities within regions.
Mesosystem	Community level	Constituent community groups, sub-cultures, connections, values, preferences, intersectionality, community networking, employment, housing, mutuality, physical environment, services available, transport, education, etc.
Microsystem	The immediate environment individuals live in.	Individuals and families that constitute the community. Inclusion or exclusion of people in the community.
Chrono-system	Changes over time	Trends in issues such as age, employment, physical environment, technology, services, internal and external perceptions of the community.

descending sphere of influence; while global issues can impact a community, it is rare to observe this impact in the reverse direction. The mesosystem of community is most critical as it fosters the complexity of the community's diverse array of interplaying, non-linear constituent microsystems. Within the context of the ecological model, the boundaries are flexible and adaptable, and issues may be represented within multiple systems. For example, the effect of events at the global level can filter into other system levels. As demonstrated, the individual is immersed in a nested system that represents a confluence of influence. The impact of global, macro or mesosystems' changes can have a ripple effect on communities (mesosystem) and individuals (microsystem). The global system represents global events that can filter down and disrupt the conditions and context of lower levels. For instance, the collapse of the Lehman Brothers bank on September 15, 2008, impacted individual countries' banking systems, triggering an economic crash. This, in turn, led to businesses' closure and, ultimately, many communities experienced unemployment and resource limitations (funding support, employment moratoriums, infrastructure development delays), which affected individuals and families. Furthermore, decisions of powerful nations concerning economic (i.e. tariffs) or social (i.e. foreign aid) issues, or areas such as visa restrictions, can reverberate within other countries' fiscal balance, development supports or international migration related to issues such as conflict or employment. Another example of a global impact is the COVID-19 pandemic. Strict public health protocols led to limitations in everyday life and the cessation of familiar activities such as free movement, socialization, employment and community socialization and integration activities. Some of these impacts continue, for example, flexibility in working from home; however, others reflect the negative effects, particularly related to marginalized groups (Maizel et al., 2024; Cannon et al., 2024).

On a macro level, the impact of wider government policies (and political systems) directs public services and expectations related to ideologies, education, crime, housing, social protection, legislation, regulation, economic systems, etc. The macro level is akin to the blueprint of culture, values and directions and can be reflected in popular media, although this may be moderated by authoritarian political systems. Macrosystem changes can be reactive (as in the example above) or proactive, for example, in relation to policy directions for issues such as human rights. The macrosystem creates a pattern of interactions within the sub-systems and shapes social exchange (Crawford, 2020).

The exo-system represents a regional or multifaceted level of connection and is comprised of communities that share some common boundaries or characteristics. This could be a geographic region or some other form of synergies that connect communities. Communities may not be directly involved at this level (but may have some representation), but decisions at this level can impact the context of individual communities within the ecosystem's sphere of influence. This could be a county council, a health region, a political electoral area or a religious diocese. For example, such entities provide governance in areas such as regional planning, local resource allocation, waste management, environmental protection or infrastructure (i.e. roads, transport). The relationship remains reciprocal; for example, a local community representative brings the needs of the community to lobby for resources, while the finite nature of these resources can impact the quality of the environment for members of the individual community.

The mesosystem represents the community and its interactions, relationships as well as the interplay of people, groups and institutions that constitute the community. It is the intersection of multiple microsystems within the community, which can result in synergistic or conflicting relationships or contexts (Kaushik et al., 2023). The mesosystem spans from characteristics of age, gender, industry, employment, educational institutions, physical environment and local infrastructure, governance, experience of equity and marginalization, services, to local transport. It also includes experiences of mutuality, history and people's transience or longevity in residence. As a community, individuals experience identity and belonging in constituting themselves but also in how that community is viewed by external stakeholders.

The microsystem is the basic building block of community and is where most individual interactions and experiences occur (Christensen, 2016; Kaushik et al., 2023). It is comprised of individuals, families, neighborhoods and groups in direct face-to-face experience. The zone of influence within the microsystem can reflect issues of power, impacting the social, economic and environmental context and involvement of the community in relation to a myriad of issues such as governance, quality of life, conflict and modes of resolution. Changes in the microsystem are termed ecological transitions, for example, the impact of unemployment or promotion; these modify the context of the individual and family and even groups (Crawford, 2020). As our focus is community, the chronosystem illustrates the changes and dynamic transitions of the community over time. It is important that the socio-historical and political context is considered, as this can explain the community's present reality, perceptions and experiences. When working with communities, it is also important to understand past and current affiliations, adaptations, change, conflict, development, resources and identity.

Later development of the ecological theory led to renaming it as the ecological systems theory, which integrated complex, reciprocal interactions, termed proximal processes. Proximal processes are described in later works by Bronfenbrenner and Morris (1998) as enduring bidirectional activities with people, objects or symbols which become increasingly more complex over time and affect developmental processes. This is represented in exploring the person-context-process-time relationships (Bronfenbrenner & Morris, 1998). In the context of community, proximal processes are important as they are formative in identity, experience and the community's understandings of the world. While Bronfenbrenner and Morris (1998) state proximal processes are positive interactions, Merçon-Vargas et al. (2020) argue the importance of understanding inverse proximal processes, which can be malignant, producing dysfunctional adaptations and negatively impacting competencies, which can contribute to disadvantage. Crawford (2020) also notes the significance of ecological validity, which reflects confirming the reality of the community within community engagement activities (see Chapter 3). Furthermore, ecological niches describe the confluence of factors that converge to form favorable or unfavorable predictors of the community's development (Crawford, 2020).

Donabedian's (1966; 2005) model has been used to gauge the quality of healthcare since the mid-1960s. It is recognized as a comprehensive systematic approach for measuring quality by examining three interrelated levels in healthcare: structure, processes and outcomes (Berwick & Fox, 2016). While later work with the ecological systems theory incorporated proximal processes, this focused on the individual-person level. Despite being developed for the measurement of healthcare quality, Donabedian offers a complementary lens to look at the community's

TABLE 2.3 Donabedian's model applied to community

Level	*As applied to community*
Structure	Describes how the community is constituted and related attributes; it includes a review of the physical, demographic, environmental, geographical, social, political and economic aspects of communities. It includes service provision, access and adequacy. In this model, the relationships of the community are also mapped to the other system levels. It includes a temporal domain of the community history. As communities are heterogeneous entities, structure also includes differentiation of sub-structures within the communities in terms of advantage and disadvantage.
Processes	This describes what, how, where levels of interaction occur and examines leadership, power, privilege and issues related to underserved communities, inequities and intersectionality. It considers how decisions are made related to communities and how things get done (or not).
Outcomes	Considers the impact, outcomes and consequences of structure and processes on the community. This correlates to Bronfenbrenner and Morris's proximal processes (i.e. community unrest and conflict), although, in this context, a single event may substantially impact a community (industry closure, employment redundancies, climate change crisis) and the relationship may not be reciprocal.

composition, how things work and what the results of such arrangements are. Table 2.3 provides a breakdown of Donabedian's levels and their application to the community.

The Donabedian model (1988; 2005) can also be used to evaluate interventions. For example, the National Health Service Improvement in the United Kingdom offers service enhancement guidance underpinned by Donabedian (ACT Academy, 2019). In this guidance, balancing measures are also considered as an important additional level to identify any unintended consequences of interventions or change and to stimulate ameliorative actions.

Collecting data for community engagement and community profiling is underpinned by mixed methods, but most important is the process of engagement, which applies person-centered principles. By combining both models, areas of evidence-based improvement can be co-identified with the community as partner, aimed at both intrinsic issues within the community or related to its external influences at the exo and macro levels. While the global level has the power to filter its influence, the bidirectional level is most remote in terms of a community's influence on global activities. Thus, the current context of the community's reality may identify negative health or social care issues and together with the community, a prioritization can occur with the co-creation of a response plan, implementation and revaluation. Chapter 3 provides additional detail on operationalizing collaborations with communities.

Conclusion

In this chapter, we have traced the emergence of person-centered care and articulated central principles in its operationalization. Activities to adapt person-centeredness to the community require attention to issues of equity and addressing health disparities, which are meaningful to the community. Following on from this, two models (the ecological systems model and the Donabedian model) were selected and adapted for use to underpin collaboration with the community. Using a person-centered approach and combining both models translate to positive relationships, which use processes such as providing support, conflict management, transformational leadership and fostering equitable processes. Processes should also value the principles of deliberative democracy, accountability and transparency. Being community-driven encourages innovation, relationship-building, respect for intersubjectivity, appreciating shared history and creating new history. Community members need to be supported in negotiating power sharing, trust and facilitating mutuality. Outcomes should evidence the creation and consolidation of community collaborations, improvement in people's lives, developing community resilience and empowerment and promoting equity by engendering a sense of belonging and identity.

References

ACT Academy (2019). *NHS improvement-online library of quality, service improvement and redesign tools: A model for measuring quality of care.* Retrieved from https://aqua.nhs.uk/wp-content/uploads/2023/07/qsir-measuring-quality-care.pdf

Akinyelure, O. P., Colvin, C. L., Sterling, M. R., Safford, M. M., Munter, P., Colantonio, L. D., & Kern, L. M. (2022). Frailty, gaps in care coordination, and preventable adverse events. *BMC Geriatrics, 22*, 476. https://doi.org/10.1186/s12877-022-03164-7.

Amorocho-Daza, H., Sušnik, J., & van der Zaag, Slinger, J. H. (2025). A model-based policy analysis framework for social-ecological systems: Integrating uncertainty and participation in system dynamics modelling. *Ecological Modelling, 499*, 110943.

Berwick, D., & Fox, D. M. (2016). Evaluating the quality of medical care: Donabedian's classic article 50 years later. *The Milbank Quarterly*, *94*(2), 237–241. https://doi.org/10.1111/1468–0009.12189

Berwick, D. M., Nolan, T. W., & Whittington, J. (2008). The triple aim: Care, health, and cost. *Health Affairs*, *27*(3), 759–769.

Black, D. (1980). *Report of the working group on inequalities in health.* DHSS: London.

Blackmon, B. J., Lee, J., Bain, R., Brazeal, B., Williams, C., & Green, Y. (2022). Person-centredness in the workplace: An examination of person-centred skills, processes and workplace factors among Medicaid waiver providers in the United States. *International Practice Development Journal, 12*(2), 1–12. Retrieved from https://aquila.usm.edu/fac_pubs/21018

Brodley, E. T., & Bradburn, W. M. (2015). Did Carl Rogers' positive view of human nature bias his psychotherapy? *The Person Centred Journal, 22*(1/2), 81–112.

Bronfenbrenner, U. (1977). Toward an experimental ecology of human development. *American Psychologist, 32*, 513–531. https://doi.org/10.1037/0003–066X.32.7.513.

Bronfenbrenner U. (1979). *The ecology of human development: Experiments by nature and design.* Harvard University Press: Massachusetts.

Bronfenbrenner, U. (1995). Developmental ecology through space and time: A future perspective. In *Examining lives in context: Perspectives on the ecology of human development.* (P. Moen, P., Elder, G. H. Jr., & Lüscher, K. eds.). American Psychological Association: Washington, pp. 619–647.

Bronfenbrenner, U., & Morris, P. A. (1998). The ecology of developmental processes. In *Handbook of child psychology: Vol. 1. Theoretical models of human development* (Damon, W. (Series Ed.) & Lerner R. M. (Vol. Ed.)), (5th ed.). Wiley: New York, pp. 993–1028.

Brooker, D., & Lathan, I. (2016). *Person-centred dementia care.* Jessica Kingsley Press: London.

Brown, H. (2025). *Navigating housing challenges for older adults: The importance of person-centred care.* Retrieved from https://housingevidence.ac.uk/navigating-housing-challenges-for-older-adults-the-importance-of-person-centred-care/#:~:text=The%20Department%20of%20Health%20and,such%20as%20a%20second%20bedroom.

Buchanan, C., & Sharma, N. (2024). *People-centred and participatory policymaking.* Retrieved from https://openpolicy.blog.gov.uk/2024/11/19/people-centred-and-participatory-policymaking/

Buber, M. (1923). *I and thou.* T & Clarke: Edinburgh.

Caesens, G., Gillet, N., Morin, A. J. S., Houle, S. A., & Stinglhamber, F. (2020). A person-centred perspective on social support in the workplace. *Applied Psychology, 69*, 686–714.

Cannon, M. L., Lynelle, B., & Jessica M. F. (2024). COVID-19 pandemic impacts on community connections and third place engagement: A qualitative analysis of older Americans. *Journal of Aging and Environment, 38*(4), 381–397. https://doi.org/10.1080/26892618.2023.2225179

Caperon, L., Saville, F., & Ahern, S. (2022). Developing a socio-ecological model for community engagement in a health programme in an underserved urban area. *PloS one, 17*(9), e0275092. https://doi.org/10.1371/journal.pone.0275092

Centre for Disease Control and Prevention (CDC) (2024). *About violence prevention.* Retrieved from https://www.cdc.gov/violence-prevention/about/index.html

Chadwick, E. (1842). *Report on the sanitary condition of the labouring population of Great Britain.* House of Commons Sessional Paper: London.

Christensen, J. (2016). A critical reflection of Bronfenbrenner's development ecological model. *Problems of Education in the 21st Century,* 69, 22–28.

Crawford, M. (2020). Ecological Systems theory: Exploring the development of the theoretical framework as conceived by Bronfenbrenner. *Journal of Public Health Issues & Practice, 4*(2), 170–176.

Djukanovic, I., Hellström, A., Wolke, A., & Schildmeijer, K. (2024). The meaning of continuity of care from the perspective of older people with complex care needs–a scoping review. *Geriatric Nursing, 55*, 354–361.

Donabedian, A. (1966; 2005). Evaluating the quality of medical care. *Milbank Memorial Fund Q, 44*(3), (suppl), 166–206. Reprinted in *Milbank Quarterly, 83*(4), 691–729.

Donabedian, A. (1988). The quality of care: How can it be assessed? *Journal of the American Medical Association, 260*(12), 1743–1748.

Ekman, I. (2022). Practising the ethics of person-centred care balancing ethical conviction and moral obligations. *Nursing Philosophy, 23*(3), e12382.

Ekman, I., Ebrahimi, Z., & Olaya Contreras, P. (2021). Person-centred care: Looking back, looking forward. *European Journal of Cardiovascular Nursing, 20*(2), 93–95. https://doi.org/10.1093/eurjcn/zvaa025

Ercan, S. A., & Dryzek, J. S. (2015). The reach of deliberative democracy, *Policy Studies Journal, 36*, 241–248.

Fackenheim, E. L. (1982). *To mend the world: Foundations of future Jewish thought.* Schocken Books: New York.

Ghasemi, F. (2025). Teachers' mental health challenges and contributing risk factors: A systematic narrative review based on the socio-ecological model. *Psychology in the Schools, 62*(7), 2111–2135.

Goodwin, R. E. (2017). The epistemic benefits of deliberative democracy, *Policy Sciences, 50*, 351–366.

Gray, A., & Woods, K. (2022) Person-centred practices in education: A systematic review of research. *Support for Learning, 37*, 309–335.

Harding, E., Wait, S., & Scrutton, J. (2015) *The state of play in person-centred care: A pragmatic review of how person-centred care is defined, applied and measured.* The Health Policy Partnership: London.

Hennelly, N., Cooney, A., Houghton, C., & O'Shea, E. (2018). The experiences and perceptions of personhood for people living with dementia: A qualitative evidence synthesis protocol. *Health Research Board Open Research, 1*(18). https://doi.org/10.12688/hrbopenres.12845.1

Horrell, J., Lloyd, H., Sugavanam, T., Close, J., & Byng, R. (2018). Creating and facilitating change for Person-Centred Coordinated Care (P3C): The development of the Organisational Change Tool (P3C-OCT). *Health Expectations, 21*(2), 448–456. https://doi.org/10.1111/hex.12631

Jones, M. C., Williams, B., Rattray, J., MacGillivray, S., Baldie, D., Abubakari, A. R., Coyle, J., Mackie, S., & McKenna, E. (2018). Extending the assessment of patient-centredness in health care: Development of the updated Valuing Patients as Individuals Scale using exploratory factor analysis, *Journal of Clinical Nursing, 27*(1–2), 65–76. https://doi.org/10.1111/jocn.13845

Kaushik, D., Garg, M., & Mishra, A. (2023). Exploring developmental pathways: An in-depth analysis of Bronfenbrenner's bioecological model. *International Journal for Multidisciplinary Research, 5*(6), 1–11.

Kern, L. M., Bynum, J. P. W., & Pincus, H. A. (2024). Care fragmentation, care continuity, and care coordination-how they differ and why it matters. *JAMA Internal Medicine, 184*(3), 236–237.

Kilanowski, J. F. (2017). Breadth of the socio-ecological model. *Journal of Agromedicine, 22*(4), 295–297. https://doi.org/10.1080/1059924X.2017.1358971

Kim, Y., & Park, J. H. (2021). Factors influencing healthy living practice by socio-ecological model. *The Journal of the Convergence on Culture Technology, 7*(4), 351–361.

Kitwood, T. (1997). *Dementia reconsidered: The person comes first.* Open University Press: Buckingham.

Larson, E., Sharma, J., Bohren, M., & Tunçalp, Ö. (2019). When the patient is the expert: Measuring patient experience and satisfaction with care. *Bulletin of the World Health Organization, 97*(8), 563–569. https://doi.org/10.2471/BLT.18.225201.

Layman, D. (2016). Robust deliberative democracy. *Critical Reviews: A Journal of Politics & Society, 28*, 494–516.

Lloyd, H., Close, J., Horrell, J., Wheat, H., & Valeras, J. (2017b). *How to use metrics, measures & insights to commission person centred coordinated care*. NHSE: Redditch.

Lloyd, H., Fosh, B., Whalley, B., Byng, R., & Close, J. (2019). Validation of the person-centred coordinated care experience questionnaire (P3CEQ). *International Journal for Quality in Health Care, 31*(7), 506–512. https://doi.org/10.1093/intqhc/mzy212

Lloyd, H., Wheat, H., Horrell, J., Sugavanam, T., Fosh, B., Valderas, J. M., & Close, J. (2018). Patient-reported measures for person-centred coordinated care: A comparative domain map and web-based compendium for supporting policy development and implementation. *Journal of Medical Internet Research, 20*(2), e54. https://doi.org/10.2196/jmir.7789

Lloyd, H. M., Pearson, M., Sheaff, R., Asthana, S., Wheat, H., Sugavanam, T. P., Britten, N., Valderas, J., Bainbridge, M., Witts, L., Westlake, D., Horrell, J., & Byng, R. (2017a). Collaborative action for person-centred coordinated care (P3C): An approach to support the development of a comprehensive system-wide solution to fragmented care. *Health Research Policy & Systems, 15*(1), 98. https://doi.org/10.1186/s12961-017-0263-z

Maizel, J. L., Haller, M. J., Maahs, D. M., Addala, A., Lal, R. A., Filipp, S. L., Gurka, M. J., Westen, S., Dixon, B. N., Figg, L., Hechavarria, M., Malden, K. G., & Walker, A. F. (2024). COVID-19 impacts and inequities among underserved communities with diabetes. *Journal of Clinical & Translational Endocrinology, 36*, 100337. https://doi.org/10.1016/j.jcte.2024.100337

Marmot, M., Allen, J., Boyce, T., Goldblatt, P., & Morrison, J. (2019). *Health equity in England: The Marmot review ten years on.* Institute of Health Equity: London.

Marmot, M., Atkinson, T., Bell, J., Black, C., Broadfoot, P., Cumberlege, J., Diamond, I., Gilmore, I., Ham, C., Meacher, M., & Mulgan, G. (2010). *Fair society, healthy lives.* The Marmot Review: London.

May, R. (1982). The problem of evil: An open letter to Carl Rogers. *Journal of Humanistic Psychology, 22*(3), 10–21.

McCallum, M., Macdonald, S., & Mair, F. S. (2024). Multimorbidity and person-centred care in a socioeconomically deprived community: A qualitative study. *The British Journal of General Practice, 74*(749), e805–e813.

McCance, T., Telford, L., Wilson, J., MacLeod, O., & Dowd, A. (2012). Identifying key performance indicators for nursing and midwifery care using a consensus approach. *Journal of Clinical Nursing, 2*(7–8), 1145–1154. https://doi.org/10.1111/j.1365–2702.2011.03820.x.

McCauley, L., Phillips, R. L., Meisnere, M., & Robinson, S. K. (eds.) (2021). Person-centered, family-centered, and community-oriented primary care. In *Implementing high-quality primary care rebuilding the foundation of health care.* The National Academies Press: Washington, D.C, pp. 93–140.

McCormack, B. (ed.) (2024). *Developing person-centred cultures in healthcare education and practice: An essential guide.* Wiley: New Jersey.

McCormack, B., & McCance, T. (2017). *Person centred practice in nursing and health.* Wiley-Blackwell: Chichester.

McCormack, B., McCance, T., & Maben, J. (2013). Outcome evaluation in the development of person-centred practice. In *Practice development in nursing.* (McCormack, B., Manley, K. & Titchen, A. eds.) (2nd ed). Wiley-Blackwell: Oxford, pp 190–211.

Merçon-Vargas, E. A., Lima, R. F. F., Rosa, E. M., & Tudge, J. (2020). Processing proximal processes: What Bronfenbrenner meant, what he didn't mean, and what he should have meant. *Journal of Family Theory & Review, 12*, 321–334. https://doi.org/10.1111/jftr.12373

Munby, J. (2007). *In the matter of MM (an adult).* Retrieved from https://www.bailii.org/ew/cases/EWHC/Fam/2007/2003.html

National Institute for Health and Care Excellence (NICE) (2016). *Community engagement: Improving health and wellbeing and reducing health inequalities.* Retrieved from https://www.nice.org.uk/guidance/ng44/chapter/recommendations#asset-based-approach

Ndu, M., Ariba, O., & Ohuruogu, A. (2022). The people-centred approach to policymaking: Re-imagining evidence-based policy in Nigeria. *Global Implementation Research & Applications, 2*, 95–104.

Nolan, M., Brown, J., Davies, S, Nolan, J., & Keady, J. (2006). *The senses framework: Improving care for older people through a relationship-centred approach. Getting Research into Practice (GRiP) Report No 2.* University of Sheffield: Sheffield.

Nundy, S., Cooper, L. A. & Mate, K. S. (2022). The quintuple aim for health care improvement: A new imperative to advance health equity. *Journal of the American Medical Association, 327*(6), 521–522.

Office for Health Improvement & Disparities (2022). *Community-centred practice: Applying all our health.* Retrieved from https://www.gov.uk/government/publications/community-centred-practice-applying-all-our-health/community-centred-practice-applying-all-our-health

Phelan, A., & Kirwan, M. (2020). Contextualising missed care in two healthcare inquiries using a socio-ecological systems approach. *Journal of Clinical Nursing, 29*(17–18), 3527–3540. https://doi.org/10.1111/jocn.15391

Phelan, A., McCormack, B., Dewing, J., Brown, D., Cardiff, S., Cook, N. F., Dickson, C., Kmetec, S., Lorber, M., Magowan, R., McCance, T., Skovdahl, K., Stiglic, G., & Van Lieshout, F. (2020). Review of developments in person-centred healthcare. *International Practice Development Journal, 10*(suppl)(3), 1–29.

Phelan, A., Rohde, D., Casey, M., Fealy, G., Felle, P., Lloyd, H., & O'Kelly, G. (2017). *Patient narrative project for person centred co-ordinated care.* University College Dublin: Dublin.

Prior, A., Vestergaard, C. H., Vedsted, P., Smith, S. M. Virgilsen, L. F., Rasmussen, L. A., & Fenger-Grøn, M. (2023). Healthcare fragmentation, multimorbidity, potentially inappropriate medication, and mortality: A Danish nationwide cohort study. *BMC Medicine, 21*, 305.

Public Health England (2018). *Health matters: Community-centred approaches for health and wellbeing.* Retrieved from https://www.gov.uk/government/publications/health-matters-health-and-wellbeing-community-centred-approaches/health-matters-community-centred-approaches-for-health-and-wellbeing#the-family-of-community-centred-approaches

Public Health England & NHS England (2015). *A guide to community-centred approaches for health and wellbeing.* Public Health England: London.

Radley, D. C., Shah, A, Collins, S. R., Powe, N. R. & Zephyrin, L. C. (2024). *Advancing racial equity in U.S. health care: The commonwealth fund 2024 state health disparities report.* The Commonwealth Fund: New York.

Redding, D. (2013). The narrative for person-centred coordinated care. *Journal of Integrated Care, 21*(6), 315–325. https://doi.org/10.1108/JICA-06–2013–0018.

Robert Wood Johnson Foundation (2019). *Culture of health, sentinel community insights: Health equity.* Princeton: New Jersey.

Rogers, C. (1946) Significant aspects of client-centered therapy. *American Psychologist, 1*(10), 415–22.

Safeguarding Ireland & HIQA (2019). *Guidance on a human rights-based approach in health and social care services.* HIQA: Dublin.

Saguy, T. (2018). Downside of intergroup harmony? When reconciliation might backfire and what to do. *Policy Insights from the Behavioural and Brain Sciences, 5*, 75–81.

Salihu, H. M., Wilson, R. E., King, L. M., Marty, P. J., & Whiteman, V. E. (2015). Socio-ecological model as a framework for overcoming barriers and challenges in randomized control trials in minority and underserved communities. *International Journal of MCH & AIDS, 3*(1), 85–95.

Sallis, J. F., Owen, N., & Fisher, E. B. (2008) Ecological models of health behavior. In *Health behavior and health education* (Glanz, K., Rimer, B. K. & Viswanath, K., eds.) (4th ed.). John Wiley & Sons: San Francisco, pp. 465–485.

Santana, M. J., Manalili, K., Jolley, R. J., Zelinsky, S., Quan, H., & Lu, M. (2017). How to practice person-centred care: A conceptual framework. *Health Expectations, 21*(2), 429–440.

Sharma, T., Bamford, M., & Dodman, D. (2015). Person-centred care: An overview of reviews. *Contemporary Nurse, 51*(2–3), 107–120.

Singer, S. J., Burgers, J., Friedberg, M., Rosenthal, M. B., Leape, L., & Schneider, E. (2011). Defining and measuring integrated patient care: Promoting the next frontier in health care delivery. *Medical Care Research and Review, 68*(1), 112–127.

Slimmen, S., Timmermans, O., Lechner, L., & Oenema, A. (2024). A socio-ecological approach of evidence on associations between social environmental factors and mental health outcomes of young adults: A systematic review. *Social Sciences & Humanities Open, 10*, 101068.

Sobolewska, A., Byrne, A., Harvey, C., Willis, E., Baldwin, A., McLellan, S., & Heard, D. (2020). Person-centred rhetoric in chronic care: A review of health policies. *Journal of Health Organisation and Management, 34*(2), 123–143. https://doi.org/10.1108/JHOM-04–2019–0078.

Sugavanam, P., Close, J., Fosh, B., Byng, R., & Lloyd, H. (2018). Co-designing a measure of person centred and coordinated care to capture the experience of the patient: The development of P3CEQ. *Journal of Patient Experience, 5*(3), 201–211.

Tangcharoensathien, V., Lekagul, A., & Teo, Y. Y. (2024). Global health inequities: More challenges, some solutions. *Bulletin of the World Health Organization, 102*(2), 86–86A.

Thomas, R. K. (2021) *Population health and the future of healthcare.* Springer International Publishing: Cham.

Timmins, L., Kern, L., Ghosh, A., Urato, C., & Rich, E. (2022). Predicting fragmented care: Beneficiary, physician, practice, and market characteristics. *Medical Care, 60*(12), 919–930.

University of Gothenburg (2020). *About person-centred care.* Retrieved from https://www.gu.se/en/gpcc/about-person-centred-care#Three-key-concepts-partnership-narrative-and-documentation

Valentijn, P. P., Schepman, S. M., Opheij, W., & Bruijnzeels, M. A. (2013). Understanding integrated care: A comprehensive conceptual framework based on the integrative functions of primary care. *International Journal of Integrated Care, 13*, e010. https://doi.org/10.5334/ijic.886

Verhasselt, L. (2025). Towards multilingual deliberative democracy: Navigating challenges and opportunities. *Representation, 61*(1), 57–74.

White, F. J. (2013). Personhood: An essential characteristic of the human species. *The Linacre Quarterly, 80*(1), 74–97.

World Health Organization (2007). *People centred healthcare: A policy framework.* World Health Organisation: Geneva.

World Health Organization (2015). *Framework on integrated people-centred health services: Report EB138/37.* World Health Organization: Geneva.

World Health Organization (2016a). Framework on integrated, people-centred health services. Report by the secretariat: Sixty-ninth world health assembly. Retrieved from tinyurl.com/WHO-people.

World Health Organization (2016b). Integrated care 4 people. Retrieved from tinyurl.com/WHO-IC4P.

World Health Organization (2018). *Continuity and coordination of care. A practice brief to support implementation of the WHO Framework on integrated people-centered health services.* World Health Organization: Geneva.

World Health Organization (2023a.) *Patient safety.* Retrieved from https://www.who.int/news-room/fact-sheets/detail/patient-safety#:~:text=Key%20facts,dollars%20each%20year%20(1).

World Health Organization (2023b). *Global health observatory*. Retrieved from https://www.who.int/data/gh

World Health Organization (2025). *Integrated people centred care.* Retrieved from https://www.who.int/health-topics/integrated-people-centered-care#tab=tab_1

3

COMMUNITY ENGAGEMENT, PROFILING AND ACTION PLANNING

Amanda Phelan

Introduction

Building on the principles of person-centered care as applied to a community, this chapter outlines strategies for collaboration with communities to maximize health and quality of life. Health inequalities have become a marker of poor well-being in communities. As early as 1842, Chadwick demonstrated how the poor sanitary conditions of the "laboring" classes influenced mortality and morbidity rates. In 1980, the Black report demonstrated widening health inequalities but also pointed to the influence of social determinants of health and the variation in health outcomes due to factors such as socio-economic status, race and the region where people lived. In the 21st century, inequalities persist (Molero, 2018; European Commission, 2023; Bambra, 2024) (also see Chapter 4). To address such inequalities, consideration of local needs is a fundamental point of departure in community profiling to ensure the diversity of contexts within which people live is examined and communities are enabled to develop meaningful and pragmatic responses that inductively map to activities supporting human flourishing.

The Concept of Need

Need is a difficult concept to define, and priorities can differ depending on who is asked. Thus, need identification is not value-free as it draws from strong voices in the community, parameters of policy imperatives, professionals/experts, various evidence bases and recognized gaps in service provision. Community-based needs are important to consider, as gaps may result in social problems. Yet, needs are contextualized within frames of resources and supply and demand, particularly when considering possible responses available in practical terms. While

DOI: 10.4324/9781032662657-4

person-centered needs assessment is a common focus when caring for individuals (Phelan et al., 2021), depth and complexity increase when needs are considered within the community context. As such, complexity theory can apply, as like organizations, communities are complex, adaptive and emergent systems (Carroll et al., 2023). Derived from the general systems theory, complexity theory observes the relationships between members that produce collective behaviors and interactions (Sammut-Bonnici, 2015; Klocek et al., 2024).

One commonly known framework of need is Maslow's hierarchy of needs. Maslow (1943) conceptualized a progressive hierarchy of needs, based on meeting fundamental physiological requirements to achieve self-fulfillment. The basic physiological needs (food, water, breathing, homeostasis) must be satisfied before humans are motivated to move to the second level (safety), then the third tier (love and belonging), the fourth tier (esteem) and, finally, the fifth level of self-actualization. While based on the individual, Maslow's hierarchy can be applied to the community as demonstrated in Figure 3.1 and the accompanying descriptors (Table 3.1).

Although Maslow (1943) initially argued that needs should be sequentially fulfilled (levels 1–5), some critics challenge the linear nature of this progression (Henwood et al., 2015). However, for the community, the diverse nature of individuals, families and constituent groups translates to a dynamic context, with a constant and varied flux in need between levels and within communities. This again resonates with complexity theory with numerous interacting elements, non-linearity, adaptations and emergence from constituent interactions (Jerab, 2025).

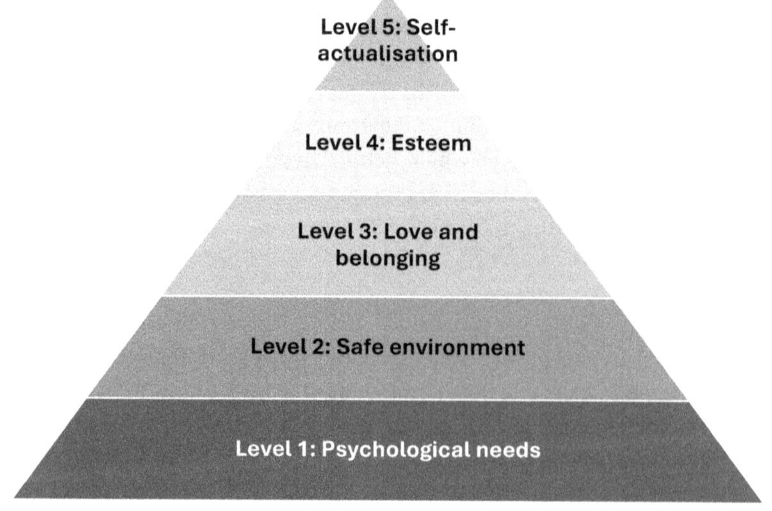

FIGURE 3.1 Maslow's hierarchy of needs

TABLE 3.1 Descriptors of Maslow's hierarchy of need applied to community

Level	*Application to community*
Level 1-Physiological needs	Access to and capacity to afford food, adequate shelter (housing), clean water, clean air, asbestos-free, smoke-free, minimal or no pollutants, optimal health for individuals in the community.
Level 2-Safe environment	Facilitate community socialization, low crime rates, psychologically safe environments and physical safety when mobilizing. Neighborhood cohesiveness, adequate income that protects against social deprivation, good health and social care support systems.
Level 3-Love and belonging	Social capital, connectedness, fostering mutuality, community groups and supportive environment for individual and group identity (church, culture, place, ethnicity, age). Equality and equity in community, shared goals and values.
Level 4-Esteem	Respect and value for all members and groups, positive identity, pride and affinity in community.
Level 5-Self-actualization	The opportunity for the community to grow, adapt, flourish and maximize potential resulting in enhanced social capital.

Bradshaw's (1972) taxonomy has also been used to assess need. This framework illustrates how needs can be articulated by different groups and how needs are based on inductive or deductive arguments. Bradshaw (1972) described four levels of need demonstrated in Table 3.2.

While this conceptualization has the advantage of viewing need from the community's perspective, comparing needs with other areas and benchmarking against normative standards can be challenging. For example, felt or expressed needs may

TABLE 3.2 Bradshaw's taxonomy of need

Category	*Description*
Felt need	Defined by the individual or group's "want". May not be expressed. Need can be defined by experience, perception or circumstances.
Expressed need	Need which is articulated by the individual or group. Represents felt need being communicated. Can be presented as a demand.
Comparative need	Need which is identified by comparison to another similar community.
Normative need	Professionally defined based on policy, or normative standards expected. If the standard falls short, a need is identified.

be over-inflated or may be conflicted with available resources (financial, environmental or human resources). Expressed need represents felt need converted to a demand. In this context, care must be taken to assess expressed needs. Is the need representing an issue shared by many sectors of the community, for example, safety on local roads, or does the need represent a bias in favor of particular groups within the community? Another reality may reflect that some sections of the community have not developed modes of self-advocacy and, therefore, have not translated felt need into expressed need. Comparative needs may be constrained by resources, while normative needs may be defined by benchmarking against a particular standard, which may also be impacted by both fiscal and situational factors. Despite such concerns, community needs assessment maps to real-world gaps, may lead to outcomes of policy, systems or environmental (physical, social) change (CDC, 2024) and commences with community profiling. Using the combined model of ecological systems (Bronfenbrenner & Morris, 1998) and Donabedian (1966; 2005) detailed in chapter 2 (Figure 2.1), we approach community profiling within a multiple systems context with a concurrent focus on structure, processes and outcomes. In working with communities, it is important to appreciate the community's (and sub-sets of the community) values, diversity and intersectionality.

Community Profiling

Working with communities means considering the diversity of people and working in partnerships to improve people's lives through connected citizenry (Lansing et al., 2023). Moreover, the importance of community engagement has been demonstrated in responses to COVID-19 (Marston et al., 2020; Caperon et al., 2022) and its aftermath (World Health Organization, 2023). It is important to engage with all groups to identify needs and sustainable responses; however, Public Health Scotland (2024), drawing on the work of McCartney and Hoggett (2023), observes that a simple focus on geography can be misleading, given that only half of people with a low income live in geographically deprived areas. Instead, proportionate universalism is based on actively targeting deficits, proportionate to the degree of need (Public Health Scotland, 2014). While national and regional plans and policies, which generally reflect international standards and best evidence (global-macro- and exo-system levels), provide guidance and aim to benchmark requirements in areas such as health, social care, environment, social protection and education, there is also a recognition that these are framed as generic expectations. In this context, the umbrella approach of policy needs to be supplemented with a recognition that local communities (meso-system) have wide and complex variations that are influenced by structural issues such as (un)employment, socio-economic groups, demographics, health status, town planning, environment (built, green spaces), transport infrastructure, housing, access to health care and other services, crime, community cohesion or conflict and a sense of affiliation (Mannarini & Fedi, 2009). Consequently, individual community needs differ, and systems' world directives may not offer lived experience solutions for the collective (van der Vlegel-Brouwer et al., 2023). As we have seen in models of person-centered care, individuals have a unique and distinct lifeworld, which has both history and context. Similarly, communities reflect the rich diversity of individuals; thus, developing flourishing communities draws on person-centered principles related to working with people as equal partners in co-creating responsive and ethical plans to identify resources and capacity to meet local needs. Partnership engagement empowers communities to improve their health and to become self-determining (Brunton et al., 2017). As such, community profiling and community development reflect a democratic process where reciprocity and transactional collaboration are key. Community profiling may be described as:

> A comprehensive description of the needs of a population that is defined or defines itself, as a community, and the resources that exist within that community, carried out with the active involvement of that community itself, for the purpose of developing an action plan or other means of improving the quality of life of the community.
>
> *(Hawtin & Percy-Smith, 2007: 5)*

Community profiling has several advantages, such as identifying health status and inequities within the community, observing key trends, disentangling a community's complexity, providing information on resources and direction on needs and priorities and providing real-time public health insights for the community (Bynner & Whyte, 2016). Profiling reflects the assessment phase and demands a deep commitment to understanding the perspectives and experiences of community members. It is a participatory methodology to explore the myriad aspects of a community (and sub-communities), including its social determinants of health, interconnections and relationships with a view to co-creating ways to enhance the lives of people in the community. Community profiling is often associated with geographical boundaries, but profiling is not limited to this focus and can represent any type of community where there is some form of affiliation (NICE, 2016).

Understanding Community Members

Working with communities means authentic engagement as equals within the partnership. In this regard, using a transformational leadership approach is key when working with community members. It is important that leadership is based on a shared vision of well-being within a positive and culture-change environment. Walton and Huey (1993) argue that transformational leaders need to demonstrate idealized influence, inspirational leadership, intellectual stimulation and individual stimulation. In this way, leading in community profiling and subsequent actions is underpinned by inspiring change, tapping into people's motivations and engendering trust (Bakker et al., 2023).

Historical and current taken-for-granted inequalities need to be rendered visible to reveal barriers to achieving optimal community well-being. Diversity across communities can translate to differences in opinions; thus, allowing time to engage with community members to identify goals and navigate conflicts is critical. This starts with acknowledging the variety of human experiences and creating conditions to vindicate the right to participation and inclusion as much or as little as desired (NICE, 2016). Relationship building is core to this process, which in turn supports the identification and navigation of meaningful goals, based on lifeworld issues. A useful model for developing partnerships with communities is described as reciprocal innovation (Sors et al., 2023), where partnerships are founded on reciprocity, learning and mutuality, bi-directional co-creation and collaboration and generating high-quality innovations. A key component of such partnerships is empowering communities to unlock their agency in identifying what matters to them; in other words, what mutual goals can be identified for the community. However, caution is needed not to over-promise and to manage realistic expectations related to change and impact (NICE, 2016). Community collaboration and engagement can achieve better health outcomes and underpin the development of practical and sustainable interventions by setting goals and ensuring that plans are appropriate and ethical (Berkeley et al., 2018). Research has demonstrated that engagement with healthcare by various groups can be influenced by suspicion and mistrust (Bazargan et al., 2021; Goodwin et al., 2022). For example, in a recent Pew report, Funk (2024) observes that 55% of Black Americans have had a negative experience with healthcare providers. Research regarding Gypsy, Traveller and Roma interactions with healthcare services also demonstrates discrimination and mistrust (Power, 2004; McFadden et al., 2018; Quirke et al., 2022). Discrimination, unconscious bias and poor encounters with formal agencies, such as health and social care, exacerbate existing mistrust and further alienate such populations (Vela et al., 2022; Sanofi, 2023). Such groups experience higher social inequities, particularly in the context of the intersectionality of identity (Bracho & Hayes, 2020), and have poorer health outcomes than other population cohorts (David & Derthick, 2018; Kennedy et al., 2023; USDHHS, 2022), pointing to the need to work to create meaningful collaborative spaces stimulating partnerships to address their determinants of health.

An authentic collaboration with community members also demands clarity of aim in the engagement process. Professionals undertaking community profiling and related engagement must demonstrate shared values in developing trusting, fostering collective community flourishing and have a genuine interest in the community's reality and lifeworld (Langsing et al., 2023; WHO, 2023). Even within communities, there is a diversity of perspectives, so collecting data, working with various groups, articulating plans, gaining consensus, planning implementation and evaluation is time-intensive (Hawtin & Percy-Smith, 2007). Some community members may be new to a geographical area, while others have lived there to old age. People from various religions and countries may share core beliefs but interpret and live those beliefs differently; some being more orthodox than others. Thus, approaches to community profiling demand "homework". As detailed later in this chapter, prior insights into the characteristics of the group demonstrate interest and commitment but also show an openness to learning about how the community operates and contribute to the avoidance of stereotyping (Irwin, 2020; Selekman, & Zavadivker, 2021). Moreover, being innovative translates to partnering with non-traditional sectors, which enables unique opportunities for wider perspectives and community development (Rhodes et al., 2021). The focus of building such partnerships is community engagement and collective empowerment to create an enabling environment, mapping to the principles of the Ottawa and Geneva Charters (WHO, 1996, 2021). Moreover, work at the community level has potential for further social innovation for broader systemic impact. This translates to scaling across (connecting across the community and beyond, which includes scaling up to impact macro systems and scaling out impacting the exo-system) and scaling deep (addressing issues of marginalization, intersectionality or equity) (Riddell & Moore, 2015; Boyle et al., 2024).

Promoting positive communities also involves a navigation of context related to the physical environment, economy, political perspectives and social circumstances. For community profiling, it is necessary to take an emic and etic view. Drawn from anthropology (Pike, 1954), the emic perspective focuses on lived experience, drawing from interpretivist theory, which involves talking to people about their lives, taking note of the environments they live in, and the structural conditions that influence their lives. Although the researcher may not be able to immerse themselves in the context fully, a careful reconstruction of a community provides in-depth insights into people's lives. An etic perspective provides an outsider's view of the reality of the community. This can incorporate the views of others regarding that community and include its history. This information is also complemented by data on the community; that is, the realist perspective (van Grootel et al., 2017) which provides insights into characteristics and measurements of the community that can be observed and collectively described (Berkeley et al., 2018). For example, for a specific area, what is the demographic and geographical composition of the area? what are the statistics of the area concerning crime, health, unemployment, schools and access to services? Are there recreation areas and public transport systems to match demographics and needs? What are external views of the area (i.e. a nice place to live or an impoverished/unsafe area)? All these descriptors impact communities and their social identity, as well as influencing how communities flourish or stagnate.

Community Profiling for Positive Health

The Center for Disease Control and Prevention (2018) consider community health needs assessment and health improvement planning as encompassing:

'...assessment that identifies key health needs and issues through systematic, comprehensive data collection and analysis.'

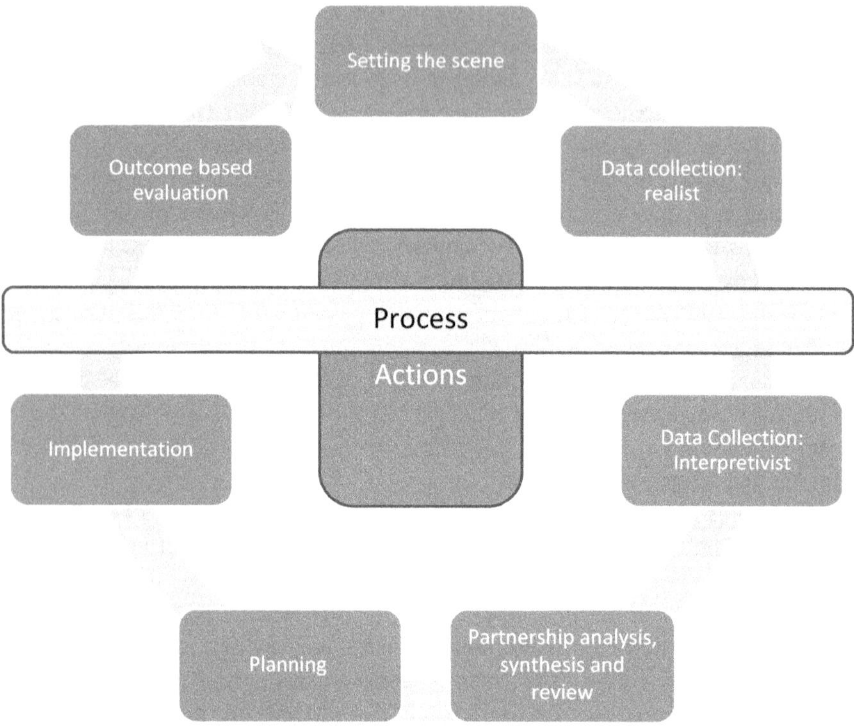

FIGURE 3.2 Community profiling approach using a participatory action research model half page

Other descriptions that describe the process of engagement include approaches within community-based participatory research and community-based engaged research (Wallerstein et al., 2020) which are founded on addressing social inequities. Figure 3.2 demonstrates the community profiling approach within a participatory action research model with a dual and continuous focus on process and action to bring about social change (Arcidiacono et al., 2016; van der Vlegel-Brouwer et al., 2023).

Process: The Importance of Being Earnest

The Clinical and Translational Science Awards Consortium et al. (2011) emphasize the value of preparation for effectiveness in engagement. This assists with the rationale for the inaugural meeting with stakeholders and agenda preparation. Within this transitional period, where planning occurs for reflection and change (RWJF, 2022), a key aim is to provide a focus for community meetings and persuade people of the value of mutual engagement. Additionally, it should be recognized that human conflict is normative (Porter-O'Grady, 2004), as such initial meetings may reveal insights into community differences, othering (Rohleder, 2014; Akbulut & Razum, 2022) or potential conflicting priorities. Accordingly, facilitating explorations of people's experiences of health translates to multiple narratives where issues of power, politics, conflict and well-being are framed (RWJF, 2022). Knowledge of such divergence enables preparation and provides scope for negotiation, potentially navigating a mutually acceptable resolution plan that benefits the community. While a neutral and transparent approach is imperative when working with community groups, power and privilege relationships need to be acknowledged and addressed (Hawtin & Percy-Smith, 2007; Rhodes et al., 2021; Bassidj & Hassan, 2022) to create inclusive, safe environments. Equally, power relationships can also be evident in community engagement itself, with facilitators being positioned in a privileged position, portraying communities as needing to be rescued. This may be implied through a lack of clarity of how community engagement works, the facilitator taking control of the process, the language used or undemocratic practices being promoted or tacitly tolerated. Addressing such issues takes courage to confront the status quo and skills of mediation, communication, relationship building, supporting partnerships and transparency. Communication strategies focus on integrating community knowledge, empowering the community and having the community involved at all levels with explicit ownership of actions (Wallerstein et al., 2020). A key aspect of community engagement is diverse representation, member commitment and enabling due diligence to the roles and responsibilities within the collective planning, implementation and evaluation of actions. This includes the appraisal of all stakeholders' competency and capacity to execute roles and avoiding an overestimation of ability. Thus, support for building capacity in individuals and organizations is an important aspect of the process (Knuttel et al., 2019). Building mutuality can be a delicate and time-consuming activity involving breaking down barriers between traditional divides; however, with skillful and supportive interactions, this work will reap sustainable collaborations and positive outcomes. Outputs of such collaborations have the potential to generate culture-centered interventions, foster partnership synergies, commitment and develop tailored plans for action in developing community well-being (Arcidiacono et al., 2016; Wallerstein et al., 2020).

Action: Setting the Scene

Community profiling may be inductive, where initial work is developed from an identified need in the area or group. A community or group may decide to approach external people to elicit expertise in collectively developing plans. This leads to networking with the key stakeholders to explore perspectives and response planning. A second approach is when a community or group is approached by others to identify and create plans to meet their needs. This may occur due to a secondment to a community as a work or study placement. An example is the Community Engagement module supported by the Irish University Association, where students work with community groups on a credit-bearing unit of study (IUA, 2023) or the myriad partnerships between educational institutions in the United States and communities (Kuttner et al., 2019). Universities and other organizations that have a core aim of public good are termed "anchor organisations", which can create local synergies, stimulate positive social change and champion local issues of concern (RWJF, 2019b) (see Chapter 12).

Scene setting is the most crucial step of community profiling. Drawing on McCormack and McCance's person-centered care framework (PCCF) (2017), applying a person-centered care approach starts with competencies that demonstrate commitment and valuing partnership approaches. Moreover, as previously noted, there is a need to acknowledge and address power differentials in such relationships (Gaventa & Cornwall, 2015) in working *with* rather than *on* people in the community to effect transformations and social change (Arcidiacono et al., 2016). In this sense, approaches draw on participatory action, leveraging stakeholders' collaborations through authentic, democratic engagement with all sectors of the community. Community profiling, or community diagnosis (Arcidiacono et al., 2016), commences with building and supporting partnerships. The contextual "homework" information is valuable in preparation for engagement with the community; this reflection before engagement demonstrates interest and values the community's complexity and diversity. By informally gathering baseline information on context, collaboration or conflicts between sectors of the community, important issues can be illuminated, and this should incorporate the history of relationships to understand the present situation. Such preparation also provides an alert to sensitive areas or points to sources of mutuality within the community. To prepare for the initial meeting, a brief review (rather than a depth analysis as per later process-related work) of published data is useful.

Information based on context may be sourced from:

- Recent annual reports related to various organization(s) (structure, turnover, membership, finances, projects and outcomes).
- Small area population statistics (population characteristics) – a broad review.
- Public coverage of the community (any newspaper reports/other commentaries) (public overview of the area).
- Area policy and planning reports.
- Local government management and reports.
- Political representation and previous interaction with community issues.

Practical data can also be gathered to assist initial conversations and instigate relationship building. This supports an understanding of the stakeholders and their lifeworld, which can be further developed in subsequent data collection stages. Preparation can include preliminary conversations with leaders in the community to discuss the objectives of crossing boundaries, co-creation and shared power of group participants. These can comprise organizational leaders, religious leaders, community group chairs/leads and local councillors and politicians. Considering the perspectives of these key stakeholders enables insights into issues related to health inequities and provides an understanding of drivers of disparities within the community (RWJF, 2019a). Initial discussions may reveal individuals or groups' marginalization, influence or status (gender, ethnicity, status, educational level, socio-economic group, historic standing) positions, which are valuable for further planning. Having insights through these opening conversations can illuminate areas of tension and collaboration, culture, motivations, pockets of exclusion and oppression, as well as general community concerns. This process can also point to policy-practice gaps and the strengths/weaknesses of social capital.

Convening the Collaboration

An overview of the initial information provides a landscape perspective to build the collaboration group and to advance community well-being and capacity. Care should be taken to convene a steering group that is representative of the community, which includes organizations, key stakeholders, voluntary and statutory groups and residents. Barriers to participation can be due to historical and structural contexts that preclude some groups' voices, thus rendering them marginalized (RWJF, 2019a). People may have various motivations for joining the steering group. For example, it may be for personal gain, community gain or responsible citizenship, or because they are strategic leaders or invited stakeholders, or because they can leverage change (Brunton et al., 2017). Failing to have a comprehensive representative group can exacerbate marginalization and may lead to a loss of confidence from some sectors in the community; the group may therefore be viewed as elitist (Kuttner et al., 2019). A community should be visualized as a multi-level embedded complex system comprised of numerous intersecting parts, which can be complementary or oppositional. Thus, community profiling should reflect such diversity while making health and social context a shared value (RWJF, 2019b).

The initial baseline information discussed with the group should provide a foundation for building knowledge of the community. While building on the individual ecological systems perspective (Bronfenbrenner, 1977; 1979; 1995; Bronfenbrenner & Morris, 1998) and integrating Donabedian's (1966; 2005) model, a preliminary understanding of the community is enabled. The foundations of community partnerships need to be made explicit and include considerations related to issues of equity and power inequalities, while supporting shared respect, common goals, sustainability, mutual benefit, relational trust, transformational approaches and applying an asset/strengths-based approach (Kuttner et al., 2019). Questions generated should enable democratic facilitation of members' voices and seek to be representative of the group rather than a sector(s) in the group. When the initial meeting is held, clarity of focus, the preliminary action of profiling the area and eliciting any gaps in community representation should occur. It is also important that the steering group management structure is identified, and roles and responsibilities clarified.

As mutual ownership of the process is key, having the group nominate and elect key management roles contributes to partnership agendas. This process is central to subsequent steps in generating actions and interventions. Ownership of the process should also translate to delineating the activities and seeking implementation support for agreed actions and interventions from steering group members. Equally, evaluation needs to demonstrate impact at various levels, where successes can be celebrated and challenges met with revised plans.

While the questions below are general prompt areas, skilled facilitators can probe further responses to further explore their consequences and impact on the community.

- What is important in the community?
- How involved are people in the community?
- Is there mutuality or division in the community?
- What is the desired outcome?
- What needs to change?
- Who or what is needed to enable transformation (decision makers)?
- What can we leverage (resources) within the community?
- What needs to be done on other levels (structural, relational, environmental, external stakeholders, funding, lobbying)?

These questions focus on the aim of the steering group and point to a need to generate more in-depth knowledge of the context of the community. This activity stimulates the next phase of community profiling, which further refines the realist and interpretivist context of the community. Volunteers may be recruited to assist in data collection or hosting events, and local awareness raising. Decisions related to potential liaisons with colleges/universities may open opportunities for students to participate in the process, while linking with universities could provide valuable research support in terms of data collection and analysis (see Chapter 12). Consideration should also be given to applying for local government community funding to support the process (Hawtin & Percy-Smith, 2007).

Data Collection (Realist Actions)

Data collection for community profiling is diverse and incorporates multiple forms of knowledge. Such further information can be sourced:

1. *Small area population statistics:* Provides useful information on the community. This review involves a deeper consideration and is also helpful to identify community issues, for example, through comparison of local data with national and international trends, providing context and indicators of need. Mapping the area to the social determinants of health explores community development and engagement to maximize health and involves identifying relevant aggregate information to begin the story of the community. Data from Small Area Health

Statistics Units (see example: https://www.imperial.ac.uk/school-public-health/epidemiology-and-biostatistics/small-area-health-statistics-unit/ Piel et al., 2020; Strömberg et al., 2023) is key. Such information is useful in balancing the health needs of communities. Linking health outcomes to social and economic data can draw on data from, for example, deprivation indexes to refine health policies at a local level and maximize the effectiveness of interventions (Teljeur et al., 2019; Pobal, 2023).
2. *Local government reports and future plans for the area.*
3. *Information on schools, (un)employment, strong cultural foci.*
4. *Links/isolation from other areas.*
5. *Community access to services/recreation.*
6. *Further linking community contexts to Bronfenbrenner & Morris's (1998) ecological systems models and Donabedian model (1966; 2005).*

Data gathered in a local area can be compared to similar regions, national data and international data (i.e. Central Statistics Office, Eurostat, WHO data, UN data). This enables the identification of needs and priorities for interventions, which can be framed within Mazlow's (1943) hierarchy or Bradshaw's (1972) taxonomy of need. It is crucial to use existing data to inform insights into the community, for example, through small area population statistics, education reports, historical books and articles, government department reports, data from local organizations and data concerning the social determinants of health. Social determinants of health provide an understanding of non-medical influences on health (CDC, 2023). These include factors such as environment, income and social protection, education, access to healthcare and quality of healthcare, community support, housing, food security, conflict and violence and social inclusion. Another aspect for consideration is related to supply and demand. An area that has new housing estates may have an influx of young families, thus demand for school places may outstrip supply. Equally, this places pressure on infrastructure such as public transport and recreational areas. New industries in the area may attract people to buy houses in the locality, but this may create a scarcity of housing stock and inflate house prices. Alternatively, the closure of factories or other sources of employment may decimate a community as unemployment may rise and impact individuals, families and local businesses, as well as the vibrancy of the area. Through a careful review, community profiling enables consideration of goals related to health equity (WHO, 2018) for the populations within the community.

Data Collection (Interpretivist Actions)

Following on from the baseline realist action within data collection about the area is a more abstract action of understanding how the community works. This can encompass several steps constituting a listening, observing and learning focus.

1. *Walk the walk and talk the talk:* A key aspect of understanding a community is to spend time getting to know it. This involves environmental scanning; walking

around the area and speaking to people. This begins the development of mutuality, the foundation of trusting relationships and the concurrent development of relationships with key stakeholders. Methods of collecting data are presented in Table 3.3 and range from informal observation to more structured modes of eliciting information.

Using a strengths (assets)-based approach. While the application of a strengths-based approach is more commonly used in individual health and social care approaches, its principles are applied in terms of exploring the assets or resources that the community has. This leads to a review of issues such as adaptation

TABLE 3.3 Data collection

Observation	Walking around an area enables a sense of both the "feel" of the area and the "look" of the area. For example, does the area feel safe or connected? The look of the area also gives some insights into the social determinants of health. Issues such as physical environment (well-kept versus neglected, green spaces, playgrounds, conditions of houses, shops, schools, safety, transport). This includes issues related to access and mobility. For example, are the paths safe for older people walking or wheelchairs? Are buildings accessible? If there are public parks, do they have benches for people to sit on and encourage socialization? Can be supplemented by video or photos which may be used to present findings, generate discussion and illuminate further data collection requirements.
Semi-structured interviews	Interviews are a common method of data collection, and it is easier to negotiate the meeting as it maps to the participants' availability and preferred venue. Interviews are also useful when community members want to discuss sensitive areas such as conflict, racism, gender issues and violence. Some people prefer to discuss their perspectives confidentially and may be more forthcoming than in a group-based environment. Interviews may be based on emic (from living in the community, what is the perspective?) or etic, Or etic drawing on the perceptions of key people living outside the community (politicians, leads in local authorities, etc.)
Convening of groups	Focus groups, community assemblies, town hall meetings, world café.
Surveys	Can be distributed to community members to elicit perspectives and identify context and need. Surveys have the advantage of enabling large numbers of respondents to have a say, while maintaining anonymity.

TABLE 3.4 Social capital and community (adapted from University of Minnesota Extension, 2024)

Social capital		
Elements	*General meaning*	*Community application*
Bonding	Bonding relates to like-minded people who share beliefs, culture or other commonalities.	Residents have close connections that create mutuality and cohesion
Bridging	Bridging is where people who have different values, culture, race, perspectives, orientations, etc., connect with each other.	Residents have broader connections that expand potential and opportunities
Linking	Linking describes connections between individuals/communities and people at a different hierarchical level i.e. elected representatives.	Residents have connections to organizations, governance bodies and systems that facilitate resources, change and development.

to the non-linear contexts within the community, effecting change and valuing the social capital that exists. New connections can promote positive relationships to illuminate opportunities for planning and implementation of change. Leveraging social capital involves three concepts as detailed in Table 3.4 (also see Chapter 5).

Within theories of person-centered care, there is a priority on the relational (Nolan et al., 2006; McCormack & McCance, 2017). Similarly, social capital emphasizes that people's relationships/networks constitute important resources enabling societal functioning and are underpinned by engagement, trust and efficacy (University of Minnesota, Extension, 2024). While bonding is seen as being useful for "getting by" founded on homogeneous interests (Gittell & Vidal, 1998), bridging is essential for "getting ahead" (Putnam, 2000). Community profiling also provides data for linking, and information can contribute to actions such as prioritizing lobbying activities for additional resources. Mahoney (2008) sees people who assist citizens in lobbying as instigators who impact the work of interest groups (mobilizers). An example of using a social capital approach was used by Ayed et al. (2021) to review the structural aspects of community supports for homeless people; findings examined what services are available and if they are accessible for this population. Cognitive dimensions were also considered, and these were described as important barriers when homeless people tried to access services (Ayed et al., 2021). Consequently, leveraging social capital can improve quality of life outcomes (Muir & Reynolds, 2009) by supporting the structural, relational and cognitive domains within the community (Makridis & Wu, 2021).

In summary, the key to building a comprehensive knowledge base about a community is ensuring data from diverse sources is sourced to enable intersectoral planning and collaboration for mutual well-being (RWJF, 2019b). Using the ecological systems model (Bronfenbrenner & Morris, 1998) and Donabedian's model (1966; 2005) facilitates a depth consideration of the whole community context. Collecting data for profiling comprises both quantitative and qualitative data to generate sensitive insights into the various nuances of the community. Quantitative data provides realist facts and figures to support context, while qualitative data enables an interpretative depth seeking to understand what life is like in the community and what matters to the community. Careful consideration of the type and variety of data collection methods is important, and approaches should be mapped to the best way to ensure the representation of diverse voices. Recruitment to participate in the various forms of data collection should involve mobilizing the leadership in the steering group to cascade information down to members of the broader community. Actions such as the use of church newsletters, local newspapers, shop windows, hosting local events and leveraging social media may be used to maximize the multiplicity of voices. In areas of diversity in terms of language, efforts should be made to include people, using translators or digital supports to facilitate involvement in the data collection phase.

Data Synthesis

Presenting Data

Real-time data should be collated in a way that represents the community and is grounded in the everyday reality of lived experience, reflecting community diversity, but as this is a partnership with community stakeholders, data should also be presented in an easily understandable format. For instance, data could be represented in graphs and pie charts which need to be explainable in plain language, but information overload should be avoided (Hawtin & Percy-Smith, 2007). In addition, communication should accommodate people who may have literacy challenges or provide translation for people who may not understand the dominant language in the community/used within the collaboration and findings' material.

Planning and Implementation

Making the linkages with the ecological systems and under the domains of structure, process and outcomes seeks to identify factors and relationships which contribute to community well-being or hinder it. In this way, the identification of actions can be targeted at discrete points and multiple levels. This allows issues to be considered comprehensively rather than in isolation and applies a jigsaw approach to describe issues of complexity within the community's reality. Consequently, once data has been presented back to the group, planning for action will occur. A core aim of convening the community steering group is to consider priorities for action and planning steps to achieve goals. In this context, creativity is essential to pool resources to overcome barriers and address multi-faceted issues identified as important in and to the community (RWJF, 2020a, 2020b). There may be some conflict at this point as different groups have subjective agendas, so careful mediation and neutral discussion are imperative to navigate conflict and develop a team strategy. The use of emotional intelligence to manage teams has garnered increasing support in managing team conflict and successful collaborations (Jamshed & Nauman, 2022; Coronado-Maldonado & Benítez-Márquez, 2023). To support confidence in the engagement, plans should be built on SMART principles.

Specific: Activities should be clear with key steps identified. Clarity is needed on who is responsible, how the action is being implemented and what is the desired outcome.

Measurable: Activities should be quantifiable in terms of measuring progress toward goals.

Achievable: Goals should be realistic and be possible within the identified time.

Relevant: Goals should align with the community's desired outcome.

Time: Time management for the activities should be explicit, monitored and reported back to the steering group.

Planning is closely related to the capacity to achieve goals to enhance people's quality of life in their community (WHO, 2020). There may be a variety of options to consider, so each should be reviewed with the aim of inclusive discussion, enabling a democratic selection of a suitable plan. While being ambitious is desirable, having an unattainable plan leads to disillusionment and despondency. Thus, the strategic plan should be inclusive of the steering group's collaborative input and identify the key objectives, steps to completion and people responsible. Essentially, this includes the identification of structural actions that the Robert Wood Johnson Foundation (2022) identifies as both changing structures and shifting actions leading to sustainable, transformative change. Identifying required resources and barriers is an important preliminary step. This may include applying for financial assistance through grants or other funding sources. Funding may target purchasing materials to achieve goals (for example, enhancing a recreational public space) and/or accessing expertise to assist in goal achievement (for example, an architect for the design of a public space).

Implementation of the plan should be supported by the steering group, with key leads nominated as responsible for completing prescribed steps. This also promotes ownership and self-determination. As the plan is implemented, a major aspect is to schedule feedback to underpin continuing trust, communicate progress or identify emerging challenges (Langsing et al., 2023). Failure is not the lack of success of a plan but the lack of flexibility and redirection if the original plan faces challenges. Having clear and regular communication pathways is a key factor in the successful implementation of plans and continued collaborative relationships (Magezi et al., 2021). As such, part of the planning should include a meeting schedule. Meetings should enable each goal leader to provide feedback and allow a discussion of progress in the context of deliverables, timeframes and "next steps". Also, as members of the steering groups are essentially representatives of the community, plans should include the dissemination of processes and outcomes to the broader community as an implementation action. Continued trust in the collaboration is underpinned by the steering group's monitoring of progress and evaluation in terms of reaching goals and timelines. It is important to acknowledge barriers that may present in multiple and competing community narratives, funding issues, power dynamics, political apathy and commitment fatigue. Unachieved goals should be analyzed for barriers in progress and matched with realistic realignment. Achieved goals consolidate the collaboration and should be celebrated; such successes can stimulate further community engagement and progress.

As with person-centered care, outcomes should be evaluated in terms of the achievement of goals and their well-being impact on the community. However, how the community has subjectively experienced the collaborative process is also important. Issues related to the provision of support, ensuring inclusion and diversity, democratic contributions, fostering psychological safety, building and sustaining collaborations and relationships are also key outcomes in the process. Levels of collaboration and their effectiveness can be measured (see Marek et al., 2014; Wilder Foundation, 2018; DeDerr, 2019), while stakeholder feedback can also enhance the evaluation of the partnership and collaboration. Addressing any challenges in the collaborative process is fundamental to sustaining relationships and to further progressing actions to enhance community well-being.

Conclusion

Community profiling is a complex process that, drawing from the principles of person-centered care, demands the creation of cultures of collaboration and shared ownership. The foundation of community profiling is creating trust and fostering partnerships across diverse groups in the community, as well as transformational leadership approaches. When working with communities, collecting data, creating equitable steering groups, articulating action plans, implementing plans to reach goals and evaluation may be time-bound. Thus, diligent oversight, skilled mediation and early action plans for emerging challenges are important. Successful collaborations can lead to sustainable, equitable partnerships that continue to focus on further community engagement and development. From this vantage point, communities can be empowered to work toward creating environments supporting human flourishing and more equitable, harmonized integration of systems and outcomes for their members (RWJF, 2019b).

References

Akbulut, N., & Razum, O. (2022). Why othering should be considered in research on health inequalities: Theoretical perspectives and research needs. *SSM - Population Health, 20*, 101286.

Arcidiacono, C., Tuozzi, T., & Procentese, F. (2016). Community profiling in participatory action research. In *Handbook of methodological approaches to community-based research* (eds Jason, L. J. & Glenwick, D. S.). Oxford University Press, Oxford, pp. 355–364.

Ayed, N., Hough, S., Jones, J., Priebe, S., & Bird, V. (2021). Community profiling: Exploring homelessness through a social capital lens. *European Journal of Homelessness, 15*(2), 37–64.

Bakker, A. B., Hetland, J., Olsen, O. K., & Espevik, R. (2023). Daily transformational leadership: A source of inspiration for follower performance? *European Management Journal, 41*(5), 700–708. https://doi.org/10.1016/j.emj.2022.04.004

Bambra, C. (2024). The U-shaped curve of health inequalities over the 20th and 21st centuries. *International Journal of Social Determinants of Health and Health Services, 54*(3),199–205. https://doi.org/10.1177/27551938241244695

Bassidj, S., & Hassan, M. (2022). *Community development practices: From Canadian and global perspectives.* Retrieved from https://ecampusontario.pressbooks.pub/communitydevelopmentpractice/chapter/chapter-3-theories-approaches-and-frameworks-in-community-work/

Bazargan, M., Cobb, S., & Assari, S. (2021). Discrimination and medical mistrust in a racially and ethnically diverse sample of California adults. *Annals of Family Medicine, 19*(1), 4–15.

Berkeley, A. F., Skinner, D., & Murphy, J. W. (2018). Defining community in community health evaluation: Perspectives from a sample of non-profit Appalachian hospitals. *American Journal of Evaluation, 39*(2), 237–256.

Black, D. (1980). *Inequalities in health: Report of a research working group.* DHSS, London.

Boyle, E., De Bhailís, D., & Kelliher, M. (2024). Scaling deep: Societal impact through a new approach to regional development. *Societal Impacts, 4*, 1–5. https://doi.org/10.1016/j.socimp.2024.100083.

Bracho, C. A., & Hayes, C. (2020). Gay voices without intersectionality is White supremacy: Narratives of gay and lesbian teachers of color on teaching and learning, *International Journal of Qualitative Studies in Education, 33*(6), 583–592.

Bradshaw, J. (1972). A taxonomy of social need. In *Problems and progress in medical care* (McLachlan, G. ed.). Seventh series NPHT/Open University Press. pp. 71–82.

Bronfenbrenner, U. (1977). Toward an experimental ecology of human development. *American Psychologist, 32*, 513–531. https://doi.org/10.1037/0003-066X.32.7.513.

Bronfenbrenner, U. (1979). *The ecology of human development: Experiments by nature and design.* Harvard University Press, Massachusetts.

Bronfenbrenner, U. (1995). Developmental ecology through space and time: A future perspective. In *Examining lives in context: Perspectives on the ecology of human development.* (P. Moen, Elder, G. H. Jr., & Lüscher, K. eds.). American Psychological Association, Washington, pp. 619–647.

Bronfenbrenner, U., & Morris, P. A. (1998). The ecology of developmental processes. In *Handbook of child psychology: Vol. 1. Theoretical models of human development* (Damon, W. (Series Ed.) & Lerner R. M. (Vol. Ed.)), (5th ed.). Wiley, New York, pp. 993–1028.

Brunton, G., Thomas, J., O'Mara-Eves, A., Jamal, F., Oliver, S., & Kavanagh, J. (2017). Narratives of community engagement: A systematic review-derived conceptual framework for public health interventions. *BMC Public Health, 17*, 944.

Bynner, C., & Whyte, B. (2016). *What works in community profiling? Initial reflections from the WWS project in West Dunbartonshire.* Retrieved from https://core.ac.uk/download/pdf/42372129.pdf#

Caperon, L., Saville, F., & Ahern, S. (2022). Developing a socio-ecological model for community engagement in a health programme in an underserved urban area. *PloS one, 17*(9), e0275092. https://doi.org/10.1371/journal.pone.0275092

Carroll, Á., Collins, C., McKenzie, J., Stokes, D., & Darley, A. (2023). Application of complexity theory in health and social care research: A scoping review. *BMJ Open, 13*, e069180. https://doi.org/10.1136/bmjopen-2022-069180

Centres for Disease Control and Prevention (CDC) (2023). *Social determinants of health.* Retrieved from https://www.cdc.gov/public-health-gateway/php/about/social-determinants-of-health.html?CDC_AAref_Val=https://www.cdc.gov/publichealthgateway/sdoh/index.html

Centres for Disease Control and Prevention (CDC) (2024). *Community needs assessment.* Centers for Disease Control and Prevention, Atlanta, GA.

Chadwick, E. (1842). *Report on the sanitary condition of the labouring population of Great Britain.* Houses of Parliament Sessional Paper, London.

Clinical and Translational Science Awards Consortium, Community Engagement Key Function Committee Task & Force on the Principles of Community Engagement (2011). *Principles of community engagement.* (second edition). NIH. Retrieved from https://ictr.johnshopkins.edu/wp-content/uploads/2015/10/CTSAPrinciplesofCommunityEngagement.pdf

Coronado-Maldonado, I., & Benítez-Márquez, M. D. (2023). Emotional intelligence, leadership, and work teams: A hybrid literature review. *Heliyon, 9*(10), e20356. https://doi.org/10.1016/j.heliyon.2023.e20356

David, E. J. R., & Derthick, A. O. (2018). *The psychology of oppression.* Springer Publishing Company, New York.

Derr, A. (2019). *Measuring the intensity of collaboration in a network.* Retrieved from https://liveplymouthac-my.sharepoint.com/:w:/r/personal/helen_lloyd-1_plymouth_ac_uk/_layouts/15/Doc.aspx?sourcedoc=%7B756E0B8A-6996-41BE-A951-62DD3D3C7029%7D&file=Chapter%203%20Community%20engagement%2C%20profiling%20and%20action%20planning.docx&action=default&mobileredirect=true

Donabedian, A. (1966; 2005) Evaluating the quality of medical care. *Milbank Memorial Fund Q, 44*(3), (suppl), 166–206. (Reprinted in *Milbank Quarterly, 83*(4), 691–729.

European Commission (2023). *Widening health-related inequalities.* Retrieved from https://knowledge4policy.ec.europa.eu/foresight/widening-health-related-inequalities_en

Funk, C. (2024). *Black Americans views of and engagement with science.* Pew Research Center, Washington, DC.

Gaventa, J., & Cornwall, A. (2015). Power and knowledge. In *The SAGE handbook of action research* (Bradbury, H. ed.). Sage, Thousand Oaks, CA, pp. 465–471.

Gittell, R., & Vidal, A. (1998). *Community organizing: Building social capital as a development strategy.* SAGE, London.

Goodwin, N., Brown, A., Johnson, H., Miller, R., & Stein, K. V. (2022). From people-centred to people-driven care: Can integrated care achieve its promise without it? *International Journal of Integrated Care, 22*(4), 17, 1–4.

Hawtin, M., & Percy-Smith, J. (2007). *Community profiling-a practical guide.* McGraw Hill, Berkshire.

Henwood, B. F., Derejko, K. S., Couture, J., & Padgett, D. K. (2015). Maslow and mental health recovery: A comparative study of homeless programs for adults with serious mental illness. *Administration & Policy in Mental Health, 42*(2), 220–228.

Irish Universities Association (2023). *Engaged research for impact: A policy briefing for Higher Education Institutions-Society and Higher Education addressing societal challenges together.* IUA, Dublin. Retrieved from www.iua.ie/wp-content/uploads/2023/12/Campus-Engage-Engaged-Research-Policy-Briefing-for-HEIs-Published-3.pdf

Irwin, H. (2020). *Communicating with Asia.* Routledge, London.

Jamshed, S., & Nauman, M. (2022). Mapping knowledge-sharing behavior through emotional intelligence and team culture toward optimized team performance. *Team Performance Management, 29*(1/2), 63–89.

Jerab, D. (2025). *An overview of complexity theory and characteristics of complex adaptive systems.* Retrieved from SSRN- https://dx. doi.org/10.2139/ssrn.5094533

Kennedy, F., Ward, A., Mockler, D., Villani, J., & Broderick, J. (2023). Scoping review on Physical Health Conditions in Mincéirs - Irish travellers. *BMJ Open, 13*(8), e068876.

Klocek, A., Premus, J., & Řiháček, T. (2024) Applying dynamic systems theory and complexity theory methods in psychotherapy research: A systematic literature review. *Psychotherapy Research, 34*(6), 828–844. https://doi.org/10.1080/10503307.2023.2252169

Kuttner, P. J., Byrne, K. A., Schmit, K., & Munro, S. (2019). The art of convening: How community engagement professionals build place-based community-university partnerships for systemic change. *Journal of Higher Education Outreach and Engagement, 23,* 131–160.

Lansing, A. E., Romero, N. J., Siantz, E., Silva, V., Center, K., Casteel, D., & Gilmer, T. (2023). Building trust: Leadership reflections on community empowerment and engagement in a large urban initiative. *BMC Public Health, 23*(1), 1252. https://doi.org/10.1186/s12889-023-15860-z

Magezi, A., Abaho, E., & Kakooza, J. B. (2021). Effective project communication and successful consortia engagements. *International Journal of Innovative Science and Research Technology, 6*(6), 1474–1483.

Mahoney, C. (2008). The role of interest groups in fostering citizen engagement: The determinants of outside lobbying. In *Politics beyond the state: Actors and policies in complex institutional settings.* (Deschouwer, K. & Jans, M. T. eds.). Institute for European Studies, Brussels University Press, Brussels, pp. 109–138.

Makridis, C. A., & Wu, C. (2021). How social capital helps communities weather the COVID-19 pandemic. *PloS one, 16*(1), e0245135.

Mannarini, T., & Fedi, A. (2009). Multiple senses of community: The experience and meaning of community. *Journal of Community Psychology, 37*(2), 211–227.

Marek, L. I., Brock, D.-J. P., & Savla, J. (2014). Evaluating collaboration for effectiveness: Conceptualization and measurement. *American Journal of Evaluation, 36*(1), 67–85. https://doi.org/10.1177/1098214014531068

Marston, C., Renedo, A., & Miles, S. (2020). Community participation is crucial in a pandemic. *Lancet (*London, England), *395*(10238), 1676–1678. https://doi.org/10.1016/S0140-6736(20)31054-0

Maslow, A. H. (1943). A theory of human motivation. *Psychological Review, 50,* 370–396.

McCartney, G., & Hoggett, R. (2023). How well does the Scottish Index of Multiple Deprivation identify income and employment deprived individuals across the urban-rural spectrum and between local authorities? *Public Health, 217*, 26–32.

McCormack, B., & McCance, T. (2017). *Person-centred practice in nursing and health care: Theory and practice*, 2nd Edition. Chichester, West Sussex.

McFadden, A., Siebelt, L., Gavine, A., Atkin, K., Bell, K., Innes, N., Jones, H., Jackson, C., Haggi, H., & MacGillivray, S. (2018). Gypsy, Roma and Traveller access to and engagement with health services: A systematic review. *European Journal of Public Health, 28*(1), 74–81.

Molero, M. I. (2018). The 21st century epidemic: Inequality in health. *Archives of Nursing Research, 2*(1), 1–18.

Muir, F., & Reynolds, P. (2009). Health visiting in practice. In *Public health nursing.* (Thornbery, G. ed.). Wiley Blackwell, West Sussex, pp. 74–99.

NICE (2016) *Community engagement: Improving health and wellbeing and reducing health inequalities.* NICE guideline [NG44]. Retrieved from https://www.nice.org.uk/guidance/ng44

Nolan, M. R., Brown, J., Davies, S., Nolan, J., & Keady, J. (2006). *The senses framework: Improving care for older people through a relationship-centred approach.* Getting Research into Practice (GRiP) Report No 2. Project Report. University of Sheffield.

Phelan, A., Rohde, D., Casey, M., Fealy, G., Felle, P., O'Kelly, G., Lloyd, H., & Carroll, A. (2021). Co-creating descriptors and a definition for person-centred coordinated health care: An action research study. *International Journal of Integrated Care, 21*(1), 11.

Piel, F. B., Fecht, D., Hodgson, S., Blangiardo, M., Toledano, M., Hansell, A. L., & Elliott, P. (2020). Small-area methods for investigation of environment and health. *International Journal of Epidemiology, 49*(2), 686–699.

Pike, K. L. (1954). *Language in relation to a unified theory of the structure of human behavior. Part I.* The Summer Institute of Linguistics, Glendale, CA.

Pobal (2023) Pobal HP Deprivation Index Launched. Retrieved from https://www.pobal.ie/pobal-hp-deprivation-index/

Porter-O'Grady, T. (2004). Embracing conflict: Building a healthy community. *Health Care Management Review, 29*(3), 181–187.

Power, C. (2004). *Room to Roam England's Irish Travellers.* Retrieved from https://www.gypsy-traveller.org/pdfs/RoomtoRoam.pdf

Public Health Scotland (2014). *Proportionate universalism and health inequalities.* Retrieved from https://www.healthscotland.com/uploads/documents/24296-ProportionateUniversalismBriefing.pdf

Public Health Scotland (2024). *Health inequalities.* Retrieved from https://publichealthscotland.scot/our-areas-of-work/equity-and-justice/health-inequalities/how-can-we-reduce-health-inequalities/

Putnam, R. D. (2000). *Bowling alone: The collapse and revival of American community.* Simon & Schuster, New York.

Quirke, B., Heinen, M., Fitzpatrick, P., McKey, S., Malone, K. M., & Kelleher, C. (2022). Experience of discrimination and engagement with mental health and other services by Travellers in Ireland: Findings from the All-Ireland Traveller Health Study (AITHS). *Irish Journal of Psychological Medicine, 39*(2), 185–195.

Rhodes, S. D., Daniel-Ulloa, J., Wright, S. S., Mann-Jackson, L., Johnson, D. B., Hayes, N. A., & Valentine, J. A. (2021). Critical elements of community engagement to address disparities and related social determinants of health: The centers of disease control and prevention community approaches to reducing sexually transmitted disease initiative. *Sexually Transmitted Diseases, 48*(1), 49–55.

Riddell, D., & Moore, M. L. (2015) *Scaling out, scaling up, scaling deep: Advancing systemic social innovation and the learning processes to support.* J.W. McConnell Foundation, Montreal.

Robert Wood Johnson Foundation (RWJF) (2019a) *Culture of health, sentinel community insights: Health equity.* Princeton, New Jersey.

Robert Wood Johnson Foundation (RWJF) (2019b) *Culture of health sentinel community insights: Anchor institutions*. Princeton, New Jersey.

Robert Wood Johnson Foundation (RWJF) (2020a) *Culture of health, sentinel community insights: Rural and small communities.* Princeton, New Jersey.

Robert Wood Johnson Foundation (RWJF) (2020b) *Culture of health sentinel community insights community narrative related to health, well-being, and health equity: What frames and influences narrative?* Princeton, New Jersey.

Robert Wood Johnson Foundation (RWJF) (2022) *Culture of health sentinel community insights: How community systems are changing to advance health, well-being, and equity.* Princeton, New Jersey.

Rohleder, P. (2014). Othering. In *Encyclopaedia of critical psychology.* (Teo, T. ed.). Springer, New York, pp. 1306–1308.

Sammut-Bonnici, T. (2015). Complexity theory. In *Wiley encyclopedia of management* (Cooper, C. L., McGee, J. & Sammut-Bonnici, T. eds.). Retrieved from https://doi.org/10.1002/9781118785317.weom120210

Sanofi (2023). *A million conversations: How we're bridging the healthcare 'trust gap' with marginalized communities.* Retrieved from https://www.sanofi.com/en/magazine/social-impact/global-poll

Selekman, J., & Zavadivker, P. (2021). People of Jewish Heritage. In *Textbook for transcultural health care: A population approach* (Purnell, L. & Fenkl, E. eds.). Springer, Cham, pp. 557–588.

Sors, T. G., O'Brien, R. C., Scanlon, M. L., Bermel, L. Y., Chikowe, I., Gardner, A., Kiplagat, J., Lieberman, M., Moe, S. M., Morales-Soto, N., Nyandiko, W. M., Plater, D., Rono, B. C., Tierney, W. M., Vreeman, R. C., Wiehe, S. E., Wools-Kaloustian, K., & Litzelman, D. K. (2023). Reciprocal innovation: A new approach to equitable and mutually beneficial global health partnerships. *Global Public Health, 18*(1), 2102202.

Strömberg, U., Baigi, A., Holmén, A., Parkes, B. L., Bonander, C., & Piel, F. B. (2023). A comparison of small-area deprivation indicators for public-health surveillance in Sweden. *Scandinavian Journal of Public Health, 51*(4), 520–526.

Teljeur, C., Darker, C., Barry, J., & O'Dowd, T. (2019). The trinity national deprivation index for health and health services research, 2016. Retrieved from https://www.drugsandalcohol.ie/34675/1/Trinity-deprivation-report-11-2019.pdf

United States Department of Health & Human Services (2022). Heart disease and African Americans. Retrieved from https://minorityhealth.hhs.gov/heart-disease-and-african-americans

University of Minnesota Extension (2024). *Community social capital model.* Retrieved from https://extension.umn.edu/leadership-approach-and-models/community-social-capital-model

van der Vlegel-Brouwer, W., Eelderink, M., & Bussemaker, J. (2023). Participatory action research as a driver for health promotion and prevention: A co-creation process between professionals and citizens in a deprived neighbourhood in The Hague. *International Journal of Integrated Care, 23*(4), 13.

van Grootel, L., van Wesel, F., O'Mara-Eves, A., Thomas, J., Hox, J., & Boeije, H. (2017). Using the realist perspective to link theory from qualitative evidence synthesis to quantitative studies: Broadening the matrix approach. *Research Synthesis Methods, 8*(3), 303–311. https://doi.org/10.1002/jrsm.1241

Vela, M. B., Erondu, A. I., Smith, N. A., Peek, M. E., Woodruff, J. N., & Chin, M. H. (2022). Eliminating explicit and implicit biases in health care: Evidence and research needs. *Annual Review of Public Health, 43*, 477–501.

Wallerstein, N., Oetzel, J. G., Sanchez-Youngman, S., Boursaw, B., Dickson, E., Kastelic, S., Koegel, P., Lucero, J. E., Magarati, M., Ortiz, K., Parker, M., Peña, J., Richmond, A., & Duran, B. (2020). Engage for equity: A long-term study of community-based participatory research and community-engaged research practices and outcomes. *Health Education & Behavior: The Official Publication of the Society for Public Health Education, 47*(3), 380–390.

Walton, S. & Huey, J. (1996) *Sam Walton: Made in America: My story.* Random House, New York.

Wilder Foundation (2018). *Wilder collaboration factors inventory.* Retrieved from https://www.wilder.org/wilder_studies/collaboration-factors-inventory/

World Health Organisation (1996). *Ottawa charter.* WHO, Geneva.

World Health Organisation (2018). *Health in all policies as part of the primary health care agenda on multisectoral action.* WHO, NY.

World Health Organisation (2020). *Quality health services-a planning guide.* WHO, Geneva.

World Health Organisation (2021). *Geneva charter for wellbeing.* WHO, Geneva.

World Health Organization (2023). *The role of community engagement in restoring trust and resilience in the aftermath of the COVID-19 pandemic and beyond.* WHO, Geneva.

4

HEALTH INEQUALITIES AND THE SOCIAL DETERMINANTS OF HEALTH AND WELL-BEING

Helen Lloyd

Introduction

This chapter begins by exploring the contested meaning of the notion of "Health" and what it means to be healthy, since this has implications for what we consider to be health inequalities and the social determinants of health (SDoH). It situates these issues within a socioecological and critical systemic framework drawing on current research and evidence to consider how these problems impact the most marginalized through the social gradient of health, which was introduced in Chapter 2. This chapter attempts to highlight how macro systems such as policies and governmental approaches, alongside meso attempts of practice and community-based solutions, hold promise to address these intractable problems. The role of micro-level and individual behaviors is considered within this broader framework with a resistance to see these problems located as the sole responsibility of the individual.

Definitions and Models

Definitions of "Health" are contested. The WHO originally described "Health" as a state of complete physical, mental and social well-being and not merely the absence of disease or infirmity (WHO, 1948). This view of "Health" is undoubtably important because it encapsulates ideas around well-being and not merely the absence of disease or illness (Trebeck & Abeyasekera, 2012) and has been further developed as optimal health fitness (euexia) (Elrick, 1980). Following the publication of the Ottawa Charter for Health Promotion (WHO, 1986), this definition was expanded to link it to health promotion. This expanded notion of "Health" as a positive concept and resource for everyday life emphasizes the importance of social and personal resources, as well as physical capacities. This definition has

DOI: 10.4324/9781032662657-5

however been critiqued for being too aspirational, ambitious and idealistic, particularly in the context of chronic illness and disability (Huber et al., 2011). It is also argued that the WHO (1986) definition conflates health with happiness and fails to acknowledge the tension between different dimensions of the definition (Huber et al., 2011; Saracci, 1997).

Definitions of health in the broadest sense are now also conflated with the notions of "well-being", another contested and relatively ill-defined concept (Hone et al., 2015). Indeed, recognition of the link between well-being and health is also evidenced as important in the UK Care Act (2014). Similar to health, well-being is considered as a positive construct by the WHO and a resource for life (WHO, 2024d), that encompasses an overall evaluation of one's quality of life and life satisfaction, reflecting physical, mental, emotional, social and spiritual dimensions; a definition of which varies across academic disciplines, ages and cultures (Michaelson et al., 2012). Like health, the concept of well-being goes beyond the mere absence of illness to encompass a sense of fulfillment, purpose and contentment in various aspects of life. However, well-being is inherently subjective and can differ greatly between individuals and groups. More appropriately considered as subjective well-being (SWB), this area of research has burgeoned in recent years providing a more nuanced and enhanced understanding of the multitude of individual, social, cultural, environmental and structural forces which shape it (Diener et al., 2018). Furthermore, SWB is distinguished from happiness, which is considered a more transient and restricted to an emotional state, rather than an enduring and multidimensional holistic construct that encompasses and sense of purpose and fulfillment (Diener et al., 2018).

The work of Amarta Sen has been influential in current notions of health, considering it as a state of being that is dependent upon a decent standard of living supported by employment, participation in social activities, the pursuit of education and the enjoyment of, and engagement in, meaningful relationships and activities (Sen, 2014). This view of health visualizes human flourishing through key capabilities, and along with contributions from American Philosopher Martha Nussbaum, forms the basis upon which models of person-centered care have been formed (Ekman et al., 2011) and a capabilities framework for the assessment of Quality of Life.

Health inequalities are descriptive differences in health outcomes or access to healthcare that occur between different populations or groups within a society. The WHO defines health inequalities as "systematic differences in the health status of different population groups, which have significant social and economic costs both to individuals and societies" (WHO, 2024c). Health inequalities are often driven by disparities in a range of socioeconomic, demographic and geographical indicators known as the Social Determinants of Health (SDoH); a set of forces which intersect to cause poor health outcomes, negatively impacting the most marginalized in society. The World Health Organization defines the SDoH as "the non-medical factors that influence health outcomes" (WHO, 2024e). According to the WHO, SDoH account for some 30–55% variance in health outcomes globally, with a greater influence than that of lifestyle choices or health care provision. The Health Foundation in England emphasizes the social (or wider) determinants of health as "the social, cultural, political, economic, commercial and environmental factors that shape the conditions in which people are born, grow, live, work and age" (HealthFoundation, 2024).

An important distinction is drawn by the WHO in referring to "health inequities" rather than "health inequalities" (WHO, 2024c). This distinction places emphasis on three distinguishing features of health inequities: (1) they are systematic, that is not produced by random or by chance, (2) they are socially produced and as such they are modifiable and (3) they are fundamentally unjust. Health inequalities, on the other hand, may not always be avoidable i.e. the cause may be genetic or biological rather than socially or economically produced. However, the effect of generational trauma and epigenetic factors deeply challenge this point.

The wider SDoH can be clustered into six broad domains as depicted in Figure 4.1 below.

This figure also depicts sub-domains of the wider determinants of health that act as either positive or negative drivers on health and social outcomes. Health inequalities manifest in various forms, including variations in morbidity, mortality, life expectancy, prevalence of diseases, access to healthcare facilities and quality of healthcare received. Importantly, health inequalities highlight systemic injustices and inequities in the distribution of resources and opportunities, leading to unequal health outcomes among individuals and communities. Addressing health inequalities requires understanding and addressing the root causes that perpetuate disparities in health, with the ultimate goal of achieving health equity for all members of society.

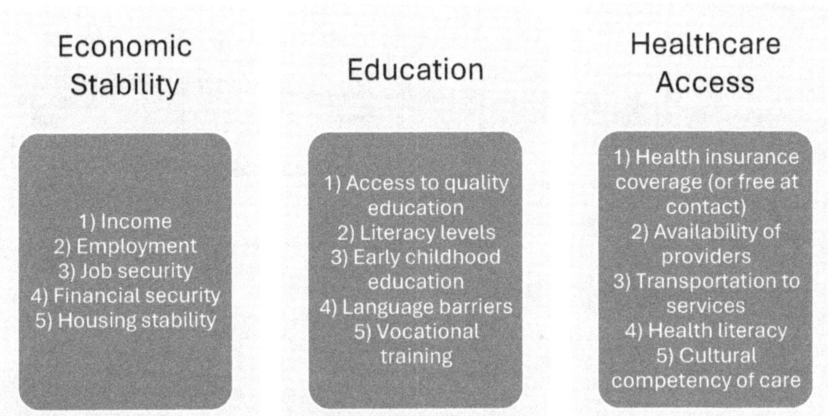

FIGURE 4.1 Wider social and structural determinants of health, adapted from WHO Social Determinants of Health (2024a)

In an attempt to understand the relationships between the wider social determinants and health outcomes, the WHO has developed an overarching program theory (Solar & Irwin, 2010), which attempts to also integrate the role of bio-psychosocial drivers of health with structural forces (see Figure 4.2). This program theory importantly attempts to highlight the relationships between the wider structural socioeconomic and political drivers and the intermediary drivers that determine health equity and well-being. Circular relationships are depicted, which repeat over successive generations and thus acknowledge temporal issues that act to compound poor outcomes for the most marginalized. The WHO framework also draws attention to the position and importance of social cohesion and social capital and the role of health systems in the amelioration of health inequity. The presence of these suggests the importance of a bio-psychosocial and ecological perspective on human health.

Recent Research

2023 saw the launch of the WHO's Health Inequality Data Repository (HIDR), a comprehensive and global collection of disaggregated data on population health and its determinants (WHO, 2023c). The HIDR contains over 11 million data points and will facilitate the monitoring of health inequity across countries and over time, according to demographic, socioeconomic and geographical factors. The launch of this data set underlines the continued commitment and importance the WHO places on global health inequity, which is further reinforced by The World

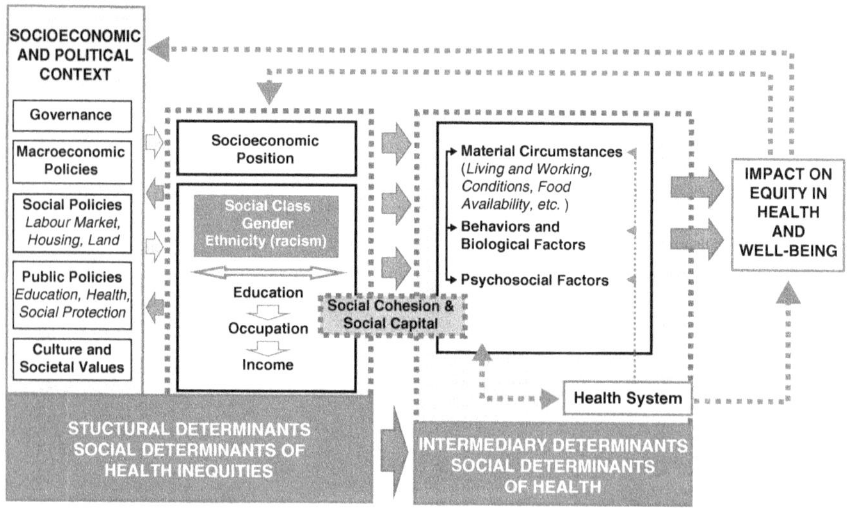

FIGURE 4.2 WHO framework of social determinants of health [World Health Organization (WHO), 2010]

Bank (Gwatkin, 2000), UNICEF (1999), and the Nations Development Programme (United Nations, 2003).

Globally, health inequities are evidenced in the following areas: mortality and morbidity, access to healthcare and workforce distribution. Current challenges also include the impact of COVID-19, the impact of climate change on health and gender-based inequalities war and conflict. The digital health divide and the rise of non-communicable diseases are emerging as significant challenges (WHO, 2024b).

Adult life expectancy rates between low- and high-income countries can differ (on average between 15 and 20 years), with a gap of 30 years between the richest and poorest nations (add WHO global observatory). Countries with high levels of both adult and child mortality have higher rates of extreme poverty and spend less per capita on healthcare, hospital beds and doctors (Ruger & Kim, 2006; WHO, 2024a). Populations within these counties are also less likely to have access to clean water, sanitation facilities and immunizations, most notably these are countries in West and Sub-Saharan Africa and Afghanistan (same citation as above).

Health inequities are also observed in the patterning of a range of communicable and non-communicable diseases. For example, cardiovascular disease, a leading cause of death and disease globally, varies both across and within counties and is significantly associated with income level (Roth et al., 2020; Ski et al., 2014). This was evidenced in a longitudinal Canadian study which revealed that heart disease increased by 27% and 37% in lower- and lower-middle-income groups compared to 6% and 12% in the higher-middle- and high-income groups (Lemstra et al., 2015).

The rise in non-communicable diseases disproportionally impacts people as they age, with more people living longer with multiple long-term conditions (Gale et al., 2014; Griffith et al., 2019). Non-communicable diseases can also impact some groups more than others, particularly those who rely on the appropriate provision of care to manage their illnesses. Access to care however is also determined by a range of factors, which for the most marginalized, often result in adverse health outcomes. Over 50% of the global population lack access to basic health services (WHO, 2023b). Forced migrants, refugees and asylum seekers, irrespective of whether they are internally or externally displaced are particularly at risk. The United Nations High Commissioner for Refugees collated statistics on forcibly displaced people in 2024 and reported that 123.2 million people were forcibly displaced; 36.8 million people were categorized refugees, 8.4 million people were seeking asylum and 73.5 million people were internally displaced (United Nations High Commissioner for Refugees, 2024). Refugees and asylum seekers often face health inequalities and poor outcomes due to little or no access to healthcare. For those who are able to access healthcare, the lack of culturally appropriate care and the poor provision of interpreters create significant barriers to access (van der Boor & White, 2020) and lead to misdiagnosis and poor treatment experiences (Schouler-Ocak & Iris T., 2023). Refugees and asylum seekers are more likely to suffer from mental ill health compared to other migrant and non-migrant groups (Priebe et al., 2016).

Healthcare workforce shortages in African, Eastern Mediterranean, South East Asia and the Western Pacific region are contributing to health inequalities in those regions. These issues are not however confined to low- and middle-income countries (LMICs), although they are likely to be most acutely felt in these areas due to poverty and a range of other systemic problems. The WHO health workforce support and safeguards list for 2023 contains the names of 55 countries in these regions that have a density of doctors, nurses and midwives below the global median of 49 per 10 000 population, representing a contributing factor to unsatisfactory universal coverage of healthcare in those regions (WHO, 2023a).

Other pressing issues in global health inequity have been recorded in severe differences in rates of maternal mortality, in particular in African countries and Afghanistan. In the Democratic Republic of Congo women have a 1/6 change of dying in childbirth compared to Iran for example where women have a 1/2372 chance of death in childbirth (Gazeley et al., 2024).

Health inequities are by no means restricted to LMICs as we have seen in the Canadian study (Lemstra et al., 2015) and as evidenced by MacKinnon et al. (2023). A recent report commissioned by the Health Foundation in England (Marmot, 2020), analyzed health equity over the 10 years since Marmot (2010) published Fair Society, Health Lives. This earlier report aimed to examine health inequalities in England and the causes of them and make recommendations for strategies to tackle them. The recommended strategies however have either failed to achieve the desired aim, or more plausibly were not implemented under ten years of austerity in the United Kingdom, with compelling links between political austerity measures and the SDoH. The results are, to directly quote Michael Marmot "shocking" (Marmot, 2020, p. 5). Key findings include the stalling of life expectancy, growth in the number of years lived in ill health, the widening of health inequalities with austerity measures and greater cuts to key public services in the most deprived areas. The associated outcomes manifest in a lowering of life expectancy in men and women in deprived areas and increases in life expectancy in the least deprived areas. Marmot (2020) also found that inequalities in life expectancy also follow a North-South divide, with people living in the North with lower life expectancies than those living in the South. Moreover, people in more deprived areas spend more of their shorter lives in ill health compared to those in more affluent areas. The poorest areas have the highest preventable mortality compared to the least preventable mortality in wealthy areas (Marmot, 2020).

Whilst life expectancy improved in many other OECD countries, it stalled and decreased in England in deprived areas in the years following 2010 and reflects a similar picture to the United States and Iceland. In the United States, this has been termed "deaths of despair", attributed to accidental poisoning, suicide and drug overdose (Rehder et al., 2021). What is important to note, is that when other countries have experienced declines in life expectancy in the past, it has been associated with war, major critical incidents or political destabilization e.g. the collapse of the Soviets Union saw life expectancy in men drop by four years (Ciment, 1999). The research cited above points to consideration of the underlying issues and factors associated with the social and structural determinant's of health and SoDH as depicted in Figure 4.2.

To understand health inequity and to plan strategies to challenge it, multisectoral efforts and commitment are required. To successfully implement effective strategies, an understanding of how the social gradient of health works to reflect health inequities is key. The "Social Gradient of health" has been well established by numerous studies (Bonaccio et al., 2016; Bray et al., 2018; Lemstra et al., 2015; Ski et al., 2014; Tillmann et al., 2017) and defined as a concept in Marmot's first edition of Fair Society, Healthy Lives (Marmot, 2010). It describes a process by which health outcomes improve incrementally further up the socioeconomic ladder, forming a "gradient" whereby individuals at each rung of the social hierarchy experience better health than those below them. In doing so, it highlights the link between social determinants such as income, education and occupational status and health disparities. Established from analysis of the Whitehall study (Wigger, 2011), it revealed that job grade was associated with poorer health and lower occupational autonomy in a longitudinal cohort of United Kingdom civil servants.

As we have seen, the social gradient of health impacts a range of health outcomes and is a global phenomenon, driven by a mix of structural and social forces ranging from material conditions such as access to resources, housing, nutritious food and healthcare. Psychosocial factors such as stress and discrimination are also important, emanating from economic insecurity or low societal status, which in turn, impacts mental and physical health. Health behaviors feed into this complex picture, but are often understood as individual lifestyle choices, when in fact there are very few choices open to people in poverty that are strongly influenced by social and economic constraints.

A key feature of the social gradient of health is that it isn't just an issue for those at the lowest levels; people's circumstances can change quickly. Redundancy, bereavement, illness and migration, for example, can cause people to slip into poverty as quickly as education, improved health and social capital can support people to thrive. For this reason, the social gradient of health affects everybody on the socioeconomic spectrum with anyone apart from the most affluent considered to be in a relatively precarious position (Marmot, 2020).

So...What Can Be Done About Health Inequity?

Inequity will only be successfully challenged and changed if equity is centered as a core societal and global value system. This requires bold modeling in leadership to create a systemic and philosophical shift from dominance and hierarchy to more equal societies and institutions. Whilst this might seem like a lofty and naïve ambition, there are examples of areas that have made progress in addressing health inequity using a whole systems approach (Marmot, 2010), in spite of the lack of political leadership to prioritize health inequalities. Before reviewing these solutions, it is worth considering the key prerequisites that support possible solutions to health inequities.

Elevating the Voices of the Excluded

Firstly "we" as a collective society of academics, practicioners, policy makers, public voices and engaged parties need to embrace our responsibility to engage in research and practice to elevate the voices of those who are disenfranchised and othered. We should consider very carefully if we are relying on dominant narratives as "truths", particularly in the United Kingdom, where the most vocal are often white British upper to middle class patients and public contributors. Taking stakeholder participation and involvement seriously and proactively is a step toward tackling inequity, since it is those who are most deprived, ill, racially minoritized and othered on the basis of gender, religion, sexual identity or disability which often suffer the most from being seldom heard. Indeed, creating equitable public and service provider partnerships to improve and implement health and social care strategies has been discussed elsewhere in this book.

Systems Thinking

What do we understand by the term "system"? Social scientists across a range of disciplines are well known for talking about systems whether they be social, cultural, religious or economic. What happens if we start to consider how these systems entwine? Bronfenbrenner's ecological system's theory (Bronfenbrenner, 1977) is particularly useful here (see also Chapter 2). First developed to map human development within an ecological relational system, it has since been helpfully employed to provide a life course understanding of the interaction between the person and their wider familial, social, structural and interconnected systems and the SDoH in a range of settings (Eriksson et al., 2018). It facilitates this by attempting to understand how health outcomes are influenced in context, highlighting the structural and social determinants for individuals and groups. Identifying where these determinants are located can help pinpoint multisector strategies to address them. Figure 4.3 below is a depiction of Bronfenbrenner's Ecological Systems Model as depicted by Guzman et al. (2023) in their paper describing a qualitative study that investigated the socioecological drivers of older people's mental health during COVID-19 in Ireland.

Fair and Targeted Allocation of Resources

Marmot (2010) made strong recommendations that to improve health inequity and tackle the social gradient of health, resources should be distributed with equity

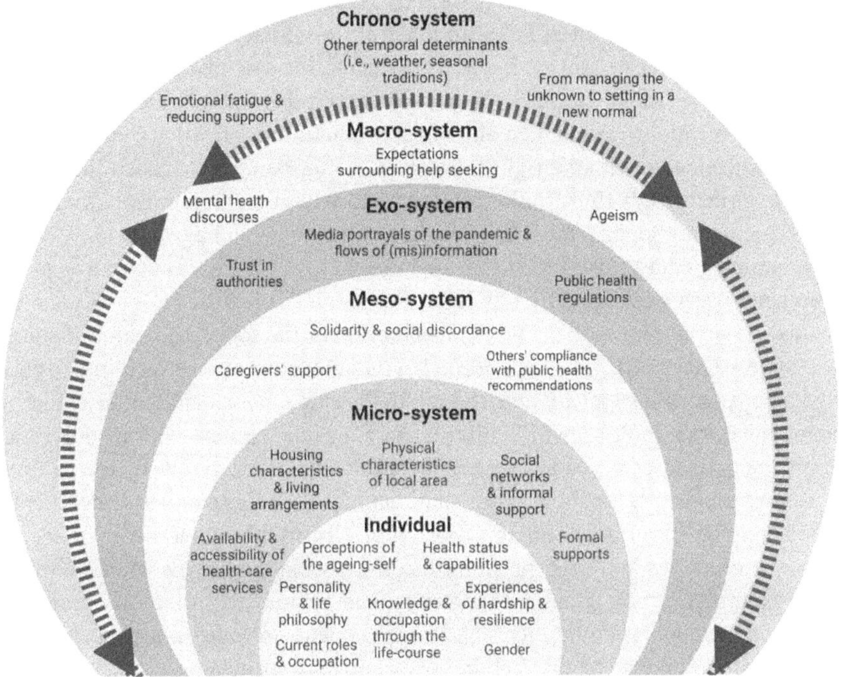

FIGURE 4.3 Bronfenbrenner's ecological model depicting factors that impacted older adults' well-being during COVID-19

based on need. This was referred to as "Proportionate Universalism". In the United Kingdom at least, this recommendation has been ignored since resource and spending allocations over the past 14 years are less focused on deprived areas than previously reported in 2010 (Marmot, 2010). Which might be reflected in the widening of health inequalities over the same period.

Understanding the relationships between the SDoH as outlined by the WHO in Figure 4.2 in an ecological systems framework, might provide a sensitive way in which to improve outcomes for those with pressing needs at scale. An approach that might best be employed by organizations such as Integrated Care Systems (ICSS), which create strategies deliverable through multisectoral provider interventions (Integrated Partnerships ICPS) to tackle health inequalities and improve local services. Reflecting the interrelationship between the structural determinants and the intermediary determinants, ICSs and ICPs, comprise NHS, local government, non-government and voluntary sector organizations and social care professionals at different levels with a level of autonomy to direct resources based in need over a given geographic footprint.

As governance and infrastructural support, Integrated Care Boards (ICBs) can create coordinated and joined up health and social systems that respond to the multifactorial nature of the SDoH. Caution is however considered since the concept of integration has often failed to materialize in real terms to improve health and social outcomes. However, integration combined with collaborative action based on equity (Lloyd et al., 2017) does hold the potential for change. This ethos holds the potential to strengthen and support community-based activities that can become sustainable with the right infrastructural support. Notwithstanding the obvious trust that needs to be built both with and within communities before health access, screening, engagement and effective treatment can be provided. A critical examination of how discrimination operates to exclude and marginalize people from health services and activities is an imperative. This needs to go beyond tick box exercises in implicit bias, to a consideration of the social and cultural context of people's lives, which moves people beyond categories to be seen intersectionally. This is a philosophical step change for health systems and cultures that are hierarchical in nature. Viewing individuals in a social context with resources and assets in a person-centered and strengths-based lens is a step toward seeing assets in communities, since people make communities (see Chapter 10). Social enterprises and non-government organizations typically do this due to their flatter management structures and their proximity to the people they work with. Below are some examples of how grass root organizations embody the principles previously discussed to support community faced improvements to some of the most marginalized, and in doing so begin to address key social determinants.

Salutogenisis: Is It One of the Keys to Tackling Health Inequalities?

The UK national health service was set up to improve the health of the nation with free at point of entry healthcare. Over the past 75 since its inception advances in technology and drug treatments have led to great improvements in the treatment of disease and ill health. These targeted advances have created a narrow conception of health as the absence of disease and not focused enough on the creation of health. The concept of Salutogenisis was conceived by Antonovsky (1979) to describe a continuum of human ill health to health in relation to stress responses. It attempts to understand the factors that support health rather than those that cause illness. In doing so, Antonovsky's work (1987) influenced a movement toward health promotion (World Health Organization, 2018), with a model of health that incorporates life experiences, considers a range of bio-psychosocial factors alongside coping responses, and in the context of an individual's access to both generalized and specific resources. It also includes a consideration of how individuals make sense both cognitively and behaviorally, of the stress challenges we face, thus creating an overall sense of coherence which determines our response (Elfassi et al., 2016). It is through our response, i.e. do we consider life to be comprehensive, manageable and meaningful, that we are more likely to achieve a status of "healthy". More recent adaptations to the model consider a Sense of Community Coherence (SOCC) and its relationship to the health of groups (Braun-Lewensohn et al., 2013; Elfassi et al., 2016).

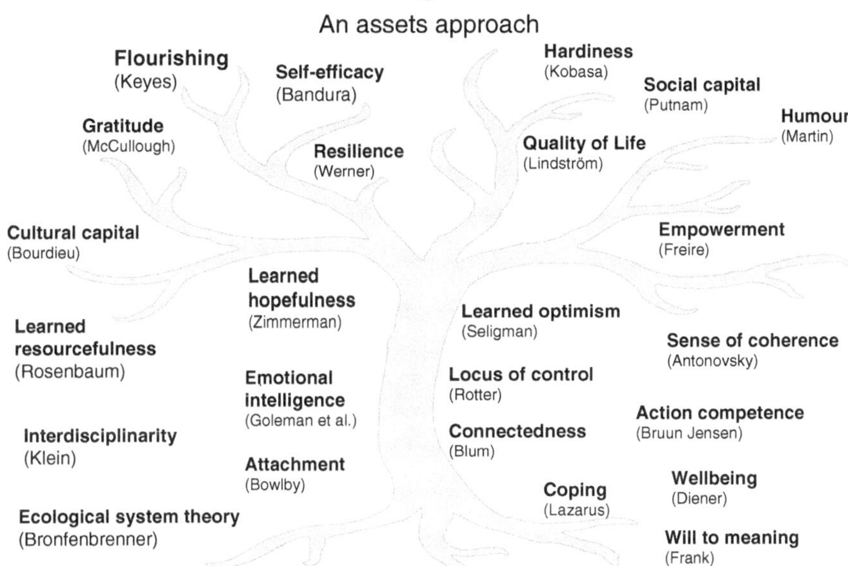

FIGURE 4.4 The model of Salutogenisis, the key domains and associated theories

Figure 4.4 depicts the model of Salutogenisis, the key domains and associated theories. As we can see, Bronfenbrenner's Ecological Systems Theory is featured alongside other theories. On examination, one can logically propose that when the accumulative load of life stressors combines with a lack of specific and generalized resources, let's call them here "Social Determinants", people experience ill health and slide down the social gradient of health.

Alt text: A tree which represents the domains and theories related to salutogenisis with the orginating author of that domain underneath. For example, "attachment (Bowlby)".

Since migration and forced displacement are key drivers of health inequality, the section that follows provides examples of how salutogenic approaches have been used to address some of the social determinants of ill health among these groups. They provide examples of how social and cultural capital, connectedness, empowerment and well-being intersect to create salutogenesis.

Examples of Salutogenic Community-Based Interventions for Refugees

Nature-Based Interventions

Over the past 20 or so years, there has been a growing interest in the role of nature to harness well-being. Whilst this research is still in its relative infancy, as a collective evidence base it shows promising findings in relation to a range of the specified domains depicted above in the representation of Salutogenisis.

Community food gardens are a form of nature-based therapy that are emerging as potential way to foster a sense of recovery in formally displaced peoples. They do this by providing an experiential learning and grounded interaction with the land and nature, and with other people in a protected space. Whilst not without their challenges, community gardens offer a route to perceptions and experiences of self-efficacy, the development of attachment and connectedness to people and place (Gómez et al., 2015; Tidball & Aktipis, 2018) in addition to improvements in physical health and nutrition (Abramovic et al., 2019; Sanchez & Liamputtong, 2017). They provide a safe space to consolidate knowledge and memories of home and integrate these with current experiences. For those for whom dialectical psychological treatment is not favored or inaccessible, the therapeutics of communal gardens offer the potential to move forward to positions of thriving or at least provide respite from the hostile situations that refugees and asylum seekers face.

In an Australian setting, Abramovic et al. (2019) explored recovery experiences in Burmese refuges. This interesting study highlighted the "more than human" aspects of recovery fostered by nature. For example, the authors demonstrate how encounters with different ecological and material engagements (e.g. soil, food) in safe spaces enable a visceral and embodied adaptive response which supports a sense of belonging and place-making which work to support recovery. A similar study in the United States by Preiss (2013) on community gardens for refugees reported improvements in well-being and a range of social and financial benefits. Community gardens also operate as a space to incorporate a sense cultural identity and belonging through offering opportunities to grow plants familiar to refugees who have lost the connection with their homeland (Strunk & Richardson, 2019).

The salutogenic effects of nature are not restricted to community gardens. Recent research has investigated Surf therapy for young asylum seekers (Britton, 2018), camping (Hurly & Walker, 2019), nature-based vocational rehabilitation (Ekstam et al., 2021) and vocational horticulture (Poulsen et al., 2020). Young refugees in Britton's study learnt to overcome difficulties and created bonds with others and the sea, whilst Hurly and Walker's (2019) study created a connection with nature and rekindled memories of home. Notwithstanding the multitude of benefits nature-based interventions confer in relation to self-efficacy, connection, attachment and belonging, as important as these findings are, perhaps the most important findings in terms of addressing inequalities were reported by Poulsen et al. (2020) and Ekstam et al. (2021), where participants developed employability, self-confidence and language skills.

In summary, nature-based interventions have the potential to operate a multitude of mechanisms to improve health and well-being. They offer a place-based asset, or a connection to natural assets, that facilitates opportunities for meaning-making and place-making for the most marginalized, with benefits for the wider community.

Peer Support

Peer support worker (PSW) models are community-based interventions whereby a person who shares an aspect of lived experience with a group of people is trained to support those people in the community. The role often incorporates signposting, listening and providing practical support (NHS, 2024). In recent years, there has been a growth in recognition of the potential for peer support to improve mental health outcomes and widen the mental health workforce in the United Kingdom at least. The evidence for PSW models across broad range of population groups and conditions remains mixed (Cooper et al., 2024). However, when focusing on some of the most marginalized groups who represent the lowest point on the social gradient of health, PSW models have reported positive benefit. A review by Gower et al. (2022a) reported that PSWs helped address refugee isolation, enhance social networks and improve access to services. Peer support models also have the potential to build self-esteem, and self-efficacy among service users, increase levels of confidence and self-awareness (Gower et al., 2022b). Community liaison workers in a study conducted by Wei et al. (2021), facilitated access to services benefiting peers by improving access to necessary resources and support systems. Ogbe et al. (2021) highlighted that peer support models offer survivors of sexual and gender-based violence opportunities for shared understanding, validation of experiences and access to information and coping strategies, reducing feelings of isolation and promoting resilience. The benefits to PSWs themselves are also documented in relation to improved employment, career development opportunities and interpersonal skills, providing ongoing training and support are helpful and supportive (Ogbe et al., 2021).

Importantly, Wei et al. (2021) highlighted that PSW models foster social support and connection outcomes by bridging the gap between peers and service providers, improving access to services and creating opportunities for community members to connect with one another. These benefits are felt for the health system in terms of providing an "integration effect" linking services users and services, but also promoting community integration between members. Similar community benefits were reported by Mahon (2022), who argues that social support and connection outcomes directly improve mental health, confidence and community integration among asylum seeking and refugee women.

Why Do These Interventions Hold Promise?

A key finding across studies of peer support work is that interventions that have been co-designed in equity with service users or potential service users and peers are the most successful (Mahon, 2022). This type of engagement and involvement ensures that interventions are grounded in the lived experience of the target group. It maximizes the potential of success because it attends to the relevance in content and ensures that the delivery of the intervention is trauma-informed. Nature- and peer-based interventions have the potential to provide safe spaces with which people can explore connections to people and places, memories and experiences, skills and knowledge. They provide access to new experiences and access to services not otherwise known. They are community assets for people who have experienced profound loss which created placed based relational meaning-making often essential for post traumatic growth and thriving. In short, they hold the potential salutogenic properties, offering attempts at a sense of coherence for the community and the individual as part of it. These types of interventions, also provide non-stigmatizing opportunities outside of traditional mental health services. As active rather than passive health promotion, people develop a sense of empowerment or self-efficacy to take control of their own narrative sense of coherence. Through engagement and participation such interventions voice the unheard and engage the disengaged. In doing so, they have the potential to begin to address some of the key impacts of health and social inequalities through increases in social can cultural capital.

Conclusion

This chapter has demonstrated that health inequalities are not merely statistical variations in health outcomes, but represent systematic, socially and structurally produced and fundamentally unjust disparities that persist across global contexts. The evidence reveals that these inequities are deeply embedded within structural and social determinants that operate at multiple levels, from macro-level policies and economic systems to meso-level community interventions and micro-level individual experiences.

The social gradient of health emerges as a critical framework for understanding how health outcomes improve incrementally with socioeconomic position, affecting not just the most disadvantaged but creating precarity across the entire social spectrum. This gradient is sustained by complex interactions between material conditions, psychosocial factors and constrained health behaviors that are often mischaracterized as individual lifestyle choices when they are, in reality, structurally determined.

Perhaps most significantly, this chapter has illustrated that addressing health inequalities requires moving beyond traditional biomedical approaches toward salutogenic interventions that focus on creating health through social capital rather than merely treating disease. The examples of nature-based interventions and peer support models for refugees and other marginalized groups demonstrate how community-based approaches can simultaneously address multiple social determinants while building individual and community resilience. These examples are elaborated with case studies in Chapter 5 on Social Capital.

The promise of these interventions are more than a sum of their parts, they provide a systemic and embedded approach to creating meaningful connections, foster empowerment and provide non-stigmatizing pathways to well-being. They exemplify how elevating the voices of the excluded and employing systems thinking can lead to innovative solutions that address root causes of ill health rather than merely treating the symptoms, and in doing so are intristically health promoting.

However, this chapter also highlights the sobering reality that without fundamental shifts in political priorities and resource allocation—guided by principles of proportionate universalism—individual interventions, however promising, cannot fully counteract the structural forces that perpetuate health inequities. The stark evidence from England's experience with austerity demonstrates how quickly progress can be reversed when political commitment to equity wanes.

Moving forward, the challenge lies in scaling up promising community-based interventions while simultaneously advocating for the macro-level systemic changes necessary to create truly equitable societies. This requires not just technical solutions, but a philosophical shift from hierarchical, to collaborative, asset-based models that recognize the interconnectedness of human flourishing with social, economic and environmental justice.

Ultimately, achieving health equity demands that we center equity as a core societal value, moving beyond the narrow confines of healthcare systems to embrace whole-system approaches that address the conditions in which people are born, grow, live, work and age. Only through such comprehensive transformation can we hope to break the intergenerational cycles of disadvantage that perpetuate health inequalities and move toward a more just and healthy world for all.

References

Abramovic, J., Turner, B., & Hope, C. (2019). Entangled recovery: Refugee encounters in community gardens. *Local Environment, 24*(8), 696–711. https://doi.org/10.1080/13549839.2019.1637832

Antonovsky, A. (1979). *Health, stress, and coping.* Jossey-Bass Inc. - References - Scientific Research Publishing. Www.scirp.org. https://www.scirp.org/reference/ReferencesPapers?ReferenceID=1480370

Antonovsky, A. (1987). Unraveling the mystery of health: How people manage stress and stay well. In *The open library* (1st ed.). Jossey-Bass. https://openlibrary.org/books/OL2733173M/Unraveling_the_mystery_of_health

Bonaccio, M., Di Castelnuovo, A., Costanzo, S., Persichillo, M., Donati, M. B., de Gaetano, G., & Iacoviello, L. (2016). Interaction between education and income on the risk of all-cause mortality: Prospective results from the MOLI-SANI study. *International Journal of Public Health, 61*(7), 765–776. https://doi.org/10.1007/s00038-016-0822-z

Braun-Lewensohn, O., Sagy, S., Sabato, H., & Galili, R. (2013). Sense of coherence and sense of community as coping resources of religious adolescents before and after the disengagement from the Gaza Strip. *Israel Journal of Psychiatry and Related Sciences, 50*(2), 110–117.

Bray, B. D., Paley, L., Hoffman, A., James, M., Gompertz, P., Wolfe, C. D. A., … & Rudd, A. G. (2018). Socioeconomic disparities in first stroke incidence, quality of care, and survival: A nationwide registry-based cohort study of 44 million adults in England. *Lancet Public Health, 3*(4), e185–e193. https://doi.org/10.1016/s2468–2667(18)30030-6

Britton, E. (2018). 'Be Like Water': Reflections on strategies developing cross-cultural programmes for women, surfing and social good. In L. Mansfield, J. Caudwell, B. Wheaton, & B. Watson (Eds.), *The Palgrave handbook of feminism and sport, leisure and physical education* (pp. 793–807). Palgrave Macmillan UK.

Bronfenbrenner, U. (1977). Toward an experimental ecology of human development. *American Psychologist, 32*(7), 513–531. https://doi.org/10.1037/0003–066X.32.7.513

Ciment, J. (1999). Life expectancy of Russian men falls to 58. *British Medical Journal, 319*(7208), 468. https://doi.org/10.1136/bmj.319.7208.468a

Cooper, R. E., Saunders, K. R. K., Greenburgh, A., Shah, P., Appleton, R., Machin, K., … & Johnson, S. (2024). The effectiveness, implementation, and experiences of peer support approaches for mental health: a systematic umbrella review. *BMC Medicine, 22*(1), 72. https://doi.org/10.1186/s12916-024-03260-y

Diener, E., Lucas, R. E., & Oishi, S. (2018). Advances and open questions in the science of subjective well-being. Collabra*: Psychology,* 4(1), 15. https://doi.org/10.1525/collabra.115

Ekman, I., Swedberg, K., Taft, C., Lindseth, A., Norberg, A., Brink, E., … & Sunnerhagen, K. S. (2011). Person-centered care--ready for prime time. *European Journal of Cardiovascular Nursing, 10*(4), 248–251. https://doi.org/10.1016/j.ejcnurse.2011.06.008

Ekstam, L., Pálsdóttir, A. M., & Asaba, E. (2021). Migrants' experiences of a nature-based vocational rehabilitation programme in relation to place, occupation, health and everyday life. *Journal of Occupational Science, 28*(1), 144–158. https://doi.org/10.1080/14427591.2021.1880964

Elfassi, Y., Braun-Lewensohn, O., Krumer-Nevo, M., & Sagy, S. (2016). Community sense of coherence among adolescents as related to their involvement in risk behaviors. *Journal of Community Psychology, 44*(1), 22–37. https://doi.org/10.1002/jcop.21739

Elrick, H. (1980). A new definition of health. *Journal of the National Medical Association, 72* (7), 695.

Eriksson, M., Ghazinour, M., & Hammarström, A. (2018). Different uses of Bronfenbrenner's ecological theory in public mental health research: What is their value for guiding public mental health policy and practice? *Social Theory & Health, 16*(4), 414–433. https://doi.org/10.1057/s41285-018-0065–6

Gale, C. R., Cooper, C., & Aihie Sayer, A. (2014). Prevalence of frailty and disability: Findings from the English longitudinal study of ageing. *Age and Ageing*, *44*(1), 162–165. https://doi.org/10.1093/ageing/afu148

Gazeley, U., Polizzi, A., Prieto, J. R., Aburto, J. M., Reniers, G., & Filippi, V. (2024). The lifetime risk of maternal near miss morbidity in Asia, Africa, the Middle East, and Latin America: A cross-country systematic analysis. *The Lancet Global Health, 12*(11), e1775–e1784. https://doi.org/10.1016/S2214-109X(24)00322-X

Gómez, E., Baur, J. W. R., Hill, E., & Georgiev, S. (2015). Urban parks and psychological sense of community. *Journal of Leisure Research, 47*(3), 388–398. https://doi.org/10.1080/00222216.2015.11950367

Gower, S., Jeemi, Z., Forbes, D., Kebble, P., & Dantas, J. A. R. (2022a). Peer mentoring programs for culturally and linguistically diverse refugee and migrant women: An integrative review. *International Journal of Environmental Research and Public Health, 19*(19). https://doi.org/10.3390/ijerph191912845

Gower, S., Jeemi, Z., Wickramasinghe, N., Kebble, P., Forbes, D., & Dantas, J. A. (2022b). Impact of a pilot peer-mentoring empowerment program on personal well-being for migrant and refugee women in Western Australia. *International Journal of Environmental Research and Public Health, 19*(6). https://doi.org/10.3390/ijerph19063338

Griffith, L. E., Gruneir, A., Fisher, K., Panjwani, D., Gafni, A., Patterson, C., Markle-Reid, M., & Ploeg, J. (2019). Insights on multimorbidity and associated health service use and costs from three population-based studies of older adults in Ontario with diabetes, dementia and stroke. *BMC Health Services Research, 19*(1), 313. https://doi.org/10.1186/s12913-019-4149-3

Guzman, V., Doyle, F., Foley, F., Craven, P., Crowe, C., Wilson, P., … & Pertl, M. M. (2023). Socio-ecological determinants of older people's mental health and well-being during COVID-19: A qualitative analysis within the Irish context. Retrieved from https://pmc.ncbi.nlm.nih.gov/articles/PMC10077967/

Gwatkin, D. R. (2000). Health inequalities and the health of the poor: What do we know? What can we do? *Bull World Health Organ, 78*(1), 3–18. Retrieved from https://www.ncbi.nlm.nih.gov/pubmed/10686729

Health Foundation. (2024). Exploring the wider determinants of health. Retrieved from https://www.health.org.uk/what-we-do/a-healthier-uk-population/useful-publications-and-resources-on-healthy-lives/exploring-the-social-determinants-of-health

Hone, L., Schofield, G., & Jarden, A. (2015). Conceptualizations of wellbeing: Insights from a prototype analysis on New Zealand workers. *New Zealand Journal of Human Resource Management, 15*(2), 97–118.

Huber, M., Knottnerus, J. A., Green, L., Van Der Horst, H., Jadad, A. R., Kromhout, D., … & Van der Meer, J. W. M. (2011). How should we define health? *Bmj, 343,* 235–238.

Hurly, J., & Walker, G. J. (2019). Nature in our lives: Examining the human need for nature relatedness as a basic psychological need. *Journal of Leisure Research, 50*(4), 290–310. https://doi.org/10.1080/00222216.2019.1578939

Lemstra, M., Rogers, M., & Moraros, J. (2015). Income and heart disease: Neglected risk factor. *Canadian Family Physician, 61*(8), 698–704. Retrieved from https://www.ncbi.nlm.nih.gov/pubmed/26836056

Lloyd, H. M., Pearson, M., Sheaff, R., Asthana, S., Wheat, H., Sugavanam, T. P., Britten, N., Valderas, J., Bainbridge, M., Witts, L., Westlake, D., Horrell, J., & Byng, R. (2017). Collaborative action for person-centred coordinated care (P3C): An approach to support the development of a comprehensive system-wide solution to fragmented care. *Health Research Policy and Systems, 15*(1). https://doi.org/10.1186/s12961-017-0263-z

MacKinnon, N. J., Emery, V., Waller, J. L., Ange, B., Preshit Ambade, Gunja, M. Z., & Watson, E. (2023). Mapping health disparities in 11 high-income nations. *JAMA Network Open, 6*(7), e2322310–e2322310. https://doi.org/10.1001/jamanetworkopen.2023.22310

Mahon, D. (2022). A scoping review of interventions delivered by peers to support the resettlement process of refugees and asylum seekers. *Trauma Care, 2*(1), 51–62. https://doi.org/10.3390/traumacare2010005

Marmot, M. (2010). *Fair society, healthy lives: The Marmot review*. The Marmot Review. https://www.parliament.uk/globalassets/documents/fair-society-healthy-lives-full-report.pdf

Marmot, M. (2020). Health equity in England: The Marmot review 10 years on. *Bmj, 368,* m693. https://doi.org/10.1136/bmj.m693

Michaelson, J., Mahony, S., & Schifferes, J. (2012). *Measuring wellbeing: A guide for practitioners*. New Economics Foundation.

NHS. (2024). Peer support workers. Retrieved from https://www.healthcareers.nhs.uk/explore-roles/psychological-therapies/roles-psychological-therapies/peer-support-worker

Ogbe, E., Jbour, A., Rahbari, L., Unnithan, M., & Degomme, O. (2021). The potential role of network-oriented interventions for survivors of sexual and gender-based violence among asylum seekers in Belgium. *BMC Public Health, 21*(1), 25. https://doi.org/10.1186/s12889-020-10049-0

Poulsen, D. V., Pálsdóttir, A. M., Christensen, S. I. et al. (2020). Therapeutic nature activities: A step toward the labor market for traumatized refugees. *International Journal of Environmental Research and Public Health, 17*(20), 7542.

Preiss, D. A. (2013). *Laying down new roots: Place attachment and well-being through community gardening among Bhutanese refugees.* (Masters). State University of New York, College of Syracuse.

Priebe S, G. D., & El-Nagib R. (2016). *Public health aspects of mental health among migrants and refugees: A review of the evidence on mental health care for refugees, asylum seekers and irregular migrants in the WHO European Region.* Retrieved from Geneve: https://www.ncbi.nlm.nih.gov/books/NBK391045/

Rehder, K., Lusk, J., & Chen, J. I. (2021). Deaths of despair: Conceptual and clinical implications. *Cognitive and Behavioral Practice, 28*(1), 40–52. https://doi.org/10.1016/j.cbpra.2019.10.002

Roth, G. A., Mensah, G. A., Johnson, C. O., Addolorato, G., Ammirati, E., Baddour, L. M., … & Fuster, V. G. B. D. (2020). Global burden of cardiovascular diseases and risk factors, 1990–2019: Update from the GBD 2019 study. *The Journal of the American College of Cardiology, 76*, 2982–3021.

Ruger, J. P., & Kim, H. J. (2006). Global health inequalities: An international comparison. *Journal of Epidemiology & Community Health, 60*, 928–936. https://doi.org/10.1136/jech.2005.041954.

Sanchez, E. L., & Liamputtong, P. (2017). Community gardening and health-related benefits for a rural Victorian town. *Leisure Studies, 36*(2), 269–281. https://doi.org/10.1080/02614367.2016.1250805

Saracci, R. (1997). The World Health Organisation needs to reconsider its definition of health. *Bmj, 314*(7091), 1409.

Schouler-Ocak, M., & Iris T., G.-C. (2023). Ethical dilemmas of mental healthcare for migrants and refugees. *Current Opinion in Psychiatry, 36*(5), 366. https://doi.org/10.1097/YCO.0000000000000886

Sen, A. (2014). *Development as freedom (1999). The globalization and development reader: Perspectives on development and global change, 525* (2nd ed.). Wiley-Blackwell.

Ski, C. F., King-Shier, K. M., & Thompson, D. R. (2014). Gender, socioeconomic and ethnic/racial disparities in cardiovascular disease: A time for change. *International Journal of Cardiology, 170*, 255–257.

Solar, O. I. A. (2010). *A conceptual framework for action on the social determinants of health. Social determinants of health discussion paper 2 (policy and practice).* Retrieved from WHO: https://www.who.int/publications/i/item/9789241500852

Strunk, C., & Richardson, M. (2019). Cultivating belonging: Refugees, urban gardens, and placemaking in the Midwest, U.S.A. *Social & Cultural Geography, 20*(6), 826–848. https://doi.org/10.1080/14649365.2017.1386323

Tidball, K. G., & Aktipis, A. (2018). Feedback enhances greening during disaster recovery: A model of social and ecological processes in neighborhood scale investment. *Urban Forestry & Urban Greening, 34*, 269–280. https://doi.org/10.1016/j.ufug.2018.07.005

Tillmann, T., Vaucher, J., Okbay, A., Pikhart, H., Peasey, A., Kubinova, R., … & Holmes, M. V. (2017). Education and coronary heart disease: Mendelian randomisation study. *Bmj, 358*, j3542. https://doi.org/10.1136/bmj.j3542

Trebeck, K., & Abeyasekera, A. (2012). Oxfam humankind index. *Wellbeing and Quality of Life Assessment, 147,* 1–15.

UK Care Act. (2014). *Care Act 2014*. Legislation.gov.uk. https://www.legislation.gov.uk/ukpga/2014/23/contents

United Nations (2003). *United Nations Development Programme Human development report 2003: Millennium development goals: A compact among nations to end poverty.* U.N. New York.

United Nations High Commissioner for Refugees. (2024). *UNHCR - Refugee statistics*. UNHCR. https://www.unhcr.org/refugee-statistics

UNICEF. (1999). *United Nations Children's Fund The progress of nations 1999.* Retrieved from New York:

van der Boor, C. F., & White, R. (2020). Barriers to accessing and negotiating mental health services in asylum seeking and refugee populations: The application of the candidacy framework. *Journal of Immigrant and Minority Health, 22*(1), 156–174. https://doi.org/10.1007/s10903-019-00929-y

Wei, K., Chopra, P., Strehlow, S., Stow, M., Kaplan, I., Szwarc, J., & Minas, H. (2021). The capacity-building role of community liaison workers with refugee communities in Victoria, Australia. *International Journal of Mental Health Systems, 15*. https://doi.org/10.1186/s13033-021-00485-9

WHO. (1948). *Constitution of the world health organization.* WHO, Geneva. Retrieved from https://iris.who.int/bitstream/handle/10665/121457/em_rc42_cwho_en.pdf

WHO. (1986). *Ottawa charter for health promotion.* WHO, Geneva.

WHO. (2018). *Health promotion in Western Pacific.* Who.int; World Health Organization. https://www.who.int/westernpacific/health-topics/health-promotion

WHO. (2023a). Global health workforce statistics update. Retrieved from https://www.who.int/publications/i/item/9789240069787

WHO. (2023b). *Tracking universal health coverage: 2023 Global monitoring report.* Washington, DC. Retrieved from https://hdl.handle.net/10986/40348

WHO. (2023c). WHO releases the largest global collection of health inequality data. Retrieved from https://www.who.int/news/item/20-04-2023-who-releases-the-largest-global-collection-of-health-inequality-data

WHO. (2024a). Global health observatory. Retrieved from https://www.who.int/data/gho

WHO. (2024b). Health inequality monitor. Retrieved from https://www.who.int/data/inequality-monitor/data

WHO. (2024c). Health inequities and their causes. Retrieved from https://www.who.int/news-room/facts-in-pictures/detail/health-inequities-and-their-causes

WHO. (2024d). Promoting wellbeing. Retrieved from https://www.who.int/activities/promoting-well-being#:~:text=Well%2Dbeing%20encompasses%20quality%20of,resources%2C%20overall%20thriving%20and%20sustainability.

WHO. (2024e). Social determinants of health. Retrieved from https://www.who.int/health-topics/social-determinants-of-health#tab=tab_1

Wigger, E. (2011). The Whitehall study. Unhealthy Work. Retrieved from https://unhealthywork.org/classic-studies/the-whitehall-study/

5

SOCIAL CAPITAL AND COMMUNITY WELL-BEING

Helen Lloyd

Introduction

Definitions, Historical and Conceptual Roots

Social Capital: The Fundamental Premise and Why It Matters

The term "capital" usually refers to a resource or asset of some form that has financial value. Capital, in this sense, is therefore an essential requirement for human survival and thriving. Social capital first emerged as a construct in the sociological literature of the 1980s to describe a network of social assets that enable people and communities to achieve goals, for themselves or for the community to which they belong (Kenton, 2024; Oxford Dictionary, 2020). Social capital is achieved through effective interpersonal relationships, which are based on a set of shared group characteristics such as identity, values and norms. Mechanisms of trust and reciprocity provide the glue by which social capital is maintained (Putnam, 2000).

Why Social Capital Matters in Contemporary Society

Chapter 4 of this book outlined the prevalent global problems with health and social inequality and how these problems have worsened in the past 15 or so years, particularly for the most deprived and vulnerablized. In these areas or communities, the erosion of social capital has resulted, in part, from years of underfunding and resource scarcity. This contributes to marginalization through barriers to existing health and social care services, unemployment, financial benefit restrictions and chronic ill health. Marginalization can be described as the process by which a person or a group is rendered insignificant, unimportant and neglected (Cambridge

DOI: 10.4324/9781032662657-6

Dictionary, 2023). In these circumstances, people and groups of people often become protective of their own resources, become mistrustful of authority figures, institutions and their fellow community members (Berger et al., 2021). For those on the margins, negative stereotypes can, over time, become internalized, leading to group and individual stigma, breeding resentment, cynicism and experiences of being othered (Phelan et al., 2014; Pickett et al., 2024; Williams, 2009).The erosion of social capital and other assets in marginalized communities results in deficits in what is termed in the sociological literature as cultural capital (Bourdieu, 1977). Cultural capital is comprised of a range of assets that a person holds, such as language skills, education, status and employment. These assets are necessary to achieve upwards social mobility in hierarchical and stratified societies, a mechanism by which to alleviate the negative impacts of the social gradient of health as outlined in Chapter 4. Social capital and projects that bring people together to address issues associated with marginalization therefore have the potential to provide systems of social support, education, employment and language skills which can both indirectly and directly improve health outcomes and improve the cultural capital of people and communities.

The importance of social capital is demonstrated by its widespread application across numerous fields, from public health to economic development, for example, social capital has been incorporated into development frameworks by the World Bank (Grootaert & Van Bastelar, 2002), recognizing its importance for poverty reduction and sustainable development.

Social Capital: Historical and Conceptual Foundations

While current understandings of social capital generally draw on the work of Robert Putnam (1993; 1995), the use of the term and its etymological origins can be traced back to the mid-1800s (Farr, 2004; Claridge, 2021). A very early reference to "social capital" (gesellschaftliche Kapital) was made by Karl Marx (1867) to refer to a collection of individual or personal capitals that might combine for communal productivity. This is perhaps unsurprising given Marx's attention to material capital is so central to his later influential theory outlined in Das Kapital (capital, Marx, 1867). Indeed, as documented by Farr (2004), political economists like Marx acknowledged the role of social associations as important contexts for generating social capital and for challenging the status quo. Such organizations included "....trusts, cartels, joint stock companies, guilds, trade unions, brotherhoods of labor, friendly societies, mutual aid societies, communes, and cooperatives" (Farr, 2004, p. 23). The emphasis placed however by the political economists of the day was less on social, and more so on material capital and the ownership of the production systems in the context of the industrial revolution.

John Dewey (1859–1952) philosopher, psychologist and educational reformer highlighted the importance of social capital over the course of his career. As a functionalist and pragmatist, he believed that people developed and adapted to their environment, and considered rational social and communal actions and a means to solve society's problems. Dewey's critical pragmatism influenced the philosophical roots of "social capital", as demonstrated by an emphasis on construction from criticism, compassion and sympathy for fellow humans and the first combination of the words "social" and "capital" together to acknowledge the human held non-material resources which could be used for the social good (Dewey, 1990).

A community setting in rural West Viginia was the location first formally referenced in relation to the term "social capital" as we currently understand it. Here Hanifan (1916) used the term "social capital" to refer to social glue which binds a unit of people together through social norms of goodwill, sympathy and support of one another through a web of social interactions and expectations. He considered social capital necessary against the backdrop of increased urbanization, poverty and isolation. His job as state educational officer for rural schools no doubt influenced his centering of educational establishments as "community centers". In these early writings, Hanifan highlighted the loss of social capital and the absence of it to create a call to action (1916).

In the late 1960s and 1970s, the counterculture movement provided a fertile anti-establishment questioning to challenge oppression and inequality. Leading theorists at the time were questioning power dynamics and examining social capital through a more critical and sociological framework. Pierre Bourdieu's (1986) contribution to the development of the role of "capital" in power frameworks cannot be underestimated. For Bourdieu, social capital was critical for explaining how social networks and social relationships determine social mobility and access to resources. Social capital, in his view, was complementary to cultural capital (a person's knowledge and skills) and economic capital (employment, assets, etc.) in securing powerful positions in society. Several components of Bourdieu's conception of social capital advanced its study and measurement. Firstly, Bourdieu considered both the size and quality of a person' social network as important. High quality (reciprocal social bonds, trust, regular contact) along with larger networks were considered key for social capital and social power. Critically, Bourdieu argued that "institutionalized" social relationships such as those achieved or facilitated through professional associations, clubs or social organizations were the ones that provided more access to social capital and advantages for social mobility. Networks like these often have rules and requirements that restrict entry, and in doing so, Bourdieu argued, were more socially divisive and thus directly contribute to social inequalities. Indeed, a key aspect of Bourdieu's (1986) conception of social capital was that social relationships and networks were much less idealized with inherent tensions across them.

In demonstrating the importance of social capital on educational performance, James Coleman (1926–1995) brought the concept into mainstream sociology in the 1980s. Coleman defined social capital functionally as resource within social structures that are necessary to support the social and educational development of children and young people. His influential educational research demonstrated that race and socio-economic status were the strongest drivers of educational outcomes, which contributed to educational desegregation policy in the United States (Andreas, 2018; Claridge, 2015; Coleman, 1990).

Robert Putman's (1993) work on social capital is widely recognized for bringing the concept into mainstream discourse and contributing to debates across multiple disciplines. His contributions have shaped both academic inquiry and policy-making, leading to important conversations about how social capital supports democratic institutions and community health. Conceptualized as a shared resource, social capital in Putman's view represented the collective capacity for participation, civic mindedness and mutual trust within communities, regions or entire nations (Putman, 1995). This differs from Bourdieu's framework, which viewed social capital more as an individual asset, while Coleman's interpretation falls somewhere between these two positions. Putnam therefore transformed social capital from an individual characteristic into a collective attribute that operates at the community or societal level. Social capital in Putman's view represents the amount of trust within a society and serves as the primary element defining contemporary political cultures. Social capital is therefore a structural element of a social systems; relationship networks, shared values and trust—that enable coordinated action and collaboration for shared benefits. Building on Coleman's work, Putnam saw social capital as a facilitator of human cooperation, suggesting that these qualities could be measured and compared across different geographic and political units.

Putnam's framework emphasizes organizational features of society, using networks, norms and trust as illustrative examples. This approach clearly establishes social capital as a community property, since the "capital" refers to social structures that shape individual behavior, rather than personal attributes that drive individual choices.

The notion of "social capital" as conceptualized by Putman is not however free from critique. Putnam has been accused of reducing complex social processes to simple measures like levels of trust, resulting in dramatic oversimplification (Foley & Edwards, 1999). Putman's theory has also been charged with invoking a circular logic where social capital is both cause and effect (Fine, 2002b). This is perhaps an unfair criticism, since trust is often cited as a generative mechanism and outcome in much realist theory building in a range of different contexts (Pawson & Tilley, 2004). Others have argued that Putman's theory lacks conceptual clarity, clear definitions and reliable measurement methods, making research difficult to compare or repeat (Woolcock, 1998). Perhaps the most significant critique is that Putman's theory overlooks how disadvantaged groups face barriers to social capital, and this lack of nuance may hide existing inequalities (Fine, 2002a). Therefore, whilst social capital may strengthen groups, it can also create barriers against outsiders and reinforce social divisions. It could also be argued that by idealizing social capital through a lens of cooperation, the theory undervalues the positive role of divergence, tension and disagreement in building social relationships.

Dimensions of Social Capital

Complex concepts like social capital can be helpfully understood in terms of dimensions. Social capital is widely considered to have three core dimensions (Nahapiet & Ghoshal, 1998): structural, cognitive and relational. Structural social capital includes social network arrangements, configurations and densities. It includes the strength of network ties (e.g. weak vs. strong ties) and their function (Brass & Burkhardt, 1992). Relational dimensions of social capital encompass trust as a core component embedded within reciprocity and social norms, interpersonal relationships and their qualities and the degree to which emotional and instrumental support is key (Coleman, 1990; Nahapiet & Ghoshal, 1998). Shared histories, stories and narratives create collective alignment and meaning-making, which in turn help to establish shared interpretations and cultural understanding. Together, these aspects create a Cognitive Dimension of social capital (Nahapiet & Ghoshal, 1998).

Social capital can also be conceptualised with three subtypes, which function differentially within each domain. These subtypes are defined as bonding, linking and bridging social capital (also see Chapter 3). Bonding social capital refers is most seen in close-knit communities, family and immediate inward social networks within the structural domain (Putnam, 2000). Bonding social capital is related to processes of cognitive alignment characterized by shared norms and shared identities, with relational deep trust and mutual support. Bridging social capital functions across groups to create cross-group connections and outward networks in a structural domain. Bridging social capital functions when there is tolerance, diversity and a shared purpose with relational and respectful cooperative ties characterised by cognitive alignment (Putnam, 2000). It supports social mobility and organizational cooperation and inter-community networks. Linking social capital is understood as the process by which resources and assets permit vertical connections and interactions across power and status hierarchies in the structural domain (Szreter & Woolcock, 2004). Within the cognitive domain, it is characterized by a trust in authority and shared expectations. In a relational sense, linking social capital is represented by a perceived legitimacy in institutions and institutional trust.

A dimensional conceptualization of social capital as presented above provides a potential to understand with greater precision and definition of how social capital functions in particular contexts to assert both positive and negative influences on health and social outcomes and health inequalities.

Understanding Community Well-Being

As outlined in Chapter 4, the concept of "well-being" like "social capital" is contested and complex, and a thorough examination of this is outside the scope of this chapter. Yet, well-being, support, trust and a sense of belonging are key elements in the positive connections people have within strong social capital contexts in communities (Ihlebæk et al., 2023; Adams et al., 2025). Building Social capital in communities therefore becomes an important lever in developing person-centered approaches in community engagement to build community well-being. This relies on the acceptance that there is an inherent ethical and practical usefulness to think beyond the individual in terms of well-being, and understand the relationships between community well-being and progress toward tackling health inequalities. Indeed, thinking beyond individual outcomes helps to acknowledge the role of structural forces on health and illness and takes a step away from notions of healing and flourishing characterized by the dominant knowledge systems of the Global North. The following current definition put forward by Wiseman and Brasher (2008) helps to acknowledge power differentials by positioning the community as identifiers of their own conditions for community well-being. It also describes community well-being in terms of objective components (e.g., infrastructure, health outcomes, income) and those that are more subjective (a sense of belonging, perceived safety): this is similar to acknowledging the unique qualities of communities described in Chapter 3.

> Community well-being is the combination of social, economic, environmental, cultural, and political conditions identified by individuals and their communities as essential for them to flourish and fulfil their potential
>
> *(Wiseman & Brasher, 2008, p. 358)*

Community well-being as defined above can be understood in finer detail through subcomponents in each dimension. For example, social well-being can be characterized through social cohesion, trust, safety, inclusion and relationships (Forjaz et al., 2011). Economic well-being is demonstrated by employment opportunities, income equality and economic stability (OECD, 2020). Health and environmental well-being are achieved through improved access to healthcare, clean air and water, green spaces (Agyeman & Evans, 2004). Cultural and spiritual well-being is created by a sense of shared identity, heritage, belonging and purpose (White, 2010), whereas political well-being is evidenced by civic participation, governance, justice and voice (Dodge et al., 2012). The overlap between dimensions and types of social capital with a dimensional understanding of community well-being is obvious.

Community well-being more recently has been informed by participatory approaches, acknowledging the role of top-down power dynamics on community-defined indicators (Atkinson et al., 2017). Other developments in conceptualizing community Well-being include the OECD's framework on regional well-being, which promotes place-based measurement of factors such as housing, jobs, access to services and civic engagement (OECD, 2020). The capabilities approach (Nussbaum, 2000; Sen, 1999) has also influenced community well-being frameworks by focusing on what individuals and groups are actually able to do and be in their environments. Thus, linking individual capabilities with those of the wider community and the interdependence of them.

Social Capital as a Well-Being Mechanism (Health, Education, Employment)

A number of systematic reviews have demonstrated relationships between social capital and well-being by targeting aspects that support it. Ehsan and colleagues (2019) explored social capital and health in a meta review of 20 studies and concluded that there was strong to moderate evidence for a positive relationship between social capital and mental and physical health. They also reported some evidence for negative relationships between social capital and health, pointing to a darker side in the relationship. Dimensionally, the evidence for relationships between social capital and health is more complicated. For example, Uphoff et al. (2013) found that for disadvantaged individuals, bonding social capital was protective of health whereas bridging and structural social capital were associated with worse outcomes for these groups. Furthermore, bridging and linking social capital were only associated with better health for more advantaged groups. Their findings suggest that higher group-level bridging social capital promoted exclusion and worse health outcomes for minorities and disadvantaged groups. These results were reversed in a review by Villalonga-Olives et al. (2017). Overall, the literature suggests that social capital has a positive effect on mental and physical health, though it would seem that the impact of it on health varies by context, group and type of social capital examined.

An international scoping review of the impact of social capital on health, education and employment (Mishi et al., 2023), also supported the findings of Ehsan et al. (2019), reporting a positive relationship between social capital and health, with high levels of social capital linked to improved mental and physical health outcomes. The authors reported that social capital was commonly measured through social support, trust, group membership and community participation and was associated with reductions in stress, supporting recovery from addiction, healthy behaviors and increasing access to resources (jobs and healthcare). However, inequality and poor social cohesion weakened these benefits, leading to worse health outcomes.

In an integrative review of the impact of family social capital (FSC) and community social capital (CSC) on the mental health of children and adolescents, McPherson et al. (2014) found that FSC, especially strong parent child relationships characterized by warmth, support and low conflict, is consistently associated with better mental health and fewer behavioral problems in children and adolescents. Authoritative parenting and cohesive, trusting extended family environments also have protective effects. Adolescents who reported positive relationships with their parent(s), with higher quality/quantity of social support networks were more likely to report higher levels of self-esteem. Conversely, parental or caregiver monitoring was linked with lower self-esteem, suggesting the need for adolescent autonomy. Family structure (e.g. two-parent households) shows some association with better outcomes but not consistently.

Specifically exploring the role of CSC on young peoples' mental health, McPherson et al. (2014) reported that access to high-quality social support networks which included peers, non-family adults and parents' own networks, was associated with positive mental health and behavior. Safe schools, supportive neighborhoods and frequent religious service attendance (as a proxy for social networks) were similarly linked to better outcomes. However, civic engagement showed little direct association.

Similar to impacts on adult health, the effects social capital on child and adolescent health vary by context and population, with the benefits of social capital less consistent in high-violence or impoverished neighborhoods (McPherson et al., 2014). This underscores the need for context-sensitive research and targeted interventions that enhance social capital while considering local conditions and subgroup differences (McPherson et al., 2014).

In examining the role of social capital on education, Helliwell and Putnam (2007) found that education boosts trust and community involvement, expanding the networks that help people thrive. Palmer and Maramba (2015), also found that educated individuals were more socially connected, with higher quality connections than those with lower levels of education. Behtoui (2016) reveals that students with families and friends who value education aim higher academically. Interestingly, they found that while some caregivers with limited education may struggle to support student success, those with peer networks and strong faculty connections benefited the most. Brouwer et al. (2016) also confirm that supportive relationships with educators offer the highest returns in confidence, motivation and achievement. Overall, the findings suggest that social capital fuels ambition, strengthens belief in one's abilities and plays a critical role in shaping educational journeys.

Social capital has also been evidenced to play a pivotal role in influencing labor market outcomes, including hiring practices and employability. Behtoui (2016) highlights its significance in both formal and informal employment dynamics. Social capital in the workplace has been shown to influence the delivery of sustainable development goals (Xu et al., 2024).

As a relational asset, social capital can advantage job seekers by facilitating access to labor market information and opportunities (Bonoli & Turtschi, 2015). However, it may also produce negative effects by creating barriers to job retention and career progression, particularly when it reinforces exclusionary hiring practices (Cheung & Phillimore, 2014). Referrals based on social ties often serve as cost-effective hiring tools for employers, though they will likely disadvantage those who lack such networks. Brady (2015) underscores the importance of weak social ties (e.g., acquaintances) over strong ties (e.g., family) in securing employment, though the impact varies by demographic and geographic factors. Bonoli and Turtschi (2015) found that foreign nationals in Switzerland maintain larger networks of former colleagues, which may indicate unstable employment. Despite this, systemic inequalities and discrimination limit the efficacy of such networks in improving job prospects. Moreover, while social networks aid employment for immigrants, factors such as language proficiency and pre-immigration qualifications are equally critical (Cheung & Phillimore, 2014).

Jay and Andersen (2018) conceptualize social capital through bonding (close personal ties), bridging (looser connections such as colleagues) and linking (relationships with those in authority) with these dimensions influencing both individual and organizational outcomes. Stone et al. (2004) expand on this framework, identifying bridging and linking as key forms of inter- and intra-organizational social capital. Cheung and Phillimore (2014) propose a tripartite measure—informal ties, generalized relationships and institutional connections—to assess social capital in the labor market. When applied to immigrant populations, Bonoli and Turtschi (2015) utilize a broad network-based approach, including ties through friends, family, ethnic groups and religious organizations.

The research to date suggests that social capital as a determinant of employment outcomes is complex, context and group specific, much like the relationships observed between social capital and health and education; while it can facilitate access, its unequal distribution and interaction with structural barriers may limit its benefits, especially for marginalized groups.

Relational Dynamics: The Importance of Trust and Reciprocity for SC and as a Fundamental Well-Being Indicator

Individual and collective well-being within communities is strongly associated with trust and reciprocity, both of which act as foundational elements of social capital (Putnam, 2000; Coleman, 1988). Effective relationships across a broad range of life domains are strongly predicated by "Trust". Whilst definitions of "Trust" vary across contexts and academic disciplines, the definition offered by Rousseau et al. (1998), provides a helpful cross-discipline view that "Trust" is a psychological state characterized by a person's acceptance of vulnerability based on positive expectations about another's intentions or behavior. This definition relates trust at an individual level but can also be extended to group level and toward institutions. "Trust" facilitates cooperation, reduces transaction costs in social and economic exchanges and enhances civic engagement (Putnam, 2000).

Communities characterized by generalized trust—where individuals believe others will act fairly—tend to experience lower crime rates, better health indicators and higher levels of life satisfaction (Helliwell et al., 2021). Institutional trust, or confidence in public systems and governance, also plays a crucial role in promoting compliance with social norms and public health measures (Chanley et al., 2000; Levi & Stoker, 2000). Both relational and institutional trust has been consistently shown by research from across the health and social sciences, to be associated with greater social cohesion, reduced stress and improved mental and physical health (Kawachi & Berkman, 2000; Helliwell & Putnam, 2004)

Reciprocity is a core component of social capital and a key mechanism through which social cohesion and trust are maintained. At its most fundamental level "Reciprocity" refers to the mutual exchange of goods, services or favors that fosters cooperation and strengthens social relations. In his seminal work "The Gift", Mauss (1954 [1925]) examined reciprocity from an anthropological and economic perspective, stressing the universal importance of the act of giving, receiving and repaying gifts to social relationships and cohesion. From a psychological perspective, reciprocity is a powerful force that induces people to return favors, thus promoting prosocial behavior and social harmony (Cialdini, 2001). Viewing reciprocity through a sociological lens, Gouldner (1960) defines it as universal norm that compels individuals to return benefits received from others, which motivates much human interaction from interpersonal to macro levels. Generalized reciprocity, characterized by Putnam (2000), describes the process where the return of a favor is not immediate or directed at the same individual and, as such, fosters social networks and collective action, strengthening community ties and long-term cooperation.

Reciprocity not only reinforces social networks but also creates a sense of belonging and security (Coleman, 1988). It contributes to well-being by creating reliable support systems during times of crisis or vulnerability (Cohen & Wills, 1985). An emphasis on individual and group reciprocity encourages altruistic behaviors, reduces social isolation and builds resilience within communities (Putnam, 2000; De Neve et al., 2018). Higher levels of well-being, including lower rates of depression, increased happiness and more equitable access to resources are reported in communities with higher rates of trust and reciprocal relationships (Helliwell et al., 2021; Kawachi & Berkman, 2000). Trust and reciprocity therefore create a potential buffer against social inequality and enhance the capacity of communities to respond to challenges collectively (De Neve et al., 2018).

In summary, trust and reciprocity are key social mechanisms that promote psychological security, social stability and public health, making them critical components of sustainable community well-being.

Cognitive Alignment: Foundational for Social Capital and Community Well-Being

Cognitive alignment is one of the key dimensions of social capital, alongside structural and relational dimensions. It encompasses the shared interpretations and systems of meaning and representation among individuals and groups (Nahapiet & Ghoshal, 1998). This facilitates a common language and a shared narrative necessary for building trust, reciprocity and collective action and behavior (Uphoff, 2000). In a reinforcing pattern, cognitive alignment creates mental models that further reinforce cultural practices and ideological structures underpinned by reliability and mutual support (Krishna & Shrader 1999). When cognitive alignment fails or fractures misunderstandings and conflicts occur, weakening the social fabric that binds communities or organizations together. In community development contexts, for example, when people share similar cognitive frameworks, this promotes collective effectiveness and strengthens their ability to tackle challenges together, ultimately supporting community health and adaptive capacity (Pretty, 2003).

Community Interventions for Displaced People: Case Studies from the Southwest of England

Community settings and third sector organizations are well placed to deliver interventions that enhance social capital for people who are marginalized or stigmatized, or for those who lack trust in statutory services. Non-government organizations (NGOs) offer a range of support services from counseling, case work, social activities and specific cultural and nature-based activities. Some offer these on a one-to-one basis, but many tend to be "group-based activities". For people who have been forcibly displaced, NGOs and Refugee Third Sector organizations are often the only contact some people have to gain support. Many organizations provide critical support and are often under-funded, oversubscribed and under researched with specific regard to refugee experiences and outcomes in England. The sparse existing research on NGO interventions demonstrates early indications toward addressing some of the social determinants of ill health witnessed in marginalized groups. For example, with evidence suggesting enhanced integration (Lewis, 2010), belonging (Stone, 2018) and socialization (Sigona, 2012). Some activities also offer opportunities for language acquisition and training opportunities to prepare refugees for employment (Morrice, 2007). Importantly, research also suggests these activities foster social capital and a refocus on post-traumatic growth and recovery (Morrice, 2007), providing opportunities for social connectedness, which is a key factor for resilience (Richards, 2015). These findings suggest that NGO activities hold the potential to lead to decreases in distress and mental health symptoms (Gallagher & Featonby, 2019) in a non-stigmatizing delivery mode (Hoeft et al., 2018). Evidence has also shown that some of these initiatives are effective in reducing potential hospitalizations (Chinman et al., 2008) and improving social functioning (Yanos et al., 2001).

Moreover, these activities have the potential to increase mutual understanding and learning among diverse communities, including UK-born residents and multi-national support networks that share knowledge and resources (Jannesari, 2022). Importantly, these activities offer important non-verbal routes to expression and connection with the self, others and the non-human world.

A diverse range of individuals, including artists, refugees and former health professionals, often work in Refugee Third Sector (RTS) groups. It is often this combination of creativity and agility, grounded in the wisdom of people with lived experience, that makes these organizations accessible for refugees. Nurturing the desire and strengths in individuals to refocus on a "new life" based on capabilities (Nussbaum, 2009; Sen, 1999), with the potential to challenge the profound disruption to personhood disruptions of forced displacement. As discussed in Chapter 4, whether explicitly intended or tacitly created, these approaches hold the potential for fostering a salutogenic approach (Antonovsky, 1996) to improve the health and well-being for refugees. They also provide a necessary bridge between health and social care organizations and refugees (Coleman & Campbell, 2009). Such initiatives meet the needs of refugees who want community-based approaches to improve their health and promote social and economic development (Arnetz et al., 2013; Misra et al., 2006).

The following sections of this chapter present examples of projects that build social capital for displaced people. All projects are based in the South West and West of England. Two are led by NGOs, and one was a funded research project to design and test an intervention.

"I am free, but I am not free": nature-based activities with a Refugee and Asylum seeker community, an ethnographic action study.

Nature-based interventions are emerging as culturally inclusive psychosocial support, yet the experiences of displaced people who engage in such activities are often underexplored. An ethnographic action research-informed approach was used to examine a nature-based program in Southwest England. Four lived experience research consultants informed the design and analysis of the study.

The research was conducted at an NGO in the Southwest of England which provides a wide range of practical, emotional and social support to members of the local displaced community. Among its initiatives are a suite of weekly nature-based activities in nearby green and blue spaces. These sessions include walking, cycling, boat trips, canoeing, visits to community gardens and time spent on local farms.

Multiple qualitative methods were used to gain a rich, contextual understanding of the nature-based program. These included participant observations, informal conversations (ethnographic interviews), formal conversations (semi-structured interviews) and a focus group. In line with participatory and ethnographic principles, the term conversation rather than interviews was agreed upon with research consultants to reduce associations with immigration or Home Office procedures. The "embeddedness" of the researcher provided a unique perspective and nuanced connection to the activities and the people who participated in them. Data was collected through five observation days, 16 conversations and one focus group, involving three staff facilitators and 30 displaced people.

Thematic framework analysis identified four key themes: to access, to connect and belong, to survive and to be me with power. Findings revealed that nature-based activities offer respite, connection and empowerment and identified the incorporation of co-production and facilitator reflective spaces. Findings also suggested that these types of interventions offer meaningful first-step support and called for greater integration of nature-based offers into public health and social policy and stronger collaboration with third sector organizations.

The findings from this study demonstrate the importance of informal networks in accessing nature-based activities and those that are built through engaging in nature-based activities. Participants relied on their existing networks (structural social capital) to learn about and access activities, which led to new cross-group networks through engagement in the activity (bridging social capital). Linking social capital was built through this project by the access it provided to people in roles of "authority" or leadership. These individuals held local knowledge and knowledge of systems and processes. Importantly, some of those with authority roles were people with whom refugees could relate through lived experience since they had previously been service users and were now volunteers or facilitators. Cognitive alignment between participants was built by sharing in new place-based experiences together and the creation of meaning and memories of these human and non-human interactions. Nature-based activities therefore created opportunities to bond, connect and belong together creating relational social capital. Learning new skills (e.g. cycling, surfing, gardening) and becoming confident and proficient created trusted experiences and feelings of empowerment. For people who have lost their home, jobs, family and friends, finding opportunities to feel "a family" creates strong experiences of bonding social capital. Against a backdrop of hostile immigration policies and public mistrust, these activities created safe psychological spaces for people to build social capital, collective action and reciprocity.

Ethnographically Informed Research Exploring the Impact of Embedding Trauma-Informed Principles in a Befriending Program for Refugees

This study explored the impact of embedding trauma-informed principles (TIP) within a refugee befriending program, where refugees were paired with local volunteers. Befriending is a widely used approach, largely adopted by the voluntary sector and designed to foster meaningful social connections for a range of populations such as individuals with mental health difficulties, elderly populations and refugees.

The NGO service in which the research was conducted is based in the Southwest of England and offers a variety of services and resettlement support to the local refugee community. An embedded clinical researcher integrated TIP into the befriending program through comprehensive training for befrienders, including a dedicated session on managing the ending of befriending relationships, the provision of regular reflective sessions and the establishment of a supportive peer network via WhatsApp. Befrienders supported refugees over a six-month or more period by providing emotional and practical support, with pairs attending community-based social activities. Ethnographic Action informed research was used through completing interviews, observations and a focus group. Participants included five befrienders and seven refugees, alongside observational data.

Thematic and framework analyses identified five key themes: the relationship, safety for befrienders, inclusivity, supporting befriendees with integration and challenges of befriending. TIP enhanced understanding of how community-based, trauma-informed interventions can support refugee recovery and resilience. The study offers practical recommendations to improve the effectiveness, inclusivity and sustainability of such programs. However, it was limited by the absence of perspectives from refugees who disengaged early from the program, limiting the diversity of perspectives that were represented.

Introducing trauma-informed approaches to the befriending scheme described above brought numerous benefits for befrienders and befriendees and helped establish social capital in several ways. Befrienders were more attuned to their privilege and power as a consequence of their trauma-informed training, making conscious efforts to support the empowerment of their befriendee. They did this by for example undertaking activities together such as a pottery making course that were new to both parties and by also encouraging choice and decision making in the befriendee. These activities and approaches developed trust and reciprocity for bonded relationships. This form of bonded social capital often was the only form of emotional support experienced by some of the befriendees, who were often isolated outside of this relationship. The befriending scheme also created inclusive practice at both individual and community levels. Befrienders learnt more about their befriendees culture during one-to-one meetings but also shared in activities focused on culturally grounded experiences around food, dance or music. Community events created opportunities for bridging social capital and the very nature of the befriending scheme provided practical bonding and linking social capital. The latter was evidenced by the knowledge sharing that befrienders used to support their befriendees integration through access to leisure, education and community activities. The reciprocity and trust so important for social capital were at the heart of the befriending program.

Routes to Wellness: Co-Designing a Peer-Led Community Approach to Support the Mental Health of Refugees

This study co-designed a peer-support worker (PSW) model for refugees to support their mental health in the community. The team who led the research was formed before funding was secured and involved key stakeholders with existing knowledge and experience of providing mental health provision and services for refugees. Both statutory and non-statutory services were involved. People with lived experience of forced displacement were also part of the team and all parties identified the need for this project and supported the development of the research bid.

A method of participatory research was used called experience-based co-design. This approach incorporates narrative storytelling to help guide a co-design approach to service development. Central to this is the identification of emotional touchpoints to direct service improvement that reflects what matters most to users and providers. "Touchpoints" capture personal and subjective experiences that are significant in relation to their service needs and health concerns. Touchpoint data in this research was transformed into a range of written, visual, digital media and creative media to inform discussions relating to the content of the PSW model.

People with lived experience and service providers took part in conversations and group conversations to explore how displaced people think about, experience and express mental distress and related issues, both generally and in relation to any interactions they may have had with services. It was this data that was used to create emotional "touchpoints". Following this phase, ten multilingual workshops with all stakeholders considered the analysis of touchpoints and the implications of these for PSW service delivery. Workshops determined the content, approach and structural components of the model and the PSW training. The evaluation framework used to test whether the PSW model was helpful was also co-designed. The PSW model was presented and discussed at a celebration event, where people from services and the community were introduced to the PSW role.

PSW were trained in narrative interaction, goal setting, safeguarding, confidentiality, NHS mental health provision and trauma-informed practice. They received supervision and mentoring support from partner organizations. PSWs were people with lived experience of forced displacement. The model was tested over nine months. PSWs were approached to support people in the community who required support for mental health issues, through community settings and through drop-ins at NGOs. They worked with people to access basic material needs, mental and physical health services, provided social networks and linked them to community groups and activities. They provided a trusted sense of hope and validation.

The above study was funded by the UK's National Institute for Health and Social Research Health Services Development Research funding stream. The project unfolded over three phases, but prior to securing the funding, the team met with NGO members and people with a refugee background to understand their priorities for research, which led to the idea for the project described above. During phase 1, researchers spent time getting to know the communities and service providers to build trust and support for the research. The team regularly met with people with lived experience of forced displacement to guide the research processes, consider language and power and to practice trauma-informed and ethical research practice. Language and approach were considered carefully when data collection ensued. Natural groups were considered for focus groups and people were provided with the opportunity for single or mixed sex focus groups. Interpretation was necessary with skilled interpreters trained in the specifics of research practice. The trust and community that began to develop around the project was consolidated through phase 2 where workshops were convened to design the intervention based on the findings from phase 1. The sharing of food, experiences, music and the use of creative processes facilitated trust building and social bonding that evolved over the design of the intervention. People with lived experience were invited to help organize and feedback the results of previous workshops and help plan and deliver the celebration events. Creative role play scenarios and other interactive activities were used to explore key themes of peer-support work and positioned people with lived experience as directors of the unfolding scene or active in the development of the model. These deliberate acts to challenge power dynamics helped gain the trust of all who attended. At the end of phase 2, a group of individuals with lived experience came together to create a testimonial video about how taking part in the research had led to positive changes in their lives. This ranged from reductions in stigma of mental illness and being able to support people in the community, a renewed sense of purpose and hope, the desire to help others and seek work, feeling socially connected, feeling valued and heard. This is remarkable given that the intervention trial was yet to be launched and attests to the power of genuine community participatory methods of research. This video and others made by the team can be accessed via the project's website create a hyperlink https://www.plymouth.ac.uk/research/psychology/routes-to-wellness.

The transformative potential of the project was realized when people transitioned from participants in phase 1, to co-designers in phase 2 and then to trained and paid PSWs in phase 3. NGOs, NHS and local council workers all attested to the value of the peer-support model which has now been commissioned by the regional Integrated Care Board. Findings from the study evidence increased social capital across multiple domains (bonding, bridging, linking) and benefits to physical and mental health, better access to education, health, work and community activities. Importantly, people reported increases in quality of life, reduced levels of distress, enhanced social networks and better knowledge of and access to appropriate support. The Routes to Wellness Study created a community and set of social networks for people who were otherwise lonely and isolated. Transformation was not restricted to people who received support, but also experienced by the PSW, the research team and the services who supported the work. Thus, this suggests that community well-being can be supported through meaningful civic engagement between the academy and the community.

Conclusion

The concept of social capital has evolved from Marx's early references to "gesellschaftliche Kapital" through Dewey's pragmatic philosophy to frameworks by Bourdieu, Coleman and Putnam. This evolution reflects a growing understanding and acknowledgment that social relationships constitute a form of capital that enables both individual and collective achievement and integral to social mobility, health and well-being. The dimensional framework (structural, relational and cognitive) is useful for contributing a nuanced understanding of how social capital operates in practice.

Accumulating evidence from across the health and social sciences demonstrates that social capital's relationship with well-being is complex and context dependent. While systematic reviews show generally positive associations between social capital and health, education and employment outcomes, the benefits vary significantly by the type of social capital (bonding, bridging, linking), the populations or groups studied (advantaged vs. disadvantaged groups), the social context (e.g. high-violence vs. safe neighborhoods) and how the construct is examined and measured. Notably, for disadvantaged populations, bonding social capital appears protective while bridging and linking social capital may sometimes be associated with worse outcomes, suggesting potential exclusionary effects.

Evidence does however strongly suggest that trust and reciprocity are fundamental mechanisms through which social capital promotes well-being. These relational dynamics create psychological safety and security, reduce transaction costs in social exchanges and enable collective action. Communities characterized by generalized trust demonstrate better health indicators, lower crime rates and higher life satisfaction.

In addition to trust and reciprocity, shared narratives, values and cultural understanding (cognitive alignment) are essential for building and maintaining social capital. This dimension facilitates common language, shared meaning-making and the capacity for collective action, which are all crucial for community well-being and cohesion.

Interventions and strategies that enhance or develop social capital in particularly marginalized communities have great transformative potential for those involved. The case studies from Southwest England demonstrate that well-designed community interventions can effectively build social capital among displaced populations. Key elements include sensitivity and attention to trauma-informed approaches that acknowledge power dynamics. Generalized community training in trauma-informed approaches could be particularly powerful in violent or deprived neighborhoods with a high prevalence of trauma. Participatory methods that position community members as experts hold immense potential to create place-based and -relevant interventions to meet people's needs. The movements in citizen science and public involvement in policy and planning attest to growing importance of these methods for creating linking and bridging social capital. Key to these efforts will be investment in safe spaces to create this type of social capital that meets people in their specific environments to understand the local context of communities lived reality. Such efforts create great opportunities for skills development and empowerment.

A central theme of this book and this chapter, argues that academics and policy makers should conceptualize community well-being as more than individual outcomes, acknowledging the collective capacity of communities to identify and pursue conditions necessary for flourishing. Conditions which include improvements across social, economic, environmental, cultural and political dimensions. Community interventions should be context-sensitive and acknowledge local power dynamics and that different types of social capital may be needed for different populations and circumstances. Participatory approaches that engage community members as co-designers are more likely to be transformative and effective in efforts to enhance community well-being. Investment in social capital development could be a cost-effective approach to addressing health inequalities providing the ethos, balance and investment is aligned and shared by all relevant stakeholders. This is important because as outlined in this chapter, social capital can have a dark side and produce negative effects, potentially reinforcing exclusion and inequality. This highlights the importance of designing interventions that promote inclusive forms of social capital rather than those that strengthen in-group bonds at the expense of broader social cohesion. In conclusion, social capital represents a powerful but complex mechanism for promoting community well-being, with particular promise for addressing health inequalities when approached thoughtfully and inclusively.

References

Adams, N. N., MacIver, E., Douglas, F., & Kennedy, C. (2025). Social capital and improved wellbeing: A qualitative investigation of the Wild Things! *Silver Saplings Adventures Programme* in Rural North-East Scotland. *Journal of Gerontological Social Work*, 1–23. https://doi.org/10.1080/01634372.2025.2488020

Agyeman, J., & Evans, B. (2004). "Just sustainability": The emerging discourse of environmental justice in Britain? *The Geographical Journal*, *170*(2), 155–164. https://doi.org/10.1111/j.0016-7398.2004.00117.x

Andreas, S. (2018). Effects of the decline in social capital on college graduates' soft skills. *Industry and Higher Education*, *32*(1), 47–56. https://doi.org/10.1177/0950422217749277

Antonovsky, A. (1996). The salutogenic model as a theory to guide health promotion. *Health Promotion International*, *11*(1), 11–18. https://doi.org/10.1093/heapro/11.1.11

Arnetz, J., Rofa, Y., Arnetz, B., Ventimiglia, M., & Jamil, H. (2013). Resilience as a protective factor against the development of psychopathology among refugees. *The*

Journal of Nervous and Mental Disease, *201*(3), 167–172. https://doi.org/10.1097/nmd.0b013e3182848afe

Atkinson, S., Bagnall, A., Corcoran, R., & South, J. (2017). What is community well-being? Conceptual review. Info@whatworkswellbeing, https://whatworkswellbeing.org/resources/what-is-community-wellbeing-conceptual-review/

Behtoui, A. (2016). Beyond social ties: The impact of social capital on labour market outcomes for young Swedish people. *Journal of Sociology*, *52*(4), 711–724. https://doi.org/10.1177/1440783315581217

Behtoui, A., & Neergaard, A. (2015). Social capital and the educational achievement of young people in Sweden. *British Journal of Sociology of Education*, *37*(7), 947–969. https://doi.org/10.1080/01425692.2015.1013086

Berger, J., Herz, H., Hüfner, J., & Sutter, M. (2021). Inequality, fairness and social capital. *European Economic Review*, *132*, 103642.

Bonoli, G., & Turtschi, N. (2015). Inequality in social capital and labour market re-entry among unemployed people. *Research in Social Stratification and Mobility*, *42*, 87–95. https://doi.org/10.1016/j.rssm.2015.09.004

Bourdieu, P. (1977). Cultural reproduction and social reproduction. In J. Karabel, & A. H. Halsey (Eds.), *Power and ideology in education* (pp. 487–511). Oxford University Press. - References - Scientific Research Publishing. Www.scirp.org. https://www.scirp.org/reference/ReferencesPapers?ReferenceID=1303718

Bourdieu, P. (1986). *The forms of capital*. UCG - Univerzitet Crne Gore. https://www.ucg.ac.me/skladiste/blog_9155/objava_66783/fajlovi/Bourdieu%20The%20Forms%20of%20Capital%20_1_.pdf

Brady, G. (2015, Summer). Network social capital and labour market outcomes: Evidence for Ireland. *The Economic and Social Review*, *46*(2), 163–195. https://www.esr.ie/article/view/339

Brass, D. J., & Burkhardt, M. E. (1992). Centrality and power in organizations. *Networks and Organizations: Structure, Form, and Action*, *191*(215), 198–213.

Brouwer, J., Jansen, E., Flache, A., & Hofman, A. (2016). The impact of social capital on self-efficacy and study success among first-year university students. *Learning and Individual Differences*, *52*, 109–118. https://doi.org/10.1016/j.lindif.2016.09.016

Cambridge Dictionary. (2023). *MARGINALIZATION | meaning in the Cambridge English Dictionary*. Dictionary.cambridge.org. https://dictionary.cambridge.org/dictionary/english/marginalization

Chanley, V. A., Rudolph, T. J., & Rahn, W. M. (2000). The origins and consequences of public trust in government. *Public Opinion Quarterly*, *64*(3), 239–256. https://doi.org/10.1086/317987

Cheung, S. Y., & Phillimore, J. (2014). Refugees, social capital, and labour market integration in the UK. *Sociology*, *48*(3), 518–536. https://doi.org/10.1177/0038038513491467

Chinman, M., George, P., Dougherty, R. H., Daniels, A. S., Ghose, S. S., Swift, A., & Delphin-Rittmon, M. E. (2014). Peer support services for individuals with serious mental illnesses: Assessing the evidence. *Psychiatric Services*, *65*(4), 429–441. https://doi.org/10.1176/appi.ps.201300244

Cialdini, R. B. (2001). The science of persuasion. *Scientific American*, *284*(2), 76–81. https://www.jstor.org/stable/26059056?seq=1

Claridge, T. (2015). Coleman on social capital–rational-choice approach. *Social Capital Research*. https://www.socialcapitalresearch.com/coleman-on-social-capital-rational-choice-approach/

Claridge, T. (2021). Evolution of the concept of social capital. *Social Capital Research*, 1–5. https://www.socialcapitalresearch.com/evolution-of-the-concept-of-social-capital/

Cohen, S., & Wills, T. A. (1985). *Stress, social support, and the buffering hypothesis*. Psycnet.apa.org. https://psycnet.apa.org/record/1986-01119-001

Coleman, J. S. (1988). Social capital in the creation of human capital. *American Journal of Sociology*, *94*(94), 95–120.

Coleman, J. S. (1990). *Foundations of social theory*. The Belknap Press of Harvard University Press.

De Neve, J.-E., Ward, G., De Keulenaer, F., Van Landeghem, B., Kavetsos, G., & Norton, M. I. (2018). The asymmetric experience of positive and negative economic growth: Global evidence using subjective well-being data. *The Review of Economics and Statistics*, *100*(2), 362–375. https://doi.org/10.1162/rest_a_00697

Dewey, J. (Ed.). (1900). *The elementary school record* (Vol. 1). University of Chicago Press.

Dodge, R., Daly, A. P., Huyton, J., & Sanders, L. D. (2012, August 28). The challenge of defining wellbeing. ResearchGate; *International Journal of Wellbeing*. https://www.researchgate.net/publication/233740458_The_challenge_of_defining_wellbeing

Ehsan, A., Klaas, H. S., Bastianen, A., & Spini, D. (2019). Social capital and health: A systematic review of systematic reviews. *SSM - Population Health*, *8*(1), 100425. https://doi.org/10.1016/j.ssmph.2019.100425

Farr, J. (2004). Social capital. *Political Theory*, *32*(1), 6–33. https://doi.org/10.1177/0090591703254978

Fine, B. (2002a). They f**k you up those social capitalists. *Antipode*, *34*(4), 796–799. Academia.edu. https://www.academia.edu/download/40824809/scantipode.pdf

Fine, B. (2002b). It ain't social, it ain't capital and it ain't Africa. *Studia Africana*, *13*, 18–33. https://www.africabib.org/rec.php?RID=288979435

Foley, M. W., & Edwards, B. (1999). Is it time to disinvest in social capital? *Journal of Public Policy*, *19*(2), 141–173. https://doi.org/10.1017/s0143814x99000215

Forjaz, M. J., Prieto-Flores, M.-E., Ayala, A., Rodriguez-Blazquez, C., Fernandez-Mayoralas, G., Rojo-Perez, F., & Martinez-Martin, P. (2011). Measurement properties of the Community Wellbeing Index in older adults. *Quality of Life Research*, *20*(5), 733–743. https://doi.org/10.1007/s11136-010-9794-2

Gallagher, J., & Featonby, J. (2019). *Hope for the future: Support for survivors of trafficking after the national referral mechanism*. British Red Cross.

Gouldner, A. W. (1960). The norm of reciprocity: A preliminary statement. *American Sociological Review*, *25*(2), 161–178. https://doi.org/10.2307/2092623

Grootaert, C., & Van Bastelar, T. (2002). Understanding and measuring social capital: A multidisciplinary tool for practitioners. In *openknowledge.worldbank.org*. Washington, DC: World Bank. https://openknowledge.worldbank.org/entities/publication/8f069a0b-b4a4-5c05-bee7-d52c5b583716

Hanifan, L. J. (1916). The rural school community center. *The ANNALS of the American Academy of Political and Social Science*, *67*(1), 130–138. https://doi.org/10.1177/000271621606700118

Helliwell, J. F., Huang, H., Wang, S., & Norton, M. (2021). World happiness, trust and deaths under COVID-19. *World Happiness Report*, *2021*, 13–57.

Helliwell, J. F., & Putnam, R. D. (2004). The social context of well–being. *Philosophical Transactions of the Royal Society of London. Series B: Biological Sciences*, *359*(1449), 1435–1446. https://doi.org/10.1098/rstb.2004.1522

Helliwell, J., & Putnam, R. (2007). Education and social capital. *Eastern Economic Journal, 33*, 1–19. https://doi.org/10.1057/eej.2007.1

Hoeft, T. J., Fortney, J. C., Patel, V., & Unützer, J. (2018). Task-sharing approaches to improve mental health care in rural and other low-resource settings: A systematic review. *The Journal of Rural Health, 34*(1), 48–62. https://doi.org/10.1111/jrh.12229

Ihlebæk, C., Katralen, H., Nordbø, E. C. A., & Skipstein, A. (2023). The role of social capital for wellbeing in people with long-term illness and disease. *Nordic Journal of Wellbeing and Sustainable Welfare Development, 2*(2), 53–67. https://doi.org/10.18261/njwel.2.2.5

Jannesari, M. T. (2022). Predictors of international entrepreneurial intention among young adults: Social cognitive theory. *Frontiers in Psychology, 13*. https://doi.org/10.3389/fpsyg.2022.894717

Kawachi, I., & Berkman, L. (2000). Social cohesion, social capital, and health. *Social Epidemiology, 174*(7), 290–319.

Kenton, W. (2024). *What is social capital? Definition, types, and examples*. Investopedia. https://www.investopedia.com/terms/s/socialcapital.asp

Krishna, A., & Shrader, E. (1999). Social capital assessment tool. In *Conference on social capital and poverty reduction* (Vol. 2224). The World Bank.

Levi, M., & Stoker, L. (2000). Political trust and trustworthiness. *Annual Review of Political Science, 3*(1), 475–507. https://doi.org/10.1146/annurev.polisci.3.1.475

Lewis, H. (2010). Community moments: Integration and transnationalism at "Refugee" parties and events. *Journal of Refugee Studies, 23*(4), 571–588. https://doi.org/10.1093/jrs/feq037

Marx, K. (1867). *Capital: A critique of political economy. Volume I: The process of production of capital*. Giuseppe Castrovilli.

McPherson, K. E., Kerr, S., McGee, E., Morgan, A., Cheater, F. M., McLean, J., & Egan, J. (2014). The association between social capital and mental health and behavioural problems in children and adolescents: An integrative systematic review. *BMC Psychology, 2*(1). https://doi.org/10.1186/2050-7283-2-7

Mishi, S., Sibanda, K., & Anakpo, G. (2023). The concept and application of social capital in health, education and employment: A scoping review. *Social Sciences, 12*(8), 450–450. https://doi.org/10.3390/socsci12080450

Misra, T., Connolly, A. M., & Majeed, A. (2006). Addressing mental health needs of asylum seekers and refugees in a London Borough: Epidemiological and user perspectives. *Primary Health Care Research & Development, 7*(03), 241–248. https://doi.org/10.1191/1463423606pc293oa

Morrice, L. (2007). Lifelong learning and the social integration of refugees in the UK: The significance of social capital. *International Journal of Lifelong Education, 26*(2), 155–172. https://doi.org/10.1080/02601370701219467

Nahapiet, J., & Ghoshal, S. (1998). Social capital, intellectual capital, and the organizational advantage. *Academy of Management Review, 23*(2), 242–266.

Nussbaum, M. (2009). The capabilities of people with cognitive disabilities. *Metaphilosophy, 40*(3–4), 331–351. https://doi.org/10.1111/j.1467-9973.2009.01606.x

Nussbaum, M. C. (2000). *Women and human development: The capabilities approach*. Cambridge University Press.

OECD. (2020). *OECD regional well-being: A user's guide*. OECD Publishing.

Oxford Dictionary. (2020). *Social capital | Definition of social capital by Lexico*. Web.archive.org. https://web.archive.org/web/20200411204827/https://www.lexico.com/en/definition/social_capital

Palmer, R. T., & Maramba, D. C. (2015). The impact of social capital on the access, adjustment, and success of Southeast Asian American college students. *Journal of College Student Development, 56*(1), 45–60. https://doi.org/10.1353/csd.2015.0007

Pawson, R., & Tilley, N. (2004). *Realist evaluation.* https://www.copasah.org/uploads/1/2/6/4/12642634/realistic_evaluationpawson.pdf

Phelan, J. C., Lucas, J. W., Ridgeway, C. L., & Taylor, C. J. (2014). Stigma, status, and population health. *Social Science & Medicine*, *103*(1), 15–23. https://doi.org/10.1016/j.socscimed.2013.10.004

Pickett, K., Gauhar, A., & Wilkinson, R. (2024). *The spirit 15 level at the enduring impact of inequality*. https://doi.org/10.15124/yao-de9s-7k93

Pretty, J. (2003). Social capital and the collective management of resources. *Science*, *302*(5652), 1912–1914. https://doi.org/10.1126/science.1090847

Putnam, R. D. (1993). The prosperous community: Social capital and public life. *The American Prospect, 13*, 35–42.

Putnam, R. D. (1995). Bowling alone: America's declining social capital. *Journal of Democracy, 6*, 65–78.

Putnam, R. D. (2000). *Bowling alone: The collapse and revival of American community*. Simon & Schuster.

Richards, L. (2015). For whom money matters less: Social connectedness as a resilience resource in the UK. *Social Indicators Research, 125*(2), 509–535. https://doi.org/10.1007/s11205-014-0858-5

Rousseau, D. M., Sitkin, S. B., Burt, R. S., & Camerer, C. (1998). Not so different after all: A cross-discipline view of trust. *Academy of Management Review*, *23*(3), 393–404. https://doi.org/10.5465/AMR.1998.926617

Sen, A. (1999). *Development as freedom*. Oxford University Press. https://www.c3l.uni-oldenburg.de/cde/OMDE625/Sen/Sen-intro.pdf

Sigona, N. (2012). Globalisation, rights and the non-citizen. *Sociology*, *46*(5), 982–988. https://doi.org/10.1177/0038038512451527 (Original work published 2012)

Stone, D. (2018). Refugees then and now: Memory, history and politics in the long twentieth century: An introduction. *Patterns of Prejudice*, *52*(2–3), 101–106. https://doi.org/10.1080/0031322x.2018.1433004

Stone, W., Gray, M., & Hughes, J. (2004). Social capital at work. *The Economic and Labour Relations Review*, *14*(2), 235–255. https://doi.org/10.1177/103530460401400206

Szreter, S., & Woolcock, M. (2004). Health by association? Social capital, social theory, and the political economy of public health. *International Journal of Epidemiology*, *33*(4), 650–667. https://doi.org/10.1093/ije/dyh013

Uphoff, E. P., Pickett, K. E., Cabieses, B., Small, N., & Wright, J. (2013). A systematic review of the relationships between social capital and socioeconomic inequalities in health: A contribution to understanding the psychosocial pathway of health inequalities. *International Journal for Equity in Health*, *12*(1), 54. https://doi.org/10.1186/1475-9276-12-54

Uphoff, N. (2000). Understanding social capital: Learning from the analysis and experience of participation. *Social Capital: A Multifaceted Perspective*, *6*(2), 215–249.

Villalonga-Olives, E., Kawachi, I., Almansa, J., & von Steinbüchel, N. (2017). Longitudinal changes in health related quality of life in children with migrant backgrounds. *PLOS ONE*, *12*(2), e0170891. https://doi.org/10.1371/journal.pone.0170891

White, S. C. (2010). Analysing wellbeing: A framework for development practice. *Development in Practice*, *20*(2), 158–172. https://doi.org/10.1080/09614520903564199

Williams, W. R. (2009). Struggling with poverty: Implications for theory and policy of increasing research on social class-based stigma. *Analyses of Social Issues and Public Policy*, *9*(1), 37–56. https://doi.org/10.1111/j.1530-2415.2009.01184.x

Wiseman, J., & Brasher, K. (2008). Community wellbeing in an unwell world: Trends, challenges, and possibilities. *Journal of Public Health Policy*, *29*(3), 353–366. https://doi.org/10.1057/jphp.2008.16

Woolcock, M. (1998). Social capital and economic development: Toward a theoretical synthesis and policy framework. *Theory and Society*, *27*(2), 151–208. https://www.jstor.org/stable/657866

Xu, J.-M., Cao, M.-G., Gao, Q.-C., Lu, Y.-X., & Stark, A. T. (2024). Nurses' workplace social capital and sustainable development: An integrative review of empirical studies. *Journal of Nursing Management*, *2024*(1). https://doi.org/10.1155/2024/8362035

Yanos, P. T., Rosenfield, S., & Horwitz, A. V. (2001). Negative and supportive social interactions and quality of life among persons diagnosed with severe mental illness. *Community Mental Health Journal*, *37*(5), 405–419. https://doi.org/10.1023/a:1017528029127

6

THE GENERATIVE COMMUNITY

An Asset-Based Community Development Approach to Well-Being

Cormac Russell

Introduction

Neighborhood belonging, social connectedness and community control are key determinants of health and well-being and are influenced by social conditions that depend on local action (Blodgett, Birch, Musella, Harkness, & Kaushal, 2022; Stansfield, South, & Mapplethorpe, 2020). However, in England, for example, only one in four Community Life Survey respondents agreed that they can influence decisions in their local areas (UK Department for Digital, 2021). Similar trends have been observed in other OECD countries and beyond where, according to the 2019 Edelman Trust Barometer, four out of five citizens feel that "the system" is not serving their interests (OECD, 2024a).

Steven Pinker argues that such levels of disaffection are unwarranted given that global life expectancy and general well-being are at historic highs and attributes this progress to the values of Enlightenment, which he views as the primary catalyst (Pinker, 2018). In contrast, James C. Scott argues that at least some Enlightenment values have mutated into various forms of Taylorism and high modernism, evident in instances of social engineering and command and control management approaches by some state institutions, which have proved counterproductive to community well-being (Ellerman, 2005). While aggregate life expectancy increased in OECD countries pre-COVID-19, the pandemic has wiped out much of these gains (OECD, 2024b). In addition, pre-COVID-19 life expectancy had already been rising faster for the affluent than the most economically marginalized; currently, this trend is accelerating (OECD, 2024b). The health gap between socioeconomic groups is worsening globally, often exacerbated by wars (Garry & Checchi, 2020), climate crises (World Economic Forum, 2024), neoliberal policies (Poirier, Sethi, Haag, Hedges, & Jamieson, 2022) and economic instabilities

DOI: 10.4324/9781032662657-7

(Benatar, Gill, & Bakker, 2011). Consequently, initiatives to tackle social injustice and close the gap in health inequalities (Heimburg, Prilleltensky, Ness, & Ytterhus, 2022), including life expectancy, illness, subjective and objective health and well-being (Foot & Hopkins, 2010), are increasing in most OECD countries.

While evidence for the link between social cohesion and health is growing, policies and practices that seek to create and develop healthy and sustainable communities at the local level are only just emerging (WHO, 2024). The paucity of place-conscious pedagogy in public health and population health policy and practice (Baker et al., 2023) can risk severely limiting the health-creating capacities of local associations (McKnight, 1996; Russell, 2020).

In *Health is Made at Home, Hospitals are for Repairs*, Nigel Crisp, a former head of the National Health Service (NHS) in England, contends that health cannot be secured solely through better access to healthcare services, regardless of how well funded and irrespective of whether these services are related directly to health, including mental health or the broader political and social determinants of health (Crisp, 2020). As the understanding of the limitations of services and the importance of community cohesion, neighborhood belonging and social capital in relation to health continues to grow, there is a strong consensus among scholars and practitioners alike that universal access to healthcare remains essential and should be provided at a "scale and intensity proportionate to levels of disadvantage" (Prilleltensky, Scarpa, Ness, & Di Martino, 2023).

Heimburg et al. (2022) and Prilleltensky et al. (2023) both advocate for policies and practices that lead to more just, equitable and inclusive societies, including access to health services. Furthermore, they emphasize the importance of community development principles and practices at the grassroots level of society. Others have argued that beyond the immediate relief action provided by services, fairer societies are created by implementing structural changes that result in lasting reforms within the dominant social order while offering reconciliation to those who have been unfairly treated and harmed (Russell, 2019). Prilleltensky (2012) claims there can be no wellness without fairness. However, many health-related interventions engage in health marketing (Morgan & Ziglio, 2010) while neglecting to support people at risk of not having valued social roles.

This chapter will argue that more strengths-based and equity-oriented community development practices should be cultivated to precipitate generative, connected communities at a scale that allows people to experience a sense of "at-homeness" or "neighbourhood" (Fifolt & McCormick, 2019). Here, we view generative communities as contexts or arenas where community members collectivize to cultivate growth and bring about change in their field. By prioritizing a place-conscious pedagogy for addressing health inequality, the neighborhood becomes a primary unit of change (Bissonnette, Wilson, Bell, & Shah, 2012) as community members collaborate to foster generative relationships with each other, their local economy and environmental and cultural contexts. Generative communities also argue that external resources should supplement, rather than supplant, their own generative capabilities. Furthermore, this chapter will assert that while change must happen at all levels of society, given what we now know about social determinants of health, communities must be enabled to become a centripetal force toward wellness for all.

The Challenge: Navigating the Spaces between Rights and Realities and Policies and Practices

Nurturing health-promoting communities that are culturally sensitive to embrace the contributions of marginalized individuals involves a fusion of community development and inclusion efforts (Russell, 2021).

To explain, a person may leave prison with a strong commitment to reintegrate into society and utilize their talents. However, it cannot be assumed that their community will readily welcome them and their contributions and forgive their past transgressions. In theory, it is easy to argue that the extent to which one is valued by others greatly impacts one's overall health and well-being. However, implementing this in ways that reach individuals who have been labeled, rejected by their communities and essentially relegated to institutions is much more challenging. Merely offering professional-led "care in the community" programs to marginalized individuals is insufficient. Instead, it is crucial to prioritize sustainable community development practices that enable socially isolated people to contribute to the well-being of the broader community.

Plena Inclusion is a movement in Spain that serves as an excellent example of inclusive practices. They promote a hyper-local form of inclusion of people with intellectual and developmental disabilities through an initiative called *Mi Casa.* Article 19 of the United Nations Convention on the Rights of Persons with Disabilities recognizes the right of persons with disabilities to choose their place of residence and to be included in their chosen community. *Plena Inclusion* accompanies hundreds of people with disabilities every day to help them pursue their "good life" outside of institutionalized settings in villages, small towns and neighborhoods across Spain. However, enforcing these rights *in a self-organising complex system like a village or neighbourhood* remains challenging. Inclusion cannot be mandated or engineered; it must be invited and nurtured. To this end, the community support staff of the *Mi Casa* initiative act as connectors between local communities and their latent hospitality and the individuals they support. They apply this asset-based community development (ABCD) approach, understanding that persons with intellectual disabilities often go unnoticed or unappreciated by their neighbors, and that the best way to address this is through fostering meaningful connections between them through gift exchange.

A Review of Evidence-Based Trends

Internationally, there is a growing movement toward implementing place-based, community-centered development approaches to health. While a full literature review is beyond the scope of this chapter, we include a range of evidence-informed policies that foreground the efficacy of neighborhood belonging and community cohesion as pathways toward population health and inclusion for all:

1 Health, including mental health and well-being, as a public good (Benatar et al., 2011), is a social and political phenomenon leading to the concept of *Social Determinants of Health.* "Health" cannot simply be produced by a clinician in the absence of thriving communities. Health and well-being are contingent on the depth and quality of social connectedness, economic and environmental security and principles of social justice. For example, the WHO defines self-care as "the ability of individuals, families and communities to promote health, prevent disease, maintain health, and to cope with illness and disability with or without the support of a health worker" (WHO, 2022). While such definitions are powerful reminders of the healing power of self-efficacy, it is important to frame such thinking in a wider political and social milieu (Marmot, 2020; Prilleltensky, 2012).
2 Choice and control matter for individuals and communities. The Marmot Review (Marmot, 2010) and its ten-year follow-up report (Marmot, 2020) both argue that having control over one's life is critical to an individual's health and well-being. Indeed, according to the World Happiness Report, having the freedom to make choices is one of the six factors that explain the variation in national well-being between countries (Helliwell et al., 2024). Pink (2011) notes that a preponderance of scientific research on human motivation underscores a "deep human need to direct our own lives, to learn and create new things, and to do better by ourselves and our world".
3 The What Works Centre for Wellbeing, the leading authority in the United Kingdom on well-being, recognized that drivers toward well-being are not solely subjective but include drivers of community well-being outcomes, including neighborhood belonging, community cohesion and support networks (Cairns, Maguire, Abdallah, Zeidler, & Tiplady-Startin, 2022).
4 Robert Putnam emphasizes the importance of social capital citing declining social capital in America as "one of the nation's most serious public health challenges" (Putnam, 2001).
5 Putnam's findings are echoed by a Brigham University Study involving 3 million participants, which found that increased social connection was linked to a 50% reduced risk of premature death. These findings highlight the value of social connections for lonely people, as opposed to activities and programs (Holt-Lunstad, Smith, Baker, Harris, & Stephenson, 2015). Xia and Li (2018) reported that people who are socially isolated have a 29% higher risk of coronary heart disease, a 32% higher risk of stroke, 64% higher risk of dementia and a 30% higher chance of premature death.
6 A growing preponderance of research suggests that neighborhood belonging, social connectedness and community control are key social and political determinants of health influenced by social conditions and can be addressed by local

action (Stansfield et al., 2020). However, in England, only one in four of the Community Life Survey respondents agrees that they can influence decisions in their local areas (UK Department for Digital, 2021).

7 Using ABCD as a lens to advance community-centered balanced care pathways toward health is in step with UK trends toward more community-centered approaches. For example, NHS England's Five Year Forward View and Nesta's Realizing the Value research program advocate for the value of pursuing personalized and community-centered approaches (The Health Foundation (UK), 2016). In tandem with community-centered approaches, personalized care sits at the heart of the NHS ten-year plan. However, there is a growing recognition that person-centered and community-centered outcomes will not result solely from therapeutic or strength-based practices with individuals. More community development work must be undertaken within the everyday context of people being helped to achieve community-centered health creation. This is why the ground-breaking report, *A Glass Half Full* (Foot & Hopkins, 2010), argued that municipalities, Health Trusts and Voluntary Housing Organizations must play an active role in precipitating more supportive communities through ABCD and other strengths-based community development processes instead of more conventional deficit-based approaches.

8 Yishun Health in Singapore has reimagined its approach to health through an ABCD approach and shares its insights from the field in the documentary *Caring Communities - Production and Participation by People* (https://issuu.com/yishunhealth/docs/caring_communities, 2022). Their findings demonstrate the preventive value of animating non-medical "community nodes", where community members engage in and often lead activities of their own choosing that are consequentially health-creating.

9 The European Community-based Mental Health Service Providers (EUCOMS) Network supports shifting from the biomedical model to a holistic model of community-based mental healthcare. Evidence shows that high-quality services should encompass the protection of human rights, a public health approach, the promotion of the recovery journey of those being served, the evaluation of the effectiveness of the development of a wide network of community support and of supplementary services, as well as the incorporation of the person being supported and peer expertise in civic participation and service planning and delivery (Keet et al., 2019).

These emergent policy trends and supporting evidence affirm that general wellness across populations cannot be achieved without fairness (Scarpa, Di Martino, & Prilleltensky, 2021), and sustainable wellness cannot exist without community. Therefore, to tackle health inequality in an equitable and sustainable way, societies must enable equitable access to services in or close to their local communities, with support for and investment in more community-owned and community-led health-creating assets. ABCD approaches have the potential to significantly contribute to the latter while remaining cognizant of the former.

ABCD

Before delving into the relationship between ABCD and generative community well-being, we must address some important considerations. Firstly, it should be noted that ABCD does not substitute for investing in improving services or addressing the root causes of health disparities.

Secondly, marginalized and low-income communities will require initial investment and ongoing equity investment to achieve the outcomes described below, which will take time to flourish.

For instance, in Flint, Michigan, where tens of thousands of residents were exposed to dangerous levels of lead and outbreaks of Legionnaires' disease, which killed at least 12 people and left a significant number of other residents with long-term life-limiting conditions, community organizing and unconditional basic income for first-time mothers are being combined with a comprehensive array of primary care and family welfare supports. The overall aim is to restore well-being for all, and in particular to eradicate child poverty, while returning a sense of power and control back to local residents who have endured decades of injustice, appalling health inequalities and negligence from various state and commercial institutions.

Community involvement in service design, decision-making and improving health knowledge will be vital. In the face of such significant breaches of trust by various institutions, supporting civic participation and racial equity necessitates substantial community development and reconciliation. Still, reforming institutional policies and practices is not the sole purpose of community development and restorative practices more generally. For communities such as Flint, restoring social cohesion and collective efficacy at the neighborhood level is also of vital importance.

Furthermore, the understanding of risk, needs and the challenges associated with prioritizing resources must not serve as excuses for bureaucratic opacity, wasteful allocation of resources or paternalistic attitudes. Instead, they should be regarded as realities that require a steadfast commitment to nurturing democratic, equity-centered, person-centered and community-centered practices and policies.

Lastly, policies and practices should ensure that those on the margins of society are valued and actively supported to participate and contribute meaningfully in society, while respecting their rights, not just to receive services and support as forms of relief action but also to actively participate in and contribute to the well-being of their communities and society as a whole.

Community and Institutions: Two Different Operating Systems

ABCD, as described in this text, argues that two essential components are necessary to advance societies toward wellness and fairness. The first is institutions, while the second is associations. These two elements, while often coterminous, can be considered as distinct operating systems. Well-functioning institutions have the capacity to produce goods and services while maintaining quality control. Consequently, they ensure that the needs of consumers can be consistently and impartially addressed on a large scale. Money plays a decisive role in maintaining the cohesion of this institutional operating system.

On the other hand, associations are primarily focused on providing care and mutuality, relying on the capabilities of their members and the level of trust they have in one another. Associations tend to function optimally on a smaller, local scale. Beyond a certain size, it becomes challenging for associations to maintain the necessary depth of interpersonal relationships required to nurture and sustain trust. At that point, a centralized administration and coordinating system are often required, resembling an institutional model. Trust is the relational adhesive that holds associations together, rather than funding or command and control systems. Association members do not perceive themselves as passive consumers; by definition, as members, they actively contribute to the well-being of their association.

Most social and economic problems arise from the utilization of an inappropriate operating system to address a specific issue, e.g. when employing medical solutions to tackle social problems. In humanistic psychology, this phenomenon is referred to as the "law of instrument" or "Maslow's hammer", which is derived from Abraham Maslow's observation that: "If the only tool you have is a hammer, you tend to see every problem as a nail". Relating this analogy to health, if the sole tool at one's disposal is an institution's service or intervention program, one is inclined to perceive every societal problem as a deficit requiring such a service or program. An ABCD approach allows us to escape "Maslow's hammer" through a process of discovering, connecting and mobilizing another invaluable and irreplaceable instrument for effecting societal and political change through the civic and democratic power and functions of associations. Unfortunately, in traditional healthcare approaches, associational life, if recognized at all, is often perceived as a problem to be remedied from outside in. Still, we contend that it is an essential power source for functioning democracies and local well-being, possessing crucial generative capabilities waiting to be valued and organized as key actors (Tocqueville & Reeve, 1835).

The ultimate challenge presented by ABCD is to establish the appropriate relationship between institutions and associations. Associations are best placed to understand what they need from external actors once they have discovered, connected and mobilized their local resources. In other words, residents of a local community can only grasp the supplementary value of institutions once they have comprehended the generative nature and capacity of their own community.

Deficits and Damage or Asset, Capabilities and Desire?

ABCD identifies six key "community-building blocks" otherwise known as assets (McKnight & Russell, 2022) in every local community:

1 The skills of residents
2 The power of local associations
3 The resources of public, private and non-profit institutions

4 The physical resources and ecology of local places
5 The economic resources of local places and reciprocal exchange in more general terms
6 The stories and heritage of local places.

Case study: Blueprint for Peace (Milwaukee)

Progress, in order to be achieved and sustained, must involve the external restructuring of our service institutions, similar to the actions taken by the Milwaukee Police Department, as partners in the implementation of the non-violent peacebuilding strategy known as the Blueprint for Peace. The Office of Violence Prevention in the Milwaukee Health Department collaborated with the Prevention Institute to facilitate the development of the Blueprint, which is based on the Institute's Adverse Community Experiences and Resilience (ACER) framework. Through this planning process, in 2017, a Blueprint was co-created to prevent various forms of violence and promote the adoption of a public health approach as a viable and complementary strategy to the criminal justice approach for ensuring public safety.

Informed by an understanding of community trauma and resilience, this process has fostered a stronger commitment to neighborhood leadership and collaboration across different sectors to promote peace. Essentially, it involves a process of shifting authority and resources from the enforcement-focused aspect of policing to the neighborhoods that are most affected by trauma, viewing this through a public health lens. By enabling these neighborhoods to organize themselves into associations of associations (i.e., a network of associations) with appropriate light touch supports, a three-pronged response is created. The first level is community-led, the second involves partnerships between communities and relevant external assistance and the third pertains to the actions that institutional helpers must take to support communities.

Previous theories on addressing violence in Milwaukee had reversed the roles of these three levels, prioritizing an enforcement-first approach that placed the responsibility for safety solely in the hands of the police. Not surprisingly, the results demonstrated the counterproductive nature of expecting the police to unilaterally establish peace. The Blueprint for Peace teaches us that when we reverse the roles within the principal-agent-arena (noting that this does not create a dichotomy but rather establishes a more effective dynamic) by adopting a public health approach through an equity lens that emphasizes community involvement and recognizes neighborhoods as central arenas for peacebuilding, improvements occur and are sustained. The strength of this approach lies not only in how neighborhoods have organized themselves but also in how city institutions have restructured themselves externally to serve the local peacebuilding capabilities of neighborhoods better, while supplementing rather than replacing these capacities with institutional support that amplifies the common good.

The Neighborhood as the Primary Unit of Change (Sampson, 2011)

Similar to Milwaukee's Blueprint for Peace, ABCD efforts focus on generating positive change and start by recognizing neighborhoods as the primary unit of transformation (McKnight, 2010). By prioritizing the neighborhood as the locus of change, it becomes possible to identify, connect and mobilize individuals, organizations and the various cultural, environmental and local economic assets within and across place-based communities. The key lies in the relationships among these different domains, rather than any specific technique, model or isolated approach. This is why working within small communities is crucial for fostering citizen-led action and, ultimately, for promoting deeper democracy and environmental sustainability, both critical factors in ensuring the well-being for all – by all.

Community-Led Functions and the Limits of Engagement

Most of the community engagement strategies employed by external agencies, rather than embracing place-based community-building approaches, persist in being highly segregated and ineffectual. This is primarily due to their premature attempt to engage communities in the services and programs they have designed before the community-building process has commenced. Consequently, community engagement endeavors overly prioritize specific target groups, such as "at-risk youth" or "elderly individuals with frailty", labels that prove to be fundamentally non-generative rather than fostering connections between diverse parts of the community across conventional divisions and standard fault lines (Russell, 2022).

As John McKnight terms it (McKnight, 1996), the principal fallacy of such engagement approaches is the "institutional assumption". Like "Maslow's hammer" (Maslow, 1966), it propels some institutional leaders to believe that solving intractable socioeconomic challenges is primarily contingent on external experts or agencies intervening with institutional solutions to ameliorate the miserable lives of deficit communities. The challenge confronting institutions facilitating community-driven transformation is first to renounce such assumptions and instead pose questions that assume competence and value lived experience civic innovation. Such as:

- Where are we replacing, controlling and overwhelming the power of people to be healthful?
- How can we listen better to what people in citizen and community space think they can do to co-create wellness and what they think would be helpful from outside?
- What is within the hands of people and in their power to change?
- How can institutions collaborate to supplement those civic powers and desires?

Although place-based communities are inherently limited and susceptible to external influences, it is still important to highlight that when effectively organized, they possess the capacity to serve as primary sources (Russell, 2020) of:

1. Health and well-being.
2. Safety.
3. Stewardship for local ecologies and biospheres.
4. Safe food production and consumption.
5. Local economic development.
6. Raising our children and young people.
7. Aging well in place/locale.
8. Enriching neighborhood and local life and community spirit.
9. Civic action toward deeper democracy.
10. Response to natural disasters and emergencies.
11. The curation of knowledge and sharing of wisdom, culture and heritage, natural care in general, such as parenting, love of a significant other, friendship, and fellowship, particularly for people who have been marginalized.
12. Our capacity to live creatively with suffering for which no medical cure exists.
13. Our capacity to live well with the unknown and unknowable.
14. The power to organize collectively at neighborhood scale as well as within other domains to demand changes to unjust systems and structures.-

All 14 expressions of solidarity play critical roles in interdependent community and civic life functions. The small scale of local places creates an environment that fosters the emergence and generativity of these expressions. The neighborhood scale serves as an ideal platform for community-building and organizing. Within this scale, various associations, comprised of citizens with different passions related to the 14 functions mentioned above, can collectively contribute to civic life and the co-creation of wellness. By leveraging community-building support, these diverse associations in a neighborhood can intertwine and form a complex network, acting as an association of associations. The collective power of this network surpasses the impact of its individual parts, resulting in a stronger and more potent whole. This association of associations, guided by a shared vision and a culture of diversity, acts as the scaffolding for a generative community.

When such civic functions are consistently carried out, individual citizens and communities as a whole are strengthened, as is the wider local democratic system. This is because individuals exercise their civic authority every time they engage in these functions. Consequently, this has a significant impact on overall well-being, as it serves as a mitigating measure against certain health disparities and fosters the promotion of health from a non-biomedical perspective. This should come as no surprise, as previously mentioned, as our social and political circumstances directly influence our health. At the same time, it is equally true that social circumstances are largely influenced by the resources and opportunities available within our local communities, while our political circumstances manifest within and beyond our neighborhoods. Citizenship cast within this frame is more than voting or sporadic participation in a civic forum or citizen jury. Along with their neighbors, citizens are also co-creators and principal actors of the 14 functions mentioned above, which, when concentrated within the scale of neighborhoods, can have significant well-being impacts that are both experienced locally and are also influential at the city, regional and national levels and sometimes beyond.

The distribution of equity-based resources and opportunities among neighborhoods results from political choices manifested through various structures such as laws, policies, practices and norms (Popay, Whitehead, Ponsford, Egan, & Mead, 2021). These structures are far from benign and many are directly responsible for creating health inequities, as they provide advantages to a minority while simultaneously disadvantaging a significant portion of society (the majority). This disparity explains why life expectancy can differ significantly between neighboring areas. However, challenging and transforming these unjust structures is rarely accomplished through institutional reform alone. Most institutions tend to maintain the existing state of affairs. Change must therefore also manifest culturally through changing attitudes and behaviors. Hence, for social and political change to sustain itself, it requires members of oppressed communities, supported by allies, to actively organize and build the necessary power to bring about changes in the current status quo.

Six Generative Community Practices

Each of the case studies shared in this chapter highlights several recurring patterns of practice. This section will provide a brief overview of how these practices facilitate generativity at the neighborhood scale. Before delving into the details, it is important to note that, at a meta-level, they all follow a basic sequence:

1. An initial exploration of what residents can accomplish on their own as an association of citizens without any outside help by discovering, connecting and mobilizing local resources.
2. Assess what residents can achieve with some degree of external support that respects the sovereignty and agency of local residents and their associations.
3. Finally, once these local resources have been fully connected and mobilized, citizens take a collective decision regarding the level and type of support they would like external agents to contribute to complement their community-driven generativity. Put simply, through dialogue, communities define what institutions can do for them.

The order presented above, albeit crucial, is also counter-cultural. Traditional change-making often follows a reverse order, beginning with the third of the above phases and working backward, which tends to inadvertently displace citizen power and generativity. In contrast, this unorthodox community-first sequence aims to connect local resources that were previously separate and enable residents to mobilize through collective citizen action and visioning. While a community-first approach must, by nature, be emergent and culturally sensitive, there are six observable practices that communities and community development practitioners worldwide routinely embrace as they become more generative. These practices include:

1 **Discovering**: Discovering local residents who naturally connect their community through neighbor-to-neighbor and associational relationship building is a vital aspect of ABCD. Bringing together connectors representing a neighborhood's entire range of diversity can be a powerful means of building a generative community at the neighborhood scale and beyond. Community connectors are inherently committed to inclusion and grassroots relational welfare and have the ability to convene a much wider social movement to generate change at all levels of community life than many more traditional community leaders do.
2 **Hosting:** Hosting is the practice of actively welcoming neighbors, especially those who have been marginalized, through inclusive learning conversations and listening campaigns. Such practices can uncover the issues that people are sufficiently passionate about to take action on with their neighbors. Some communities find it helpful to have a community development practitioner to support these processes.
3 **Portraying:** As residents and their associations build solidarity and momentum around shared themes of concern, they often find it beneficial to create dynamic portraits of the assets they can utilize to move forward. Creating a shared and evolving asset map of primary assets that are local and within community control, secondary assets that are local but not community-controlled and tertiary assets that are neither local nor community-controlled facilitates effective decision-making and strategic planning. Hence, this practice is powerful in helping citizens identify those resources already at their disposal and determine the best approaches to connect disparate assets and leverage external resources. This is crucial for fostering generativity, as generative communities thrive by sustainably tapping into their internal resources.
4 **Solidarity Building:** Intentionally and mindfully engaging in activities together, such as sharing meals, tending a community garden or shared decision-making, can bring communities closer together. When these activities are done well, they can foster a deep sense of interconnectedness among community members. For example, instead of relying solely on voting to reach agreements, some communities choose to prioritize dialogue and relationality over efficient decision-making. By doing so, they consciously shape their relationships and emphasize solidarity among members. In situations where building solidarity is hindered by factors such as the harshness of the local built environment or a traumatic experience, community builders often seek to create "shareable moments" to

enable neighbors to develop solidarity through shared experiences and collaborative actions. Building solidarity helps to bridge divides within communities and build trust among individuals who may not have worked together or trusted each other before. Ultimately, trust serves as the glue that holds generative communities together as they work toward the common good.

5 **Celebrating:** Impromptu and ritualized community celebrations are vital for maintaining morale, showcasing promising practices and honoring the efforts and progress of community members. They also contribute to culture-building, collective healing and resiliency.
6 **Visioning:** Creating a shared vision that establishes priorities and unveils possibilities for a community's shared future is a powerful community-building practice. It ensures that the community assumes ownership of the process and becomes the main driver of the processes and the resulting actions. Inherently democratic community visioning processes also define how communities will forge mutual alliances with useful outsiders committed to supplementing, not supplanting, community priorities and capabilities.

Conclusion

This chapter examined the health-creating and preventative capacities of communities, showcasing promising practices from Singapore, Spain and America to illustrate the role of ABCD in promoting equitable community-centered approaches to well-being. Overall, this chapter demonstrates how ABCD allows practitioners to integrate person-centered and community-centered approaches. This integration involves recognizing and valuing the unique strengths of individuals and communities in line with the principles of proportionate universalism. Additionally, it requires enablement policies and practices that support citizens to contribute to the well-being of their communities, thereby fostering civic power, solidarity and meaningful connections with others. By valuing what is important to citizens and their associations, while enabling them to find meaningful social roles that matter to others, the narrative shifts from a focus on the individual to collective well-being. This aligns with a wealth of scientific research on human motivation, which emphasizes the "deep human need to direct our own lives, to learn and create new things, and to do better by ourselves and our world" (Pink, 2011).

The central idea is that well-being cannot be manipulated or imposed from above through service, program-oriented approaches, nor can it be unilaterally legislated for communities or socially isolated individuals. However, as the Blueprint for Peace initiative proves, well-being as a common good can start to be enabled by treating neighborhoods as primary units of well-being.

When the focus is on sickness, the primary actor is "the doctor"; however, when the focus is on well-being, local communities become the main actors and are therefore generative in their own right. Clinicians and allied professionals play important but supplementary roles in this context. In order to move toward a future where communities are acknowledged as valuable creators of health, it will be necessary to transfer some authority and sufficient resources from the acute ends of the healthcare system to the primary unit of well-being: generative neighborhoods. However, it is important to note that generativity typically does not occur spontaneously; it requires enablement. While it can be argued that every neighborhood has generative capacities, these capabilities have yet to be fully realized in many neighborhoods. By enabling local residents and their associations to be in charge of the generative effort to create wholeness, we can take a foundational step toward community-centered population health.

Having said that, in achieving equitable population health outcomes, it remains crucial that Marmot's principle of proportionate universalism (Marmot, 2010) serves as the foundation for all future strategies to address health inequalities. This is because a generative community cannot be solely attained through monetary means. It requires the collective efforts of a village, as well as the support of an enabling state with progressive and fair taxation policies that prioritize health as a common good.

References

Baker, R. M., Ahmed, M., Bertotti, M., Cassidy, J., Chipuriro, R., Clewett, E., & Kelly, M. P. (2023). Common health assets protocol: A mixed-methods, realist evaluation and economic appraisal of how Community-Led Organisations (CLOs) impact on the health and well-being of people living in deprived areas. *BMJ Open, 13*(3), e069979–e069979. https://doi.org/10.1136/bmjopen-2022–069979

Benatar, S. R., Gill, S., & Bakker, I. (2011). Global health and the global economic crisis. *American Journal of Public Health, 101*(4), 646–653. https://doi.org/10.2105/AJPH.2009.188458

Bissonnette, L., Wilson, K., Bell, S., & Shah, T. I. (2012). Neighbourhoods and potential access to health care: The role of spatial and aspatial factors. *Health & Place, 18*(4), 841–853. https://doi.org/10.1016/j.healthplace.2012.03.007

Blodgett, J. M., Birch, J. M., Musella, M., Harkness, F., & Kaushal, A. (2022). What works to improve wellbeing? A rapid systematic review of 223 interventions evaluated with the Warwick-Edinburgh mental well-being scales. *International Journal of Environmental Research, 19*(23). https://doi.org/10.3390/ijerph192315845

Cairns, M., Maguire, R., Abdallah, S., Zeidler, L., & Tiplady-Startin, K. (2022). *What works to improve social capital? A rapid review of the effectiveness of interventions aimed at improving social capital outcomes (neighbourhood belonging, social support network and community cohesion)*. Bristol. Retrieved from: https://uwe-repository.worktribe.com/output/10230366

Crisp, N. (2020). *Health is made at home: Hospitals are for repairs. Building a healthy and health-creating society*. Salus Global Knowledge Exchange.

Ellerman, D. (2005). *Helping people help themselves*. University of Michigan Press.

Fifolt, M., & McCormick, L. C. (2019). Advancing public health education through place-based learning: "On the Road in the Deep South". *Pedagogy in Health Promotion, 6*(2), 102–112. https://doi.org/10.1177/2373379919839076

Foot, J., & Hopkins, T. (2010). *A glass half-full: How an asset approach can improve community health and well-being.* https://www.local.gov.uk/sites/default/files/documents/glass-half-full-how-asset-3db.pdf

Garry, S., & Checchi, F. (2020). Armed conflict and public health: Into the 21st century. *Journal of Public Health (Oxford, England), 42*(3), e287–e298. https://doi.org/:10.1093/pubmed/fdz095

Heimburg, D. V., Prilleltensky, I., Ness, O., & Ytterhus, B. (2022). From public health to public good: Toward universal wellbeing. *Scandinavian Journal of Public Health, 50*(7), 1062–1070. https://doi.org/10.1177/14034948221124670

Helliwell, J. F., Layard, R., Sachs, J. D., De Neve, J.-E., Aknin, L. B., & Wang, S. (2024). *World happiness report 2024.* https://happiness-report.s3.amazonaws.com/2024/WHR+24.pdf

Holt-Lunstad, J., Smith, T. B., Baker, M., Harris, T., & Stephenson, D. (2015). Loneliness and social isolation as risk factors for mortality. *Perspectives on Psychological Science, 10*(2), 227–237. https://doi.org/10.1177/1745691614568352

Keet, R., de Vetten-Mc Mahon, M., Shields-Zeeman, L., Ruud, T., van Weeghel, J., Bahler, M., … & Pieters, G. (2019). Recovery for all in the community; position paper on principles and key elements of community-based mental health care. *BMC Psychiatry, 19*(1), 174. https://doi.org/10.1186/s12888-019-2162-z

Marmot, M. (2010). *Fair society, healthy lives. Strategic review of health inequalities in England post-2010.* https://www.instituteofhealthequity.org/resources-reports/fair-society-healthy-lives-the-marmot-review/fair-society-healthy-lives-exec-summary-pdf.pdf

Marmot, M. (2020). *Health equity in England: The Marmot review 10 years on.* https://www.health.org.uk/publications/reports/the-marmot-review-10-years-on

Maslow, A. (1966). *The psychology of science: A reconnaissance.* Harper & Row.

McKnight, J. (1996). *The careless society: Community and its counterfeits.* Barnes and Noble.

McKnight, J. (2010). Asset mapping in communities. In A. Morgan, E. Ziglio, & M. Davies (Eds.), *Health assets in a global context: Theory, methods, action* (pp. 59–76). Springer.

McKnight, J., & Russell, C. (2022). Asset-based community development. In L. Rapp-McCall, A. Roberts, & K. Corcoran (Eds.), *Social workers desk reference* (4th ed., pp. 104–105). Oxford University Press.

Morgan, A., & Ziglio, E. (2010). Revitalising the public health evidence base: An asset model. In A. Morgan, M. Davies, & E. Ziglio (Eds.), *Health assets in a global context* (pp. 3–16). Springer.

OECD. (2024a). Integrity and influence in policy-making. *OECD Topics.* Retrieved from https://www.oecd.org/governance/ethics/influence/

OECD. (2024b). Life expectancy at birth. *OECD Library.* Retrieved from https://www.oecd-ilibrary.org/sites/d90b402d-en/index.html?itemId=/content/component/d90b402d-en#boxsection-d1e18901-437bb29ef0

Pink, D. H. (2011). *Drive: The surprising truth about what motivates us.* Canongate Press LTD.

Pinker, S. (2018). *Enlightenment now: The case for reason, science, humanism, and progress.* Viking, an imprint of Penguin Random House LLC.

Poirier, B., Sethi, S., Haag, D., Hedges, J., & Jamieson, L. (2022). The impact of neoliberal generative mechanisms on Indigenous health: A critical realist scoping review. *Globalization and Health, 18*(1), 61–61. https://doi.org/10.1186/s12992-022-00852-2

Popay, J., Whitehead, M., Ponsford, R., Egan, M., & Mead, R. (2021). Power, control, communities and health inequalities I: Theories, concepts and analytical frameworks. *Health Promotion International, 36*(5), 1253–1263. https://doi.org/10.1093/heapro/daaa133

Prilleltensky, I. (2012). Wellness as fairness. *The American Journal of Community Psychology, 49*(1–2), 1–21. https://doi.org/10.1007/s10464-011-9448-8

Prilleltensky, I., Scarpa, M. P., Ness, O., & Di Martino, S. (2023). Mattering, wellness, and fairness: Psychosocial goods for the common good. *American Journal of Orthopsychiatry, 93*(3), 198–210. https://doi.org/10.1037/ort0000668

Putnam, R. (2001). *The collapse and revival of American community* (p. 37). Simon & Schuster.

Russell, C. (2019). Does more medicine make us sicker? Ivan Illich revisited. *Gaceta Sanitaria, 33*(6), 579–583. https://doi.org/10.1016/j.gaceta.2018.11.006

Russell, C. (2020). *Rekindling democracy: A professional's guide to working in citizen space*. Cascade Books.

Russell, C. (2021). Getting to authentic co-production: An asset-based community development perspective on co-production. In E. Loeffler & T. Bovaird (Eds.), *The Palgrave handbook of co-production of public services and outcomes* (pp. 173–192). Springer International Publishing.

Russell, C. (2022). Understanding ground-up community development from a practice perspective. *Lifestyle Medicine, 3*(4), e69. https://doi.org/10.1002/lim2.69

Sampson, R. (2011). Neighborhood effects, causal mechanisms, and the social structure of the city. In P. Demeulenaere (Ed.), *Analytical sociology and social mechanisms* (pp. 227–250). Cambridge University Press.

Scarpa, M. P., Di Martino, S., & Prilleltensky, I. (2021). Mattering mediates between fairness and well-being. *Frontiers in Psychology, 12*, 744201. https://doi.org/10.3389/fpsyg.2021.744201

Scott, J. C. (2020). *Seeing like a state*. Yale University Press.

Stansfield, J., South, J., & Mapplethorpe, T. (2020). What are the elements of a whole system approach to community-centred public health? A qualitative study with public health leaders in England's local authority areas. *BMJ Open, 10*(8), e036044. https://doi.org/10.1136/bmjopen-2019–036044

The Health Foundation (UK). (2016). *Realising the value*. https://www.health.org.uk/sites/default/files/RtVRealisingTheValue10KeyActions.pdf

Tocqueville, A. D., & Reeve, H. (1835). *Democracy in America*. London: Saunders and Otley, to 1840. [Pdf] Retrieved from the Library of Congress, https://www.loc.gov/item/09021576/.

UK Department for Digital, Culture, Media and Sport. (2021). *Community life survey technical report 2020/21*. https://www.gov.uk/government/statistics/community-life-survey-202021

WHO. (2022). *WHO guideline on self-care interventions for health and well-being, 2022 revision*. World Health Organization.

WHO. (2024). WHO releases new guidance on monitoring the social determinants of health equity. *WHO News*. Retrieved from https://www.who.int/news/item/19-02-2024-who-releases-new-guidance-on-monitoring-the-social-determinants-of-health-equity

World Economic Forum. (2024). *Quantifying the impact of climate change on human health*. Geneva, Switzerland. Retrieved from: https://www3.weforum.org/docs/WEF_Quantifying_the_Impact_of_Climate_Change_on_Human_Health_2024.pdf

Xia, N., & Li, H. (2018). Loneliness, social isolation, and cardiovascular health. *Antioxid Redox Signal, 28*(9), 837–851. https://doi.org/10.1089/ars.2017.7312

7

THE ROLE OF TRUST AND SENIOR LEADERSHIP SPONSORSHIP IN ENABLING PUBLIC AND PATIENT INVOLVEMENT IN HEALTH SYSTEMS

Éidín Ní Shé, Michael John Norton and Tina Bedenik

Introduction

Modern and evolving health and social care systems must be focused on learning to advance continuous improvement and innovation (Mcdonald et al., 2024). Enabling this type of culture requires senior leaders to support and engage in change initiatives (Harrison et al., 2022). Involving patients and the public in these changes provides a key mechanism to create person-centered improvements. There is a significant focus in the literature and in policy and practice on advancing understanding of what public and patient involvement (PPI) in health and social care involves and on mapping subsequent impacts (Bedenik et al., 2024; George & Kovacs Burns, 2024; Ní Shé et al., 2020; Palmer et al., 2019; Conklin et al., 2015). This focus aligns with an aim to shift the health and social care cultures to include patients/service users and their families and care networks as active partners in all aspects of health and care research, including the design, planning, decision-making and the evaluation of service improvements.

This chapter explores the evolution of the involvement of patients and service users outlining the differing terms of engagement, involvement and co-design (Table 7.1). This chapter also explores current challenges in enabling involvement in health and social care. As authors who have had experience undertaking various types of involvement, we advocate for area senior leaders and managers to pay attention to the patient/service users' voice in health provision. We stress the importance of developing trust, time and resources at the pre-commencement stage so that PPI can flourish at every stage of the research/service improvement process.

DOI: 10.4324/9781032662657-8

Background and Context

Up until the late 1960s, the idea of involvement of the patient/service user in receipt of services was not considered a viable option. The patient/service user was observed as the passive recipients of care, where services were delivered to the person based on what was seen as the only legitimate expertise, which doctors possessed at that time. In 1969, an academic by the name of Sherry Arnstein, first identified differing levels of involvement through what she conceptualized as: the ladder of participation (Figure 7.1) (Arnstein, 1969). This ladder was made of eight rungs, which were further subdivided into three phases which were then used to illustrate the various degrees of participation (Norton, 2022). Phase one: nonparticipation, takes on the two bottom rungs. Here is basically how services operated prior to the 1960 and for a time after this date also. Services viewed patient/services user as passive recipients of care. Within this space, there was a clear hierarchy with patients/service users holding no decision-making power. The next three rungs: informing, consultation and placation, encompassed varying degrees of involvement, but such involvement was also observed as tokenistic in nature.

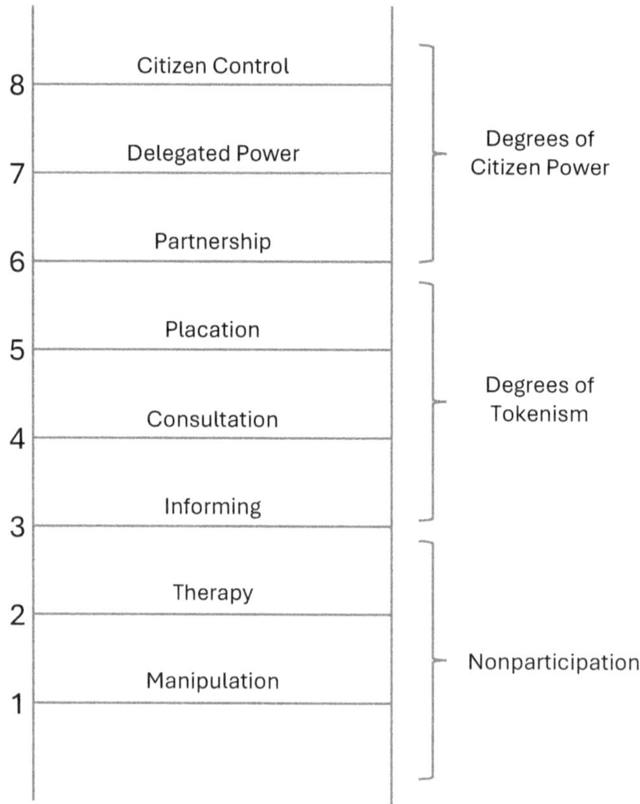

FIGURE 7.1 Arnstein's ladder of participation

In other words, patients and service users were involved in decision-making – from an observational perspective, but in actual fact had no decision-making capacity or influence. The final three rungs documents varying degrees of citizen control. It starts with a partnership where providers as well as users of services work together for the betterment of the said service. However, there is still a hierarchy evident here. This is unlike delegation where there is equal and mutual involvement of all parties, with shared power and decision-making capacity. The final rung: citizen control is the complete opposite of the first two rungs of this ladder as it documents a process whereby knowledge, power and decision-making capacity are completely taken from the provider of services and given to the patient/service user. Here, as a result, the hierarchy is reversed so it is the patient/service user that holds the decision-making power and not that of the provider of services.

This ladder of participation has changed on several occasions since Arnstein first created the concept of a ladder of participation. In recent years, the New Economics Foundation created an alternative ladder of participation. With this new ladder came a change in language for multiple rungs as our understanding of the concept of participation has grown. Of particular importance is the change of the last two rungs of the ladder to include the concepts of co-design and co-production (McMillan, 2019). Co-design and co-production are today often used interchangeably to mean the same thing (Health Service Executive, 2024). However, there are unique differences between them (Table 7.1). Additionally, the term co-creation is also used interchangeably today with that of co-design and co-production. Yet again, there are subtle differences between these three terms, but all relate to the production of an item or service. To begin with, let's explore co-production. Co-production is often observed as the parent concept in the co-family (Norton, 2022). In fact, it is considered an umbrella term, mainly because of its use within a vast array of disciplines including economics, law, management, health care and now mental health care since its conception by Elinor Ostrom in 1977 (Boyle and Harris, 2009; Brandsen and Honingh, 2015; Filipe et al., 2017, Stott and Johnson, 2018, Norton, 2022, Norton, 2022a). However, for the purposes of this text, co-production will be defined using Norton's (2022) definition. Here co-production involves:

> the creation and continuous development of a dialogical space where all stakeholders, including service users, family members, carers, supporters and service providers enter a collaborative partnership with the aim of not only improving their own care but also that of service provision.
>
> *(Norton, 2022: 27)*

Co-design differs slightly to that of co-production as it involves the meaningful participation of the end user in the innovation and revision of health care services (Silvola et al., 2023). In this way, users move from influencing delivery alone to becoming a vital component in the creation, design and evaluation of services. An example of this multimodal influence of all stakeholders is in experience-based co-design where creative tasks are considered important in the development and flourishment of trust and innovation required for the relationship to develop and grow healthy. Co-creation, on the other hand, differs slightly again from that of co-design and indeed co-production. Here, co-creation involves a process of equal partnership and the active contribution of all stakeholders, including end users in the conceptualization of ideas, design and testing of these said ideas (Fusco et al., 2023).

TABLE 7.1 Defining the differing terms of engagement, involvement and co-design

Term	*Definition*
Public and patient engagement	Research and or improvement work that is "about awareness raising, sharing, disseminating knowledge about research, and engaging patients, service users, carers, families using health and social care services, people with lived experience of health conditions (who may or may not be current patients), patient advocacy organizations, and members of the public in a conversation about research. This might be through: • Research open days or dissemination events • Through the media and social media • Science festivals" (Health Service Executive, 2021: 3).
Public and patient involvement *associated term consumer involvement*	Research and or improvement work being carried out "with" or "by" members of the public rather than "to", "about" or "for" them (UK National Institute for Health Research advisory group INVOLVE).
Co-design *associated terms of co-creation, experience-based co-design*	"Co-design is a values-based methodology. Within healthcare the process includes bringing together service users, clinical and non-clinical staff and, at times, relevant support and advocacy groups to work together to improve or refine elements of the care systems, services or processes. It is focused on the reality of healthcare contexts and of healthcare staff work environments. At its core is open reciprocal democratic dialogue where all participants contribute equally. This approach moves from consulting to enabling the involvement of all from the outset. It ensures and supports all relevant partners to be involved in defining the problem, designing the solution and monitoring and championing the implementation" (Ní Shé and Harrison, 2021).
Co-creation	A collaborative approach which allows for engagement with diverse stakeholders at all stages of a project in order to increase the impact of health interventions on the target population (Vargas, Whelan, Brimblecombe and Allender, 2022).
Co-production	Co-production refers to "the creation and continuous development of a dialogical space where all stakeholders, including service users, family members, carers, supporters and service providers enter a collaborative partnership with the aim of not only improving their own care but also that of service provision" (Norton, 2022: 27).

However, neither co-production nor co-creation within their scope examines user involvement in the research process, but co-design, on the other hand, does include user involvement in the research process. Examples of where this is noted include: Slattery et al. (2020) and Tremblay et al. (2022). In recent years, user involvement in an array of research activities has become increasingly popular. This process of co-producing research is known as PPI (Vinnicombe et al., 2023).

PPI is quickly becoming an essential aspect of the research process (Park et al., 2020). However, it is still an area of interest that is developing, particularly surrounding its definition and mechanism of action (Biggane et al., 2019; Norton, 2024). According to the Irish Health Service Executive (HSE) run office: Research and Development (2023), PPI involvement should navigate every aspect of the research process from the formulation of the research question, to the design of the methodology, through to the dissemination of knowledge and the evaluation of the inner workings of the research team, of which PPI plays a central component. In reality, this has been achievable through the integration of peer researchers – those with lived experience of a health and/or social care issue who happen to also be a researcher and also through the development and integration of lived experience advisory panels. However, PPI is not without its challenges with research suggesting barriers at both the researcher and PPI representative sides which include poor communication and lack of adequate training to incorporate PPI in research (Agyei-Manu et al., 2023).

Regardless of the above difficulties in defining the term, for the purposes of this text, we will utilize Abell and colleagues' definition of PPI which centers around the design and conduct of research in a way that is most beneficial to the individuals impacted by such research. As such, due to the claims of Biggane and colleagues, this chapter will examine the concept of involvement, particularly as it relates to the phenomenon of PPI in order to support the further development of the concept for use in health care research.

Current Challenges in Involvement

Involving diverse partners in an organization focused on improving and enabling change requires senior leaders to focus on enabling mechanisms (Bedenik et al., 2024; Harrison, 2024). The key to this is focused pre-planning and responsiveness to the changes identified. Post the COVID-19 pandemic, change fatigue has emerged as staff burnout increased and trust in their organization to respond to change decreased (Morain and Aykens, 2023). Recent work by Martin and colleagues (2024) captured via an ethnographic study the levels of co-creation in five English health and social care organizations found an increasing promotion of ideas of co-production by leaders in the system. This resulted in local contexts that were undertaking a version of co-creation. However, these initiatives were controlled and "even before co-creative interactions began, they appeared to be regulated by an implicit sense of what was acceptable and what was not" (Martin et al., 2024: 15). The work calls into focus the need for senior leaders to pay specific attention to the "discursive forms of meta-governance in delimiting the scope of co-creation" (Martin et al., 2024: 1).

PPI includes participation in the design and conduct of health and social care research to improve healthcare services, and increasingly as a response to requirements made by policymakers and health research funders (Locock et al., 2017). Challenges pertaining to such inclusion are related to the impact PPI has on the research process, as well as the people and communities impacted by such research. An earlier systematic review of the impact of PPI on research suggested that the encountered challenges are specific to different points of the research cycle (Brett et al., 2014b). Specifically, in both the early research stage when project proposals are being developed, as well as in data collection and analysis phase, PPI may result in departure from scientific methods traditionally used by researchers and thus challenge traditional power dynamics; whereas in the dissemination phase, PPI is associated with the concern about sharing findings before they are published. In addition, a systematic review of the impact of PPI on service users, researchers and communities suggested that successful implementation of PPI in research is largely contingent upon social interactions between all parties (Brett et al., 2014a). Namely, from the perspective of patients and service users, challenges revolve around feeling inexperienced, marginalized and emotionally overwhelmed, as well as facing assumptions about the lack of knowledge or, indeed, insufficient knowledge about research methodology necessary to make a meaningful contribution. On the other hand, the research community experiences issues with allocating resources to enable PPI, concerns about contributors' competence and difficulties with both accepting the views of contributors and sharing power over research. Similar issues were also identified in a systematic review of the impact of PPI on the National Health Service (NHS) in the United Kingdom (Mockford et al., 2012). The results indicated that collaboration between service users and healthcare professionals led to a change in attitudes and beliefs about the value of PPI; however, the process was difficult due to mismatched expectations about involvement, and a lack of resources and experience in building such collaborations. These results remain relevant given that the United Kingdom is considered "a leader in publishing work on PPI" (Biddle et al., 2021). A later review focused on the experiences of patient partners in research and confirmed these findings (Lauzon-Schnittka et al., 2022). Although PPI was a generally positive experience for the contributors, the study demonstrated that the challenges pertaining to team dynamics and power differentials had "the potential to make or break the experience of patient-partners" (Lauzon-Schnittka et al., 2022: 15). Interestingly, research into current trends in PPI in cancer research suggest that the aforesaid challenges about power relations were largely absent from recent studies, which may indicate a lack of critical attention to the process of PPI and in turn increases the risk of tokenism (Pii et al., 2019). In addition, this review described the lack of participation of men, ethnic minorities and socioeconomically disadvantaged social groups in PPI in research, suggesting that representativity in PPI remains a methodological concern (Pii et al.,

2019). This is not just related to cancer research, but to all disciplines in which PPI representation is a requirement of the research process and that examines different social worlds.

The Advancement of PPI Needs to Ensure Responsiveness from Senior Leaders and Managers

A key part of any responsive health system is the ability to be responsive to change that is inclusive of the relevant "actors" and addresses their needs within the local context of delivery (Rapport et al., 2022). There is much depth in the literature on the many challenges of undertaking change in the system (Clarke et al., 2024). Notably health system change has been strongly influenced by paternalistic, provider-driven and disease-focused models of service delivery, and as a result, improvement methodologies having often been singular in their dimensions of change (Greenhalgh et al., 2019). Senior leaders and managers in the system have a clear role in supporting PPI within the system (Carlini et al., 2024). Leaders and managers are central to enabling PPI in health and social care systems. The focus should be on enabling the right culture within the organization based on ongoing learning, information sharing and openness, whilst fostering creativity, innovation and critical thinking and creating a conducive atmosphere for successful PPI change initiatives (Bedenik et al., 2024). Yu and Sangiorai's (2018) outline that leaders and managers can implement proactive strategies such as setting up PPI training to support staff. Below we outline further areas that leaders and managers can focus on.

Developing Trust

Trust is argued to be the most fundamental relationship attribute in the medical arena, as well as in other areas of service provision, such as the voluntary, community sector and social care, for its propensity to influence attitudes, behaviors and clinical outcomes, as well as patients' relationships with service providers (Hall et al., 2001, 2002). It is also an essential component in research that actively encourages user involvement and PPI. In their influential paper Mayer and colleagues define trust as

> the willingness of a party to be vulnerable to the actions of another party based on the expectation that the other will perform a particular action important to the trustor, irrespective of the ability to monitor or control that other party.
>
> *(Meyer et al., 1995: 712)*

Trust and vulnerability are closely related, because trust implies an individual's acceptance to make themselves vulnerable to the actions of another party, and therefore, voluntarily gives away power (Sucher and Gupta, 2021). Trust can be a mechanism that underpins meaningful PPI; however, its multi-dimensional nature may add complexity when trying to incorporate PPI in health systems. To exemplify, interpersonal and impersonal trust signify trust in individuals, and trust based on roles, systems or reputation, respectively (Gilson, 2003, Atkinson and Butcher, 2003). Patients may have trusting relationships with their healthcare practitioners, and yet a low level of trust in the health system. Trust also reflects the direction of receiving and giving within a relationship, and it can be bi-directional or reciprocal, and unidirectional or asymmetrical (Gilfoyle et al., 2022).

Importantly, voluntary and involuntary or compulsory trust reflects the complex interplay between individual agency, power and lack thereof and dependency within the health system. Put differently, patients and service users sometimes may engender compulsory trust in the medical field because they have "no choice but to trust" (Gilson, 2003; Haddow et al., 2011). The ability to trust appears to be unequally distributed within society, since a trusting worldview is related to socio-economic characteristics and social capital, as described in chapter 5. People with higher levels of education and those in higher occupational classes seem more likely to trust, as do people who participate in social activities and avail of emotional and instrumental support resulting from interconnectedness (Li et al., 2018; Baroudi et al., 2022). This suggests that trust favors those who already benefit from the existing political, social and economic structures, which in turn raises a policy challenge related to including patients and service users that belong to underprivileged and vulnerable social groups (Gilson, 2003). This is a particularly salient point due to the benefits associated with and resulting from trust. Namely, trust can promote legitimacy of governance, support ethical outcomes and advance democratic participation (Gilson, 2003; Li et al., 2018). It facilitates workplace cooperation and sustainable partnerships (Dirks and Ferrin, 2001, 2002; Gilfoyle et al., 2022) and has a positive effect on motivation, work engagement and quality of service delivery (Six, 2018).

We previously argued that trust in health systems needs to be built on the three levels through organizational, managerial, leadership and individual practices that nurture trust with all stakeholders (Bedenik et al., 2024). On the macro level interpersonal trust can be built upon already existing trust in healthcare institutions, and on the mezzo level through organizational leadership styles and management practices that inspire trust (Ibid.). However, senior leaders and managers play an important role regarding trust-building practices on the micro level. Metz and colleagues (2021, 2022) proposed a novel theoretical model to build trust between implementation stakeholders and optimizing patient care in the context of health services. Their model is based on findings from previous research on trust and evidence use, and it suggests that the two fundamental strategies to build trusting relationships with stakeholders are technical and relational. The former relate to frequent interactions, responsiveness, demonstration of expertise and achievement of quick wins, and the latter include display of vulnerability, authenticity, engagement in co-learning and empathy-driven exchanges and bi-directional communication (Metz et al., 2022). By leaning into these attitudes and behaviors, senior leaders and managers can showcase their knowledge, reliability and competence and facilitate trust with patients and service users. Metz and colleagues' model posits the characteristics of the trustee in the center of the trust-building process and interestingly overlaps with the influential integrative model of organizational trust proposed by Roger and colleagues (1995). On this view, trust is developed through demonstrating trustworthiness through the three interrelated factors that may fluctuate over contexts: ability, benevolence and integrity. However, this earlier model also acknowledges that trust is influenced by individual's propensity to trust, which is a trait that denotes a general willingness to trust based on personality, previous experiences and background (Roger et al., 1995.). Therefore, while senior leaders and managers can create conditions of trust to enable meaningful PPI, the contributors can actively aid this process through a reflexive awareness, positive and optimistic disposition and a willingness to practice considered risk and vulnerability.

Importance of Planning at the Pre-Commencement Stage

A key enabler of enhancing trust is ensuring the inclusive involvement of PPI partners at the planning stages of a change project. Frequently PPI partners are approached for their involvement at the commencement of a project. They are often not offered any input in the design or the prioritization process, and it often occurs that the PPI partners were often spending significant time to ensure that the project is culturally appropriate for their population group and accessible (Ní Shé et al., 2019). Without focused attention on changing this culture by leaders and managers, the status quo will remain. The pre-commencement stage is where ideas are developed, or initial partnerships are explored and is often where the agenda setting occurs (Ní Shé et al., 2020). Notably this stage should focus on modes of outputs that are important to partners such as policy briefs, blogs, storyboard so it can be costed into the work. Also, clear discussions are required on evaluating and agreeing measure to capture on the PPI process undertaken. Recent research noted a gap of guidance on undertaking this pre-commencement stage, noting the phase where inequities of power concerning agenda setting were occurring (Ní Shé et al., 2020). As a potential solution, the paper stressed the need to embed value-based approaches such as respect, openness, reciprocity and flexibility from the pre-commencement. Identifying what all partners would like to achieve from the work should be prioritized (Ní Shé et al., 2020). This will enable the development of guidelines/protocols around ways of working, ensuring flexibility and clarity on data ownership and usage.

Bringing Together Diverse Group of People

A meaningful inclusion of service users, families and carers in the health and social care systems implies asking less "What is the matter with you?" and more "What matters to you?" (Berwick, 2016). Central to this process is the reconfiguration of power relationships between all stakeholders. A conscious effort to integrate patients' experiential and contextual knowledge alongside healthcare practitioners' expert knowledge challenges status quo and counters epistemic injustice often experienced by the recipients of care (Fricker, 2007; Knowles et al., 2021a; 2021b). Patient competence can be classified as originating from experiential expertise and skill-based competencies. Experiential expertise refers to "applicable knowledge drawn from experiences with health issues or other related experiences", whereas skill-based competencies describes skills such as "writing and language abilities when adapting documents for participants, or social skills when leading interviews for data collection" (Lauzon-Schnittka et al., 2022). In essence, these skills come from learned knowledge, the knowledge that one ascertains not through life experience but through academic endeavors. Incorporation of the two types of patients' competence and a diversity of views and perspectives can complement academic and scientific knowledge and allow for the democratization of health research (Lauzon-Schnittka et al., 2022). However, for this to happen, patients need to have adequate self-belief and confidence in their skillset to engage with the researchers and healthcare practitioners as equals, which can depend on the type of capital that they have. Locock and colleagues (2017) argue that economic, cultural and social capital are relevant in the context of understanding power differentials between researchers and patients; however, symbolic capital as the "perceived levels of status, prestige and respect held by individuals within and beyond immediate social networks" can also be used to equalize relationships (Locock et al., 2017:838).

Focus on Language

Language and the knowledge transferred through language equates to power (Shi et al., 2021). In health care, the knowledge one holds, based on micro, mezzo and macro factors, allows for hierarchical imbalances of power to take place. For example, one views the clinician as all-knowing due to their access and ability to utilize knowledge to treat the individual concerned. This gives the clinician a certain positionality within that social world based on respect and indeed the power associated with same. PPI involvement in health research is one mechanism of balancing hierarchal structures through the interplay of language and knowledge. A central role of PPI in health research is to make the knowledge produced from a research activity accessible to the lay population (Mc Menamin et al., 2022). In this way, through the translation of clinical knowledge to lay language, PPI allows for the patient/service user to understand a particular phenomenon and to judge on whether the application of this new knowledge to their own health situation can support meaningful recovery from a health issue. However, for the PPI representative to achieve this, a number of factors need to be addressed, including how the PPI representative's lived experiences match the research topic and their ability to advocate for the patient/service user voice in the research space based on their lived experiences.

Environment and Resources

The literature has stressed that PPI collaboration and engagement should occur in safe, accessible and inclusive spaces as identified by PPI partners (Ní Shé et al., 2019). Ensuring spaces are accessible for PPI needs should be guaranteed by the health system partners by undertaking an audit at the start of work. This should be monitored and reviewed throughout the project. It is also essential that the environment of involvement, either face to face or virtually is adequately resourced to enable participation. This includes covering the costs for internet access resourcing for community partners including the inclusion of independent facilitators. Having multiple partners working on a project can often result in tensions given the remits of different agendas that can emerge (Adshead and Dubula, 2016). It is therefore important that independent facilitators support the process of consensus. It is also important that time and adequate flexible resources are made available to celebrate success and achievements throughout a partnership. This process of feedback and celebration supports on going trust and validation of PPI efforts.

Expenses

Everyone involved in the research process should be treated equally to other members of the research team. This includes payment for expertise delivered by such individuals as well as other expenses to allow effective contributions by PPI representatives, such as childcare expenses, subsistence payments for food when out on research based excursions and so on. For traditional research staff, this works quite seamlessly. However, for patients/service users who engages in co-production, inclusive of PPI, issues can arise. According to Pizzo et al. (2015) the payment of expenses for PPI contributions is calling the efficacy and worth of PPI into question. The impact of such questioning has been noted in a 2023 commentary by De Simini and colleagues who noted that some grant applications now only seek to fund the immediate PPI representative and not the entire PPI team that supports the application. The funding of just one person to act as representative for an entire patient/service user body can lead to tokenistic practices, particularly if these individuals do not have the lived experience of the phenomenon under investigation. In the United Kingdom, the National Institute for Health and Care Research (NIHR) has provided guidance on payment for PPI representatives where protocols have been put in place to counteract such tokenistic practices (National Institute for Health and Care Research, 2023). An added complication encountered specifically by the Irish mental health services was the impact such engagement had on an individual's social welfare payment. This led to a complete abolishment of the remuneration scheme by Irish health services at that time. An abolishment that is still enforced today. Despite this, those engaged in PPI should be and are entitled to be fully reimbursed and renumerated for their time and expertise. However, the danger lies with other governmental bodies that may see such remuneration as a mechanism of employment and thus stop vital social welfare payments needed for these individuals to live in today's society. Despite this, even if such issues were addressed, the idea of financing PPI in health research remains a contentious issue as different principal investigators view activities that warrant payment differently, leading to no standardization of PPI in health research to date (Blackburn et al., 2018).

Follow Up

Ensuring clear modes of communication throughout a project is also central to enabling PPI in health systems. Developing and implementing communication protocols from the pre-commencement stage will enhance communication and understanding. Learning from an evaluation process is also key. What worked or did not work in the PPI process should be sued to benchmark progress but also enable a more "nuanced" understandings to support speed and scale (Bovin, 2019). At the end of a PPI collaboration, it's also critical that leaders and managers act on what has been agreed upon. Leaders and managers must also be open to the fact that PPI initiatives have outcomes other than initially planned is neither new nor novel but has been overlooked when thinking about PPI (Ní Shé and Harrison, 2021).

Conclusion

PPI approaches continue to be prioritized locally, nationally and internationally in enabling person-centered care. However, the performance of PPI in itself is increasing in complexity and ambiguity due to both internal and external factors. Despite this, it is clear that within research, the perspective of patients and service users on research debates is becoming important, and in some instances, like in mental health care, is expected. As a result, the role of the leader or manager in the health setting is becoming clearer in the eyes of PPI. That is to both create and enable the conditions, as described above, necessary for PPI to grow and flourish within their organization. Consequently, there are challenges to creating and embedding these conditions, which require time and attention to tease out properly. But one thing is for certain, this is what is now expected in the provision of health care (and social care?) and the creation of evidence within health services and as such, these institutions need to adapt to facilitate these changes as we move forward into the future.

References

Abell, L., Maher, F., Begum, S., Booth, S., Broomfield, J., Lee, S., … & Gray, L. J. (2023) Incorporation of patient and public involvement in statistical methodology research: A survey assessing current practices and attitudes of researchers. *Research Involvement and Engagement, 9*, 100. https://doi.org/10.1186/s40900-023-00507-5.

Adshead, M., & Dubula, V. (2016). Walking the walk? Critical reflections from an Afro-Irish emancipatory research network. *Educational Action Research, 24*(1), 115–133.

Agyei-Manu, E., Atkins, N., Lee, B., Rostron, J., Dozier, M., Smith, M., & McQuillan, R. (2023). The benefits, challenges, and best practice for patient and public involvement in evidence synthesis: A systematic review and thematic synthesis. *Health Expectations, 26*(4), 1436–1452. https://doi.org/10.1111/hex.13787.

Ärleskog, C., Vackerberg, N., & Andersson, A.-C. (2021) Balancing power in co-production: Introducing a reflection model. *Humanities and Social Sciences Communications, 8*(1), 108.

Arnstein, S. R. (1969) A ladder of citizen participation. *Journal of the American Institute of Planners, 35*(4), 216–224. https://doi.org/10.1080/01944366908977225.

Atkinson S., & David, B. (2003) Trustin managerial relationships. *Journal of Managerial Psychology, 18*, 282–304.

Baroudi, M., Goicolea, I., Hurtig, A. K., & San-Sebastian, M. (2022). Social factors associated with trust in the health system in northern Sweden: A cross-sectional study. *BMC Public Health, 22*, 881. https://doi.org/10.1186/s12889-022-13332-4

Bedenik, T., Kearney, C., & Ní Shé, É. (2024) Trust in embedding co-design for innovation and change: Considering the role of senior leaders and managers. *Journal of Health Organization and Management*, 38(9), 36–44. https://doi.org/10.1108/JHOM-07-2023-0207

Berwick, D. M. (2016). Era 3 for medicine and health care. *JAMA, 315*(13), 1329–1330. https://doi.org/10.1001/jama.2016.1509

Biddle, M. S. Y., Gibson, A., & Evans, D. (2021). Attitudes and approaches to patient and public involvement across Europe: A systematic review. *Health & Social Care in the Community, 29*(1), 18–27. https://doi.org/10.1111/hsc.13111

Biggane, A. M., Olsen, M., &Williamson, P. R. (2019) PPI in research: A reflection from early stage researchers. *Research Involvement and Engagement, 5*, 35. https://doi.org/10.1186/s40900-019-0170-2.

Blackburn, S., McLachlan, S., Jowett, S., Kinghorn, P., Gill, P., Higginbottom, A., Rhodes, B., Stevenson, F., & Jinks, C. (2018). The extent, quality and impact of patient and public involvement in primary care research: A mixed method study. *Research Involvement and Engagement, 4*, 16. https://doi.org/10.1186/s40900-018-0100-8

Boivin, A. (2019). From craft to reflective art and science: Comment on "Metrics and evaluation tools for patient engagement in healthcare organization-and system-level decision-making: a systematic review". *International Journal of Health Policy and Management, 8*(2), 124.

Boyle, D., & Harris, M. (2009). The challenge of co-production: How equal partnership between professionals and the public are crucial to improving public services. Available at: https://neweconomics.org/uploads/files/312ac8ce93a00d5973_3im6i6t0e.pdf.

Brandsen, T., & Honingh, M. (2015). Distinguishing different types of co-production: A conceptual analysis based on the classical definitions. *Public Administration Review, 6*(3), 426–435. https://doi.org/10.1111.puar.12465.

Brett, J. O., Staniszewska, S., Mockford, C., Herron-Marx, S., Hughes, J., Tysall, C., & Suleman, R. (2014a). A systematic review of the impact of patient and public involvement on service users, researchers and communities. *The Patient, 7*(4), 387–395. https://doi.org/10.1007/s40271-014-0065-0

Brett, J. O., Staniszewska, S., Mockford, C., Herron-Marx, S., Hughes, J., Tysall, C., & Suleman, R. (2014b). Mapping the impact of patient and public involvement on health and social care research: A systematic review. *Health Expectations, 17*(5), 637–650. https://doi.org/10.1111/j.1369-7625.2012.00795.x

von Busch, O., & Palmås, K. (2023).*The Corruption of Co-Design: Political and Social Conflicts in Participatory Design Thinking*. Taylor & Francis.

Bussu, S., Adrian, B., Rikki, D., & Graham, S. (2022). Embedding participatory governance. *Critical Policy Studies, 16*(2), 133–145.

Bussu, S., & Tullia Galanti, M. (2018). Facilitating coproduction: The role of leadership in coproduction initiatives in the UK. *Policy and Society, 37*(3): 347–367.

Carlini, J., Muir, R., McLaren-Kennedy, A., & Grealish, L. (2024), Transforming health-care service through consumer co-creation: directions for service design. *Journal of Services Marketing, 38*(3), 326–343. https://doi.org/10.1108/JSM-12-2022-0373

Chauhan, A., Leefe, J., Shé, É. N., & Harrison, R. (2021). Optimising co-design with ethnic minority consumers. *International Journal for Equity in Health, 20*(1), 240.

Clarke, E., Näswall, K., Wong, J., Pawsey, F., & Malinen, S. (2024). Enabling successful change in a high-demand working environment: A case study in a health care organization. *Journal of Health Organization and Management*, Vol. ahead-of-print No. ahead-of-print. https://doi.org/10.1108/JHOM-02-2023-0051

Conklin A., Morris Z., & Nolte, E. (2015) What is the evidence base for public involvement in health-care policy?: Results of a systematic scoping review. *Health Expectations, 18*(2), 153–165.

De Simoni, A., Jackson, T., Humphrey, W. I., Preston, J., Mah, H., Wood, H. E., Kinley, E., Rienda, L. G., & Porteous, C. (2023). Patient and public involvement in research: The need for budgeting PPI staff costs in funding applications. *Research Involvement and Engagement, 9*, 16. https://doi.org/10.1186/s40900-023-00424-7.

Dirks, K. T., & Ferrin, D. L. (2001). The role of trust in organizational settings. *Organization Science, 12*(4), 450–467. https://www.jstor.org/stable/3085982

Dirks, K. T., & Ferrin, D. L. (2002). Trust in leadership: Meta-analytic findings and implications for research and practice. *Journal of Applied Psychology, 87*(4), 611–628. https://doi.org/10.1037/0021-9010.87.4.611

Fillipe, A., Renedo, A., & Marston, C. (2017). The co-production of what? Knowledge, values and social relations in health care. *PLOS Biology, 15*(5), e2001403–e2001406. https://doi.org/10.1371/journal.pbio.2001403.

Fricker, M. (2007) *Epistemic Injustice: Power and the Ethics of Knowing*. Oxford University Press.

Fusco, F., Marsilio, M., & Guglielmetti, C. (2023) Co-creation in healthcare: Framing the outcomes and their determinants. *Journal of Service Management, 34*(6), 1–26. https://doi.org/10.1108/JOSM-06-2021-0212.

George, M., & Kovacs Burns, K. (2024). Co-designing healthcare quality improvement: The Kovacs Burns & George orientation guide. *Journal of Patient Experience, 11*. https://doi.org/10.1177/23743735231223854

Gilfoyle, M., MacFarlane, A., & Salsberg, J. (2022). Conceptualising, operationalising, and measuring trust in participatory health research networks: A scoping review. *Systematic Reviews, 11*, 40. https://doi.org/10.1186/s13643-022-01910-x

Gilson, L. (2003). Trust and the development of health care as a social institution. *Social Science & Medicine, 56*(7), 1453–1468. https://doi.org/10.1016/s0277-9536(02)00142-9

Greenhalgh, T., Hinton, L., Finlay, T., Macfarlane, A., Fahy, N., Clyde, B., & Chant, A. (2019). Frameworks for supporting patient and public involvement in research: Systematic review and co-design pilot. *Health Expectations, 22*(4), 785–801. https://doi.org/10.1111/hex.12888.

Haddow, G., Bruce, A., Sathanandam, S., & Wyatt, J. C. (2011). 'Nothing is really safe': A focus group study on the processes of anonymizing and sharing of health data for research purposes. *Journal of Evaluation in Clinical Practice, 17*(6), 1140–1146. https://doi.org/10.1111/j.1365-2753.2010.01488.x

Hall, M. A., Dugan, E., Zheng, B., & Mishra, A. l. K. (2001). Trust in physicians and medical institutions: What is it, can it be measured, and does it matter? *Milbank Quartely, 79*(4), 613–639. https://doi.org/10.1111/1468-0009.00223.

Hall, M. A., Zheng, B., Dugan, E., Camacho, F., Kidd, K. E., Mishra, A., & Balkrishnan, R. (2002). Measuring patients' trust in their primary care providers. *Medical Care Research and Review, 59*(3), 293–318. https://doi.org/10.1177/107755870205900300

Harrison, R., Chauhan, A., Le-Dao, H., Minbashian, A., Walpola, R., Fischer, S., & Schwarz, G. (2022 July). Achieving change readiness for health service innovations. *Nursing Forum, 57*(4), 603–607. https://doi.org/10.1111/nuf.12713.

Harrison, R., Newman, B., Chauhan, A., & Sarwar, M. (2024). Employing cofacilitation to balance power and priorities during health service codesign. *Health Expectations: An International Journal of Public Participation in Health Care and Health Policy, 27*(1), e13875. https://doi.org/10.1111/hex.13875

Health Service Executive (2021). Guide to patient and public involvement in HSE research. Research and Development. Available at: https://hseresearch.ie/wp-content/uploads/2021/12/Guide-no-8-Patient-and-Public-Involvement-in-HSE-Research.pdf

Health Service Executive (2024). *A National Framework for Recovery in Mental Health 2024–2028.* Available at: https://www.hse.ie/eng/services/list/4/mental-health-services/mental-health-engagement-and-recovery/resources-information-and-publications/a-national-framework-for-recovery-in-mental-health.pdf.

Knowles, S. E., Allen, D., Donnelly, A., Flynn, J., Gallacher, K., Lewis, A., McCorkle, G., Mistry, M., Walkington, P., & Brunton, L. (2021a). Participatory codesign of patient involvement in a learning health system: How can data-driven care be patient-driven care? *Health Expectations, 25*(1), 103–115. https://doi.org/10.1111/hex.13345

Knowles, S. E., Allen, D., Donnelly, A., Flynn, J., Gallacher, K., Lewis, A., McCorkle, G., Mistry, M., Walkington, P., & Drinkwater, J. (2021b). More than a method: Trusting relationships, productive tensions, and two-way learning as mechanisms of authentic co-production. *Research Involvement and Engagement, 7*, 34. https://doi.org/10.1186/s40900-021-00262-5.

Lauzon-Schnittka, J., Audette-Chapdelaine, S., Boutin, D., Wilhelmy, C., Auger, A. M., & Brodeur, M. (2022). The experience of patient partners in research: A qualitative systematic review and thematic synthesis. *Research Involvement and Engagement,* 8(5), 55. https://doi.org/10.1186/s40900-022-00388-0

Li, Y., Smith, N., & Dangerfield, P. (2018). Social trust: The impact of social networks and inequality. In D. Phillips, J. Curtice, M. Phillips & J. Perry (eds.), *British Social Attitudes 35*. 35th edn, London, pp. 1–25.

Locock, L., Boylan, A. M., Snow, R., & Staniszewska, S. (2017). The power of symbolic capital in patient and public involvement in health research. *Health Expectations, 20*(5), 836–844. https://doi.org/10.1111/hex.12519

Martin, G. P., Desai, A., Zoccatelli, G., Brearley, S., & Robert, G. (2024). Constraining co-creation? An ethnographic study of Healthwatch organizations in England. *Public Management Review*. https://doi.org/10.1080/14719037.2024.2308186

Mayer, R. C., Davis, J. H., & Schoorman, F. D. (1995 July). An integrative model of organizational trust. *The Academy of Management Review, 20*(3), 709–734.

McDonald, P. L., Foley, T. J., Verheij, R., Braithwaite, J., Rubin, J., Harwood, K., … & Van Der Wees, P. J. (2024). Data to knowledge to improvement: creating the learning health system. *BMJ*, 384, e076175. https://doi.org/10.1136/bmj-2023-076175.

Mc Menamin, R., Isaksen, J., Manning, M., & Tierney, E. (2022). Distinction and blurred boundaries between qualitative approaches and public and patient involvement (PPI) in research. *International Journal of Speech Language Pathology, 24*(5), 515–526. https://doi.org/10.1080/17549507.2022.2075465.

McMillan, G. (2019). Participation: Its impact on services and the people who use them. Available at: https://www.iriss.org.uk/resources/insights/participation-its-impact-services-and-people-who-use-them.

Metz, A., Albers, B., Burke, K., Bartley, L., Louison, L., Ward, C., & Farley, A. (2021). Implementation practice in human service systems: Understanding the principles and competencies of professionals who support implementation, human service organizations: Management. *Leadership & Governance, 45*(3), 238–259. https://doi.org/10.1080/23303131.2021.1895401

Metz, A., Jensen, T., Farley, A., Boaz, A., Bartley, L., &Villodas, M. (2022). Building trusting relationships to support implementation: A proposed theoretical model. *Frontiers in Health Services, 2*, 894599. https://doi.org/10.3389/frhs.2022.894599

Mockford, C., Staniszewska, S., Griffiths, F., & Herron-Marx, S. (2012). The impact of patient and public involvement on UK NHS health care: A systematic review. *International Journal for Quality in Health Care, 24*(1), 28–38. https://doi.org/10.1093/intqhc/mzr066

Morain, C. O., & Aykens, P. (2023). Employees are losing patience with change initiatives. *Harvard Business Review*, 9 May 2023. https://hbr.org/2023/05/employees-are-losing-patience-with-change-initiatives.

National Institute for Health and Care Research. (2023). *Payment for Public Involvement in Health and Care Research: A Guide for Organisations on Employment Status and Tax.* Available at: https://www.nihr.ac.uk/documents/Payment-for-Public-Involvement-in-Health-and-Care-Research-A-guide-for-organisations-on-determining-the-most-appropriate-payment-approach/30838.

Ní Shé, É., & Harrison, R. (2021). Mitigating unintended consequences of co-design in health care. *Health Expect, 24*(5), 1551–1556.

Ní Shé, É., Cassidy, J., Davies, C., De Brún, A., Donnelly, S., Dorris, E., … & O'Philbin, L. (2020). Minding the gap: Identifying values to enable public and patient involvement at the pre-commencement stage of research projects. *Research Involvement and Engagement, 6*(1), 46. https://doi.org/10.1186/s40900-020-00220-7.

Ní Shé, É., Morton, S., Lambert, V., Ní Cheallaigh, C., Lacey, V., Dunn, E., … & Kroll, T. (2019). Clarifying the mechanisms and resources that enable the reciprocal involvement of seldom heard groups in health and social care research: A collaborative rapid realist review process. *Health Expectations, 22*(3), 298–306. https://doi.org/10.1111/hex.12865.

Norton, M. (2022a). Co-production in trauma-responsive organisations. In: D. Mahon (ed.) *Trauma-Responsive Organisations: The Trauma Ecology Model.* Emerald Publishing Limited, pp. 147–158.

Norton, M. (2022). *Co-Production in Mental Health: Implementing Policy into Practice.* Routledge.

Norton, M. J. (2014) Mandating patient and public involvement in research: Is it cause for concern? *Journal of Evidence Based Healthcare, 6*, e5681. https://dx. doi.org/10.17267/2675-021Xevi-dence.2024.e5681.

Palmer, V. J., Weavell, W., Callander, R., Piper, D., Richard, L., Maher, L., ... & Robert, G. (2019). The participatory zeitgeist: An explanatory theoretical model of change in an era of coproduction and codesign in healthcare improvement. *Medical Humanities, 45*, 247–257.

Park, S., Khan, N., Stevenson, F., & Malpass, A. (2020) Patient and public involvement (PPI) in evidence synthesis: How the PatMed study approached embedding audience responses into the expression of a meta-ethnography. *BMC Medical Research Methodology, 20*, 29. https://doi.org/10.1186/s12874-020-0918-2.

Pii, K. H., Schou, L. H., Piil, K., & Jarden, M. (2019). Current trends in patient and public involvement in cancer research: A systematic review. *Health Expectations, 22*(1), 3–20. https://doi.org/10.1111/hex.12841

Pizzo, E., Doyle, C., & Matthews, R. (2015) Patient and public involvement: How much do we spend and what are the benefits. *Health Expectations, 18*(6), 1918–1926. https://doi.org/10.1111/hex.12204.

Rapport, F., Smith, J., Hutchinson, K., Clay-Williams, R., Churruca, K., Bierbaum, M., & Braithwaite, J. (2022). Too much theory and not enough practice? The challenge of implementation science application in healthcare practice. *Journal of Evaluation in Clinical Practice, 28*(6), 991–1002. https://doi.org/10.1111/jep.13600.

Research and Development. (2021) *Guide to Patient and Public Involvement in HSE Research: Knowledge Translation, Dissemination, and Impact: A Practical Guide for Researchers.* Available at: https://hseresearch.ie/wp-content/uploads/2021/12/Guide-no-8-Patient-and-Public-Involvement-in-HSE-Research.pdf.

Richards, D. P., Poirier, S., Mohabir, V., Proulx, L., Robins, S., & Smith, J. (2023). Reflections on patient engagement by patient partners: How it can go wrong. *Research Involvement and Engagement, 9*, 41. https://doi.org/10.1186/s40900-023-00454-1

Shi, C., Zhang, F., Zhu, P., & Shi, Q. (2021) How is knowledge perceived as power? A multilevel model of knowledge power in innovation networks. *Frontiers in Psychology, 12*, 630762. https://doi.org/10.3389/fpsyg.2021.630762.

Silvola, S., Restelli, U., Bonfanti, M., & Croce, D. (2023). Co-design as enabling factor for patient-centred healthcare: A bibliometric literature review. *ClinicoEconomics and Outcomes Research, 15*, 333–347. https://doi.org/10.2147/CEOR.S403243.

Six, F., Nooteboom, B., & Hoogendoorn, A. (2010). 'Actions that build interpersonal trust: A relational signalling perspective. *Review of Social Economy, 68*(3), 285–315. https://doi.org/10.1080/00346760902756487

Slattery, P., Saeri, A. K., & Bragge, P. (2020) Research co-design in health: A rapid overview of reviews. *Health Research Policy and Systems, 18*, 17. https://doi.org/10.1186/s12961-020-0528-9.

Stott, L., & Johnson, T. (2018). Co-production: Enhancing the role of citizens in governance and service delivery. Available at: https://european-social-fund-plus.ec.europa.eu/system/files/2021-06/TD4-Co-production%20-%20enhancing%20the%20role%20of%20citizens%20in%20governance%20and%20service%20delivery.pdf

Sucher, S., & Shalene, G. (2021). *The Power of Trust: How Companies Build It, Lose It, Regain It.* PublicAffairs.

Tremblay, M., Hamel, C., Viau-Guay, A., AND Giroux, D. (2022) User experience of the co-design research approach in ehealth: Activity analysis with the course-of-action framework. *JMIR Human Factors, 9*(3), e35577. https://doi.org/10.2196/35577.

Vargas, C., Whelan, J., Brimblecombe, J., & Allender, S. (2022). Co-creation, co-design, co-production for public health – A perspective on definition and distinctions. *Public Health Research Practice, 32*, 3222211.

Vinnicombe, S., Bianchim, M. S., & Noyes, J. (2023) A review of reviews exploring patient and public involvement in populations health research and development of tools containing best practice guidance. *BMC Public Health, 23*, 1271. https://doi.org/10.1186/s12889-023-15937-9.

Yu, E., & Sangiorgi, D. (2018). Service design as an approach to implement the value cocreation perspective in new service development. *Journal of Service Research, 21*(1), 40–58. https://doi.org/10.1177/109467051770935.

PART 2

Practice Innovations to Promote Community Well-being

8

SOCIAL PRESCRIBING

Can a Person-Centered Approach Also Benefit the Community?

Debra Westlake and Stephanie Tierney

Introduction

This chapter uses the case of the English National Health Service (NHS) to examine whether social prescribing can bridge the gap between healthcare, which focuses largely on the individual, and community-based initiatives, that enhance both personal and local neighborhood assets. We explore evidence in the literature and ongoing research studies, as well as policy guidance.

We start by giving a background to social prescribing and its relationship to person-centered care, then go on to address a series of questions: How does social prescribing relate to community well-being in theory and policy? What does the evidence say about how this works in practice? What are the potential opportunities and challenges to this implementation model in the NHS? Finally, we consider the implications for future practice by giving two examples.

What Is Social Prescribing and How Does It Relate to Person Centeredness?

An estimated 20% of people in England visit their general practitioner (GP) for non-medical issues (Torjesen 2016); the Low Commission found that 15% of GP visits were for social welfare advice (The Low Commission 2015). Issues such as loneliness, domestic violence, housing, employment and financial problems can impact physical and mental health and lead people to seek healthcare advice because they are not sure where else to turn for support.

Social prescribing has gained popularity in recent years as a means of addressing these social determinants of health (Marmot 2010, NHS England 2020, Lawler, Sherriff et al. 2023). Social prescribers, also known as social prescribing

DOI: 10.4324/9781032662657-10

link workers (SPLWs), well-being advisors or community connectors (Tierney, Wong et al. 2019) are employed in the English NHS to deliver social prescribing via referrals from community organizations, doctors and other health and social care professionals. They spend time listening to people's worries and hopes, in the form of a "what matters to you" conversation (Barry and Edgman-Levitan 2012), make a plan with the person to address these concerns and may introduce them to statutory or community support services and cultural experiences (Chatterjee, Camic et al. 2018, Tierney, Wong et al. 2020). Social prescribing is both a process and a pathway (Litt, Coll-Planas et al. 2023). The three-step process of referral, meeting an SPLW and subsequent connection to community services is a pathway of relationships aimed at enhancing social connectedness and well-being (Husk, Blockley et al. 2020, Westlake, Elston et al. 2022). A recent international Delphi panel study established consensus that "SP is a holistic, person-centred, and community-based approach to health and well-being that bridges the gap between clinical and non-clinical supports and services" (Muhl, Mulligan et al. 2023).

Social prescribing sits within NHS England's personalized care framework, which emphasizes tailored care through guided conversations and shared decision-making (NHS England 2019). Theoretical models of Person Centeredness existed before the NHS introduced SPLWs (Ekman, Swedberg et al. 2011, Britten, Moore et al. 2017) and the concept of linking people to community activities to enhance well-being is longstanding (Department Health and Social Care, PHE et al. 2016, Dayson 2017, Westlake, Ekman et al. 2022). However, funding and nationwide roll out of the SPLW role across English primary care is a relatively recent development (NHS England 2019). This initiative is part of a broader policy to expand and diversify primary care teams, with the goal of better addressing the complex and evolving needs of patients with long-term conditions (NHS England 2022).

Studies of social prescribing interventions have shown that the approach improves patient outcomes when it contains the components of a person-centered approach and that good practice examples of this model exist (Moffatt, Steer et al. 2017, Wood, Ohlsen et al. 2021, Cooper, Flynn et al. 2023, Tierney, Wong et al. 2024). However, evidence also shows that social prescribing implementation varies significantly, ranging from simple signposting of patients to resources, through to more holistic, relationship-centered approaches that provide ongoing, intense support and that a variety of organizational and individual resources are needed to ensure that a person-centered approach is implemented (Kimberlee 2015, Calderón-Larrañaga, Milner et al. 2021, Westlake, Elston et al. 2022). The wide variation in implementation – including the populations referred, the length and content of interventions and the training and background of SPLWs – as well as variety of measures and incompleteness and lack of reliability of data collected, has made it difficult to build a consistent measurement framework and evidence base for patient outcomes in social prescribing. In addition, appropriate outcomes for social prescribing – both for individuals and health systems – and the optimal time frame for measuring outcomes has not yet been established (Polley, Chatterjee et al. 2022). As a result, the literature presents differing conclusions – often relating to specific conditions such as those with type 2 diabetes or long-term conditions (Bickerdike, Booth et al. 2017, Kiely, Croke et al. 2022, Moffatt, Wildman et al. 2023). A realist approach, which is designed to understand how and why complex interventions, such as social prescribing, might produce certain outcomes is potentially a suitable methodology because of its focus on specific contexts (Tierney, Wong et al. 2020, 2024). Given the diversity in implementation and complex problems which social prescribing seeks to address, it may be that evaluations need to be conducted over longer time frames (Westlake, Tierney et al. 2023).

To What Extent Can Social Prescribing Contribute to Community Well-Being in Addition to Person-Centered Outcomes?

Policy and Theory

Current policy and theory suggest that social prescribing plays a dual role in promoting community well-being. On the one hand, it focuses on personalizing support for individuals, and on the other hand, it aims to balance this individual focus with broader community well-being.

Community well-being is a multidimensional concept that includes collaboration on social issues, sustainable change and asset-building at the local level (see Chapters 2 and 10). Social prescribing is considered a key public health approach to strengthening community well-being alongside its individualized care focus (Office for Health Improvement and Disparities (OHID) 2019, South, Bagnall et al. 2019, NHS England 2024). NHS England's Comprehensive Model of Personalized Care integrates social prescribing as part of its strategy, instructing Integrated Care Boards (ICBs) to address community health needs through both individual and community-centered approaches (NHS England 2019, 2020).

SPLWs are central to this model, with explicit responsibility for community development. Guidance suggests they collaborate with local partners to support, develop and sustain community groups, spending up to one day per week on this community building role (NHS England 2023). The NHS also recommends measuring the impact of social prescribing on community capacity building in primary care (NHS England 2023).

However, research evidence highlights tensions between individual-centered care and community connectedness. Some studies argue that focusing too much on individual needs can undermine social networks and interdependence within communities (Morris, Thomas et al. 2022). Before social prescribing became widespread through the NHS, it was a more community-led, "bottom-up" approach, exemplified by approaches like the Rotherham model, which emphasized local group connections (Dayson and Bashir 2014). Critics warned that scaling up social prescribing through large institutions like the NHS risked diluting the model by shifting the burden of service delivery onto communities without sufficient support (Dayson 2017).

The following section examines current evidence assessing whether these concerns are justified by firstly considering the opportunities arising from the current NHS model of social prescribing in primary care, followed by the challenges to its capacity to incorporate community well-being alongside person-centered care.

What Does the Evidence Say About How This Works in Practice? Example of the English NHS Model of SPLWs in Primary Care

Benefitting Individuals Within Communities

UNDERSTANDING THE IMPLEMENTATION OF LINK WORKERS IN PRIMARY CARE: A REALIST EVALUATION TO INFORM CURRENT AND FUTURE POLICY

This study aimed to explore how SPLW are being introduced into GP surgeries in England and to produce evidence-based recommendations on their implementation in this setting. A realist evaluation addressed the question – When implementing link workers in primary care to sustain outcomes – what works, for whom, why and in what circumstances? Realist evaluation is a theory-driven approach to understanding how and why complex interventions, such as social prescribing work (or fail) in specific contexts. The approach seeks to uncover *how* mechanisms are triggered by particular contexts to produce outcomes, providing actionable insights for refining policies or programs (Pawson and Tilley 1997). The study was conducted with SPLWs and healthcare staff in 7 GP surgeries in England. Researchers spent three weeks with SPLWs, attending meetings alongside them, observing their interactions with patients, healthcare staff and representatives from VCSE organizations. Additionally, 61 patients and 93 professionals (including healthcare staff, link workers and VCSE workers) were interviewed. Follow-up interviews were conducted with 41 patients and SPLWs 9–12 months later. The collected data were coded and analyzed to develop statements that reveal how the context surrounding the link worker activates mechanisms that contribute to both intended and unintended outcomes. SPLWs in the study were managed by both primary care and by VCSE organizations; some were subcontracted to VCSE organizations and based in the community, while others were based exclusively in doctors' surgeries.

Our study on the implementation of social prescribing in primary care (Tierney, Wong et al. 2024) (Tierney, Wong et al. 2024) found that when SPLWs recommended local community support options to patients, this significantly reduced their feelings of overwhelm and distress. SPLWs helped patients by connecting them to practical support (e.g., financial aid, housing, food banks) and opportunities to reduce isolation or encourage exercise. This guidance helped patients feel more supported and capable of managing their well-being. Even if they did not immediately use recommended community resources, knowing the options existed boosted their confidence, prompting some to seek their own solutions (Westlake, Wong et al. 2024, Tierney, Wong et al. 2024). A good understanding of available community resources was key to SPLWs being able to conduct their role effectively and provided an important bridge out of primary care and into the community, a finding echoed by other studies (Chatterjee, Camic et al. 2018). When SPLWs were from the local community or had relevant local experience, their knowledge of available resources was advantageous (Tierney, Wong et al. 2024).

Increasing Awareness of Social Solutions to Health Issues in Primary Care

Our study also found that placing SPLWs within doctors' surgeries helped raise awareness of the social determinants of health by integrating a focus on social issues into primary care. Health professionals observed that community activities positively impacted patients' health and well-being, reinforcing the value of local engagement in enhancing patient outcomes. SPLWs had the potential to challenge medical determinism and to support a more social and community-based approach to primary healthcare. This is reinforced where there is primary care buy-in to the individual SPLW and their role (Tierney, Wong et al. 2020, Hazeldine, Gowan et al. 2021, Westlake, Elston et al. 2022) and where the SPLW feels they have integrated well into primary care settings (Tierney, Westlake et al. 2025).

Increasing Social Capital

Social capital as presented in chapter 5, refers to the networks, relationships and trust within a community that enable people to collaborate, share resources and support each other (Bourdieu 1986). Studies suggest that when SPLWs create tailored social opportunities (e.g., walking groups, crafting sessions, online exercise) and provide knowledge of and access to support services within local or online communities, they enhance individuals' social assets and have the potential to increase their social capital (Tierney, Wong et al. 2020, Vidovic, Reinhardt et al. 2021). Models that integrate the individual and community approach in tandem with a population health perspective are proposed to be most effective (Younan, Junghans et al. 2020).

Some SPLWs contribute to community development by identifying service gaps and collaborating with VCSE colleagues to address them. This may involve partnerships within the SPLW's organization or across sectors. During COVID-19 lockdowns there were many examples of SPLWs creating or connecting patients to online activities in place of in-person gatherings (Chatterjee, Camic et al. 2018, Westlake, Elston et al. 2020, 2022).

Social Prescribing in Primary Care – What Are the Challenges to a Model of Social Prescribing That Incorporates Community Well-Being?

A key threat to social prescribing's success is lack of investment in community resources. The absence of strategic funding, especially post-COVID when many VCSE organizations faced financial struggles, has been identified as a major obstacle (Morris, Thomas et al. 2022, Sandhu, Alderwick et al. 2022). VCSE providers have reported an increasing number of referrals into their services by SPLWs since the national roll out of social prescribing (Westlake, Elston et al. 2022). Providers warn that without capacity building in the VCSE, social prescribing may struggle to connect individuals with appropriate community resources. As one organization puts it, there are "too many travel agents, not enough holidays" (Dudley CVS 2022).

Another obstacle is the lack of systematic methods for assessing community-level impacts in social prescribing (Vidovic, Reinhardt et al. 2021). While NHS policy recommends collecting community impact data, most measures in primary care focus on individual health and well-being outcomes, rather than social impacts, and may lead to attention being diverted from wider community engagement (National Voices 2020).

When SPLWs are based in VCSE organizations rather than doctors' surgeries, they may face conflicting demands: working holistically with individuals over time versus increasing patient turnover by limiting number and length of appointments (Tierney, 2024 forthcoming). While SPLWs have a degree of discretion about some elements of their work, the imperative to accept growing numbers of referrals for increasingly complex patients is likely to have an impact on capacity for community development work (Tierney, Westlake et al. 2025). SPLWs who lack prior knowledge of diverse community options to address individual prescriptions may struggle in their roles, as their limited time within the NHS makes it challenging to establish new connections.

Critics argue that the current model of social prescribing in the NHS may unintentionally widen, rather than reduce, health inequalities within communities. While there are examples of good practice, for example in certain areas of London (Race Equality Foundation 2024), overall there is a lack of evidence of social prescribing's impact on addressing inequalities for minoritized ethnic communities.

Building such an evidence base is likely to be hampered by limitations in data collection and analysis related to inequalities and social prescribing (Race Equality Foundation 2024). However, there is some evidence suggesting provision of SPLWs is not proportionate to need, since there are fewer FTE equivalent SPLWS in areas of high deprivation (Wilding, Sutton et al. 2024), and there is also a lack of uptake of social prescribing in certain communities – such as ethnic minority groups, men, younger people (Khan, Al-Izzi et al. 2023) and people on low incomes (Gibson, Pollard et al. 2021). The reasons for this are not yet known.

A meta-ethnography on SPLWs' experience of their role concluded that "across the studies we reviewed, there was evidence to suggest that those experiencing precarious life circumstances may not be able to engage with the intervention to the same extent as service users from more affluent backgrounds" (Turk, Tierney et al. 2024). While we do not yet fully understand why this is, plausible reasons include practical barriers for people accessing social prescribing – such as the costs of transport or memberships of clubs and societies that might be prescribed – as well as the social and cultural capital that might be required to take advantage of connections it offers (Gibson, Pollard et al. 2021). Until there is more robust evidence about who accesses and benefits from social prescribing, it will be difficult to assess how far social prescribing is contributing to building better communities if not all communities have equal exposure to the service (Khan and Tierney 2024).

A connected argument suggests that social prescribing and similar interventions, which focus on addressing individual issues and behaviors, are inherently flawed in their ability to tackle the broader social determinants of health or to effectively reduce health inequalities. It is contended that it is "aberrant logic" (Moscrop 2023) or a "fantasy" (Mackenzie, Skivington et al. 2020) for policy makers to tackle structural factors that underpin health inequalities via micro-level interventions that re-produce the status quo and do not challenge wider social and political impacts on communities (Scott-Samuel and Smith 2015). MacKenzie, Skivington and Fergie's study evaluated SPLW services in Glasgow to explore their potential to drive social change within GP practices and the broader community. The service was set up to focus on reducing health inequalities. However, they observed a "lifestyle drift" over time in practitioners' approaches, with the focus shifting from addressing systemic issues to changing individual patient behaviors (Mackenzie, Skivington et al. 2020). Although based in Scotland, these findings are relevant to social prescribing in the English NHS, as similar challenges are noted in other studies (Gibson, Pollard et al. 2021).

What, then, are the implications for the future of social prescribing in supporting both individual personalized care and the communities in which individuals live – communities that are vital to its overall success? Here we give two solutions which have been proposed: firstly, a theoretical framework from an academic partnership study and, secondly, an example of novel practice in a GP surgery in the southwest of England.

Community-Enhanced Social Prescribing (Morris, Thomas et al. 2022)

Community-Enhanced Social Prescribing (CESP) is a theoretical framework that integrates both individual and community well-being into the social prescribing model. The framework combines two evidenced models: Connected Communities (Parsfield, Morris et al. 2015) and Connecting People (Webber, Reidy et al. 2015), A recently completed feasibility trial, carried out in a number of sites across England, aimed to combine social prescribing (using the "Connecting People" model) and community building (using the "Connected Communities" model) (Webber, Bauer Annette et al. 2024). SPLWs were key facilitators within the trial, aiming to provide support to reduce loneliness and social isolation and increase availability of local resources (community building). The Connected Communities model incorporates a funding partnership to support the development of new community resources which SPLWs might connect people to, thereby overcoming some of the obstacles to an integrated model of social prescribing. The framework emphasizes reciprocal benefits: individuals not only improve their health through community connections but also contribute to building community assets through active local participation, including volunteering. Based on evidence from the feasibility trial, it is suggested that CESP might be a way forward to "improve both individual and collective outcomes", but only where corresponding funding to VCSE providers is part of the model (Morris, Thomas et al. 2022).

Proactive Social Prescribing – An Example from Southwest England

The "Lanson model" was developed at Launceston Medical Centre: a rural GP practice in Cornwall, England. The practice was one of the pioneers in employing clinical psychologists in primary care (British Psychological Society 2022). The psychologists are part of a mental health team which includes mental health nurses, occupational therapists and also SPLWs, who are managed by the lead clinical psychologist (Wood and Magill 2022). The Lanson team describe their commitment to responding to health inequalities through an approach to social prescribing which involves both "reactive" social prescribing, in which referred individuals are seen for appointments, balanced with "proactive" social prescribing which identifies and addresses unmet health and social needs through the Population Health Management program (NHS England 2023, 2024). GP data is analyzed to identify populations needing extra support. The social prescribing team are co-located at a Health Hub with local stakeholders, including adult social care and VCSE, and spend at least 50% of their worktime addressing community health needs by developing projects to fill service gaps and to securing funding and other resources for groups or individuals. The lead SPLW enjoys the autonomy and the focus on preventive work and has launched various initiatives, including volunteering programs, diabetes prevention groups and securing funding for gym memberships.

How Far Do These Examples Address Critiques to the Model of Social Prescribing That Focus on Individual Behavior Change Rather Than on Developing Community Support?

These are individual examples of good practice in which SPLWs either work alongside community builders or develop community resources themselves. Supportive GP surgeries, like the Launceston center or practices involved in the CESP evaluation, permit SPLW autonomy and flexibility in embracing these dual roles. SPLWs in less supportive GP surgeries may face referral pressures that lead to the de-prioritization of community development. There are no examples we are aware of that evidence the sustainability and scaling up of such approaches that seek to uphold the dual role of SPLWs in supporting individuals and communities. Evidencing of the CESP theoretical model is in progress (University of York 2024). However, whether such approaches demonstrate clear outcomes relating to health inequalities is not clear at present.

There is a need for research to show how best practice can be utilized alongside proposed theoretical models to build a plausible theory of how social prescribing contributes to community well-being in a meaningful way. This would include defining clear community outcomes alongside person-centered ones. Developing theory is important to help with informing intervention pathway development and to advance social prescribing in a way that supports person-centered care alongside community development. This will require funding and support for the VCSE sector as well as for SPLW schemes. Funding will be needed both to build assets (community groups and activities) as well as to adequately resource time for relationship building and collaboration across sectors (National Voices 2020). The VCSE sector should be involved in co-producing models and outcomes for what this would look like.

ICBs in England, responsible for planning and funding NHS services locally, play a key role in incorporating the VCSE sector in commissioning. Devon, a county in southwest England, offers examples of effective practice where the VCSE sector actively participates in commissioning decisions (Westlake, Elston et al. 2020). The VCSE should be involved throughout the social prescribing process – from referral through SPLW support to community connections. This approach could enhance individual well-being and strengthen community resilience, encouraging individuals to actively contribute to their communities.

Conclusion

While social prescribing has the potential to bridge individualized services and community development, its theory and practice often reveal a tension between personalization and community building. This has led to criticisms that it may inadvertently widen health inequalities by under-resourcing essential community support.

The implications for the future of social prescribing are significant. To be truly effective, social prescribing must go beyond improving individual well-being and also focus on strengthening the communities where individuals live. This means that future efforts should integrate a more community-centered approach, addressing the broader social determinants of health that influence overall health outcomes. By doing so, social prescribing can better support not only individuals but also the community structures that are crucial for sustaining long-term health and reducing inequalities within communities. This requires a fundamental shift in the focus of commissioning decisions that go beyond the needs of individuals.

References

Barry, M. J. and S. Edgman-Levitan (2012). "Shared decision making — The pinnacle of patient-centered care." *The New England Journal of Medicine* 366(9): 780–781.

Bickerdike, L., A. Booth, P. M. Wilson, K. Farley and K. Wright (2017). "Social prescribing: Less rhetoric and more reality. A systematic review of the evidence." *BMJ Open* 7: e013384.

Bourdieu, P. (1986). *The forms of capital. Handbook of theory and research for the sociology of education.* Richardson J. Westport, CT., Greenwood: 241–258.

British Psychological Society (2022). "Clinical psychology in primary care – How can we afford to be without it? Guidance for clinical commissioners and integrated care systems." https://doi.org/10.53841/bpsrep.2022.rep165

Britten, N., L. Moore, D. Lydahl, O. Naldemirci, M. Elam and A. Wolf (2017). "Elaboration of the Gothenburg model of person-centred care." *Health Expectations* 20(3): 407–418.

Calderón-Larrañaga, S., Y. Milner, M. Clinch, T. Greenhalgh and S. Finer (2021). "Tensions and opportunities in social prescribing. Developing a framework to facilitate its implementation and evaluation in primary care: A realist review." *BJGP Open* 5(3): BJGPO.2021.0017.

Chatterjee, H. J., P. M. Camic, B. Lockyer and L. J. M. Thomson (2018). "Non-clinical community interventions: A systematised review of social prescribing schemes." *Arts & Health* 10(2): 97–123.

Cooper, M., D. Flynn, L. Avery, K. Ashley, C. Jordan, L. Errington and J. Scott (2023). "Service user perspectives on social prescribing services for mental health in the UK: A systematic review." *Perspect Public Health* 143(3): 135–144.

Dayson, C. (2017). "Social prescribing 'plus': A model of asset-based collaborative innovation?" *People, Place and Policy* 11(2): 90–104.

Dayson, C. and N. Bashir (2014). The social and economic impact of the Rotherham Social Prescribing Pilot Sheffield. Main Evaluation Report. Centre for Regional Economic and Social Research. https://www.shu.ac.uk/centre-regional-economic-social-research/publications/the-social-and-economic-impact-of-the-rotherham-social-prescribing-pilot-main-evaluation-report

Department Health and Social Care, PHE and NHS England (2016). Independent report: Review of partnerships and investment in the voluntary sector - How voluntary, community and social enterprise (VCSE) organisations contribute to wellbeing, health and care. https://www.gov.uk/government/publications/review-of-partnerships-and-investment-in-the-voluntary-sector

Dudley, C. V. S (2022). "“Real, inspiring and creative”: Reflections on a social prescribing conference with a twist." https://www.dudleycvs.org.uk/real-inspiring-and-creative-reflections-on-a-social-prescribing-conference-with-a-twist/ Accessed 27/8/24.

Ekman, I., K. Swedberg, C. Taft, A. Lindseth, A. Norberg, E. Brink, J. Carlsson, S. Dahlin-Ivanoff, I. L. Johansson, K. Kjellgren, E. Lidén, J. Öhlén, L. E. Olsson, H. Rosén, M. Rydmark and K. S. Sunnerhagen (2011). "Person-centered care--ready for prime time." *European Journal of Cardiovascular Nursing* 10(4): 248–251.

Gibson, K., T. M. Pollard and S. Moffatt (2021). "Social prescribing and classed inequality: A journey of upward health mobility?" *Social Science & Medicine* 280: 114037.

Hazeldine, E., G. Gowan, R. Wigglesworth, J. Pollard, S. Asthana and K. Husk (2021). "Link worker perspectives of early implementation of social prescribing: A 'Researcher-in-Residence' study." *Health & Social Care in the Community* 29(6): 1844–1851.

Husk, K., K. Blockley, R. Lovell, A. Bethel, I. Lang, R. Byng and R. Garside (2020). "What approaches to social prescribing work, for whom, and in what circumstances? A realist review." *Health & Social Care in the Community* 28(2): 309–324.

Khan, K. and S. Tierney (2024). *The role of social prescribing in addressing health inequalities. Social prescribing policy, research and practice.* M. Bertotti. Switzerland, Springer.

Khan, K., R. Al-Izzi, A. Montasem, H. Gordon, C. Brown and J. Goldthorp (2023). "The feasibility of identifying health inequalities in social prescribing referrals and declines using primary care patient records [version 2; peer review: 2 approved, 1 approved with reservations]. *NIHR Open Research* 3: 1. https://doi.org/10.3310/nihropenres.13325.2.

Kiely, B., A. Croke, M. Shea, F. Boland, E. Shea, D. Connolly and S. M. Smith (2022). "Effect of social prescribing link workers on health outcomes and costs for adults in primary care and community settings: a systematic review." *BMJ Open* 12(10): e062951.

Kimberlee, R. (2015). "What is social prescribing?" *Advances in Social Sciences Research Journal* 2(1): 102–110. https://doi.org/10.14738/assrj.21.808

Lawler, C., G. Sherriff, P. Brown, D. Butler, A. Gibbons, P. Martin and M. Probin (2023). "Homes and health in the Outer Hebrides: A social prescribing framework for addressing fuel poverty and the social determinants of health." *Health & Place* 79: 102926.

Litt, J. S., L. Coll-Planas, A. L. Sachs, M. Masó Aguado and M. Howarth (2023). "Current trends and future directions in urban social prescribing." *Current Environmental Health Reports* 10(4): 383–393.

Mackenzie, M., K. Skivington and G. Fergie (2020). "“The state They're in”: Unpicking fantasy paradigms of health improvement interventions as tools for addressing health inequalities." *Social Science & Medicine* 256: 113047.

Marmot, M. (2010). "Fair society healthy lives." from https://www.instituteofhealthequity.org/resources-reports/fair-society-healthy-lives-the-marmot-review.

Moffatt, S., J. Wildman, T. M. Pollard, K. Gibson, J. M. Wildman, x, N. Brien, B. Griffith, S. L. Morris, E. Moloney, J. Jeffries, M. Pearce and W. Mohammed (2023). "Impact of a social prescribing intervention in North East England on adults with type 2 diabetes: the SPRING_NE multimethod study." *Public Health Research* 11(2): 1–185. https://doi.org/10.3310/AQXC8219

Moffatt, S., M. Steer, S. Lawson, L. Penn and N. O'Brien (2017). "Link worker social prescribing to improve health and well-being for people with long-term conditions: qualitative study of service user perceptions." *BMJ Open* 7: e015203.

Morris, D., P. Thomas, J. Ridley and M. Webber (2022). "Community-enhanced social prescribing: Integrating community in policy and practice." *International Journal of Community Well-Being* 5(1): 179–195.

Moscrop, A. (2023). "Social prescribing is no remedy for health inequalities." *BMJ* 381: 715.

Muhl, C., K. Mulligan, I. Bayoumi, R. Ashcroft and C. Godfrey (2023). "Establishing internationally accepted conceptual and operational definitions of social prescribing through expert consensus: A Delphi study." *BMJ Open* 13: e070184.

National Voices (2020). *Rolling out social prescribing understanding the experience of the voluntary, community and social enterprise sector.* https://www.nationalvoices.org.uk/publication/rolling-out-social-prescribing/

NHS England. (2019). "Comprehensive model of personalised care." Retrieved 26/6/24, from https://www.england.nhs.uk/publication/comprehensive-model-of-personalised-care/.

NHS England. (2019). "NHS long term plan." from https://www.longtermplan.nhs.uk/publication/nhs-long-term-plan/.

NHS England (2020). *Social prescribing and community-based support: Summary guide.* N. England.

NHS England. (2022). "Network contract directed enhanced service – Contract specification 2022/23 – primary care network requirements and entitlements." Retrieved 29/09/22, from https://www.england.nhs.uk/wp-content/uploads/2022/03/B1357-network-contract-frequently-asked-questions-2022-23-march-2022.pdf

NHS England (2023). Draft social prescribing maturity framework. Version 2.0. https://www.happyhealthylives.uk/clientfiles/files/document_library/Draft%20Social%20Prescribing%20Maturity%20Framework%20v2.0%20February%202023.pdf

NHS England (2023). Social prescribing: Reference guide and technical annex for primary care networks. https://www.england.nhs.uk/publication/social-prescribing-reference-guide-and-technical-annex-for-primary-care-networks/

NHS England. (2023). "Workforce development framework: social prescribing link workers." Retrieved 10/23, from https://www.england.nhs.uk/long-read/workforce-development-framework-social-prescribing-link-workers/.

NHS England. (2024). "Population health management." Retrieved 29/8/24, from https://www.england.nhs.uk/long-read/population-health-management/.

Office for Health Improvement and Disparities (OHID), G. U. (2019). Community centred practice; applying all our health. https://www.gov.uk/government/publications/community-centred-practice-applying-all-our-health/community-centred-practice-applying-all-our-health

Parsfield, M., D. Morris, M. Bola, M. Knapp, A.-L. Park, M. Yoshioka and G. Marcus (2015). *Community capital. The value of connected communities.* London: RSA.

Polley, M., H. J. Chatterjee, S. Asthana, M. Bertotti, L. Cartwright, K. Husk, L. Burns, S. Tierney and O. b. o. t. N. A. P. Collaborative] (2022). "Are there any medium- to long-term outcomes reported for social prescribing and, if so, what are they?" London: National Academy for Social Prescribing.

Race Equality Foundation (2024). Social prescribing, health inequalities and Black, Asian and minoritised ethnic communities. https://raceequalityfoundation.org.uk/wp-content/uploads/2024/11/Social-Prescribing-Report-REF_v5.pdf

Sandhu, S., H. Alderwick and L. M. Gottlieb (2022). "Financing approaches to social prescribing programs in England and the United States." *Milbank Quarterly* 100(2): 393–423.

Scott-Samuel, A. and K. E. Smith (2015). "Fantasy paradigms of health inequalities: Utopian thinking?" *Social Theory & Health* 13: 418–436.

South, J., A. M. Bagnall, J. A. Stansfield, K. J. Southby and P. Mehta (2019). "An evidence-based framework on community-centred approaches for health: England, UK." *Health Promotion International* 34(2): 356–366.

The Low Commission. (2015). "The role of advice services in health outcomes: Evidence review and mapping study." Retrieved 20/4/24, from www.lowcommission.org.uk/dyn/1435582011755/ASA-report_.

Tierney, S., D. Westlake, G. Wong, A. Turk, S. Markham, J. Gorenberg, J. Reeve, C. Mitchell, K. Husk, S. Redwood, A. Meacock, C. Pope and K. R. Mahtani (2024). "The consequences of micro-discretions and boundaries in the social prescribing link worker role in England: a realist evaluation." *Health and Social Care Delivery Research* 13(27):1–17. https://doi.org/10.3310/JSQY9840. PMID: 39271647

Tierney, S., D. Westlake, G. Wong, A. Turk, S. Markham, J. Gorenberg, J. Reeve, C. Mitchell, K. Husk, S. Redwood, C. Pope, B. Baird and K. R. Mahtani (2025). "Experiences of integrating social prescribing link workers into primary care in England: Bolting on, fitting in or belonging." *British Journal of General Practice: BJGP* 75(752):e195–e202. https://doi.org/10.3399/BJGP.2024.0279

Tierney, S., G. Wong and K. R. Mahtani (2019). "Current understanding and implementation of 'care navigation' across England: a cross-sectional study of NHS clinical commissioning groups." *British Journal of General Practice* 69(687): e675–e681. https://doi.org/10.3399/bjgp19X705569.

Tierney, S., G. Wong, D. Westlake, A. Turk, S. Markham, J. Gorenberg, J. Reeve, C. Mitchell, K. Husk, S. Redwood, T. Meacock, C. Pope, B. Baird and K. R. Mahtani (2024). "Patient buy-in to social prescribing through link workers as part of person-centred care: a realist evaluation." *Health and Social Care Delivery Research* 13(27): 49–66. https://doi.org/10.3310/ETND8254

Tierney, S., G. Wong, N. Roberts, A.-M. Boylan, S. Park, R. Abrams, J. Reeve, V. Williams and K. R. Mahtani (2020). "Supporting social prescribing in primary care by linking people to local assets: A realist review." *BMC Medicine* 18(1): 49.

Torjesen, I. (2016). "Social prescribing could help alleviate pressure on GPs." *BMJ* 352: i1436.

Turk, A., S. Tierney, B. Hogan, K. R. Mahtani and C. Pope (2024). "A meta-ethnography of the factors that shape link workers' experiences of social prescribing." *BMC Medicine* 22(1): 280.

University of York. (2024). "Community enhanced social prescribing." Retrieved 30/8/24, from https://www.york.ac.uk/business-society/research/spsw/community-enhanced-social-prescribing/.

Vidovic, D., G. Y. Reinhardt and C. Hammerton (2021). "Can social prescribing foster individual and community well-being? A systematic review of the evidence." *International Journal of Environmental Research and Public Health* 18(10): 5276.

Webber, M., B. Annette, D. Morris, J. Ridley and C. Peter (2024). "Community-enhanced social prescribing: A non-randomised controlled mixed methods feasibility study, NIHR." https://fundingawards.nihr.ac.uk/award/NIHR201874

Webber, M., H. Reidy, D. Ansari, M. Stevens and D. Morris (2015). "Developing and modeling complex social interventions: Introducing the connecting people intervention." *Research on Social Work Practice* 26(1): 14–19.

Westlake, D., G. Wong, S. Markham, A. Turk, J. Gorenberg, C. Pope, J. Reeve, C. Mitchell, K. Husk, S. Redwood, A. Meacock, K. R. Mahtani and S. Tierney (2024). ""She's Been a Rock": The function and importance of "holding" by social prescribing link workers in primary care in England—Findings from a realist evaluation." *Health & Social Care in the Community* 2024(1): 2479543.

Westlake, D., I. Ekman, N. Britten and H. Lloyd (2022). "Terms of engagement for working with patients in a person-centred partnership: A secondary analysis of qualitative data." *Health & Social Care in the Community* 30(1): 330–340.

Westlake, D., J. Elston, A. Gude, F. Gradinger, K. Husk and S. Asthana (2022). "Impact of COVID-19 on social prescribing across an integrated care system: A researcher in residence study." *Health & Social Care in the Community* 30(6): e4086–e4094.

Westlake, D., J. Elston, F. Gradinger, K. Husk and S. Asthana. (2020). "Social prescribing across Devon STP: Mapping and evaluating the implementation of social prescribing." Retrieved 29/8/24, from https://www.plymouth.ac.uk/rails/active_storage/blobs/proxy/eyJfcmFpbHMiOnsibWVzc2FnZSI6IkJBaHBBaE9RIiwiZXhwIjpudWxsLCJwdXIiOiJibG9iX2lkIn19--9e808d4ea11523df6e1acd893cb6b47de771cbb1/DESSPER_-_Interim_project_report_13.10.20_-_Final.pdf.

Westlake, D., S. Tierney, G. Wong and K. R. Mahtani (2023). "Social prescribing in the NHS-is it too soon to judge its value?" *Bmj* 380: 699.

Wilding, A., M. Sutton, E. Agboraw, L. Munford and P. Wilson (2024). "Geographic inequalities in need and provision of social prescribing link workers." *British Journal of General Practice: BJGP* 74(748): e784–e790. https://doi.org/10.3399/BJGP.2023.0602

Wood, E., S. Ohlsen, S.-J. Fenton, J. Connell and S. Weich (2021). "Social prescribing for people with complex needs: a realist evaluation." *BMC Family Practice* 22(1): 53.

Wood, P. and R. Magill. (2022). "We try to remove all barriers to accessing a psychologist." Retrieved 12/11/24, from https://www.bps.org.uk/psychologist/we-try-remove-all-barriers-accessing-psychologist.

Younan, H. C., C. Junghans, M. Harris, A. Majeed and S. Gnani (2020). "Maximising the impact of social prescribing on population health in the era of COVID-19." *Journal of the Royal Society of Medicine* 113(10): 377–382.

9

IMPLEMENTING PERSON-CENTERED CARE INTO A COMMUNITY SETTING

Can the Combined Use of Distributed Leadership and a Community Recovery Model Help?

Elizabeth A. Curtis and Catherine Comiskey

Introduction

This chapter is about whether the combined use of distributed leadership (DL) and a community recovery model (CRM) used within community mental health services could help with the implementation of person-centered care (PCC) to a community setting. This chapter does not provide a detailed account of either PCC, DL or a CRM given that material on these are already available in extant literature (e.g. Britten et al., 2016; Ekman et al., 2011; Spillane, 2005; Curtis et al., 2021; Harris et al., 2022, SAMHSA, 2012). Rather, its aim is twofold. Firstly, to summarize the main tenets of PCC, DL and a CRM and secondly, to report similarities between these concepts and on this basis suggest tentatively the combined use of DL and a CRM to support the implementation of PCC into a community health setting. This approach was necessary given a lack of research evidence about the combined use of DL and a CRM to support implementing PCC. To fulfill the first aim, this chapter provides overviews of research literature about the three concepts. With regard to the second aim, literature for each of the three concepts was examined for similarities, which is considered a suitable approach for combining ideas from diverse concepts. To support the use of similarity in this way, Estes (2003, p. 914) reported that ".... similarity is thought to play an important role in conceptual combination". Additionally, this chapter provides an example of a research study that combined a person-centered approach with a CRM. Although this study did not include the testing of DL in its design, aspects of DL were used during parts of the study. Any suggestion put forward in this chapter about the combined use of DL and a CRM to support implementation of PCC into a community setting is tentative given the lack of research evidence to support this. However, researchers may wish to examine empirically the utility of the idea for applications within the context of their

DOI: 10.4324/9781032662657-11

personal practices. This chapter concludes by providing information in tabular format (Table 9.1) that may be useful for those who wish to use DL together with a CRM and the Gothenburg Model of PCC. The focus of this chapter is healthcare, but due to a dearth of research on DL in this discipline, we have used literature from the fields of education and management to support content and demonstrate similarities where necessary. What follows next is an overview of literature on PCC, DL and a CRM.

Overview of Literature

PCC: Healthcare systems are constantly striving to improve patient or service user care and performance (Santana et al., 2018) and as a consequence, continue to change rapidly for both providers of care and recipients of care (Byrne et al., 2020). Changing care delivery to a PCC approach is necessary for improving both the quality of care delivered and patient safety (Institute of Medicine, 2001; Santana et al., 2018). The justification for such a change is multifactorial, but one likely reason is better access to health information and more knowledgeable and proactive patients and service users (Gardiner, 2008; Byrne et al., 2020) who regard themselves as key players within healthcare teams (Byrne et al., 2020).

PCC refers to a model of care that recognizes patients as assets with resources and therefore with potential to be "equal partners in the design and co-production of care" (Berntsen et al., 2021, p. 23). PCC is not a new concept in healthcare, but despite its prominence and many attempts at implementation, patients and health professionals alike have voiced concerns that service users are neither receiving individualized care or being treated with dignity and respect (Berntsen et al., 2021). In fact, authors such as Berntsen et al. (2021) and Agledahl et al. (2011) have reported that PCC remains inadequate in practice and that this will persist until there is acceptance of PCC as a core factor in quality care. PCC is important within healthcare because it is a core value in providing and maintaining high standards of care, and is necessary for achieving health goals set by the World Health Organization (WHO) (WHO, 2005, 2015). However, despite its importance for decades and its recognition as a core competency for health professionals (WHO, 2005), implementation of PCC remains challenging for most healthcare systems (Santana et al., 2018; Berntsen et al., 2021; Burgers et al., 2021).

The World Health Organization (2007) in their policy framework for PCC recognized the difference between the established patient-centered care and the need for the broader more holistic PCC approach. Patient-centered care they state, has been recognized as one of the six attributes of healthcare quality, the other five being safety, timelines, effectiveness, efficiency and equity. While patient-centered care addresses issues of quality, it fails to meet some of the broader health challenges, and it does not consider that before a person becomes a patient they need to be informed and empowered to protect and promote their own health. PCC goes beyond patient needs and reaches out beyond clinical settings to people, their families and their communities. It also recognizes that healthcare practitioners are people and healthcare systems and organizations are groups of people too. These people's needs also must be considered and they must be empowered to change the system for the better. This basic principle of empowerment within PCC where person includes all of those involved in the systems of care directly relates to the principles of DL (WHO, 2007).

Giusti et al. (2020) have endeavored to assess the research evidence for PCC. In their systematic review, they explored the empirical evidence underpinning the concept and practice of PCC for those with serious illnesses. They state that while PCC is recognized as a core competency for healthcare professionals and a key component of primary care delivery, there remains debate and disparity about how the concept can be understood and implemented within a wide variety of settings. They reviewed its implementation with people experiencing serious illnesses and reported that decisions within complex clinical scenarios can involve varied healthcare professions and families. Joint decision-making between these groups is crucial. This finding again emphasizes the need for DL with PCC and people, families and healthcare professionals dealing with serious illness. Giusti et al. (2020) in their review also found that PCC highlighted the importance of the involvement of family and friends and the structuring of the service and system to ensure continuity of care. Nkhoma et al. (2022) in their later systematic review exploring the impact of PCC on outcomes and costs also recognize in their definition of PCC that PCC is focused on people rather than on illness.

DL: There can be little doubt about the importance of effective leadership in nursing and healthcare (Hewison, 2020). For example, leadership is central to quality and integrating healthcare (Sfantou et al., 2017), increased employee engagement and job satisfaction (Quek et al., 2021). However, despite such robust evidence, "leadership in healthcare has, quite rightly, been subjected to biting criticism and regular revelations about scandalous failures ..." (Curtis et al., 2021, p. 256) as demonstrated in reports such as the Mazars Review (Mazars, 2015) and the Áras Attracta Swinford Review (Áras Attracta Swinford Review Group, 2016), that were published following high profile investigations into inadequate care and unnecessary patient and client deaths. More recently, a review of the internal workings of the Care Quality Commission (CQC) in the United Kingdom found significant breaches and failings by the CQC to identify unacceptable performance (Department of Health and Social Care, 2024). It is now clear that leadership must change from a heroic, concentrated configuration to a more distributed process (Harris, 2013 Ahmed et al., 2015, Cordoba et al., 2022), especially since research findings have indicated that high performing hospitals are those that foster staff participation in decision-making and practice DL (West et al., 2015). Ahmed et al. (2015) share a similar view and have called for the National Health Service (NHS) to renounce its practice of heroic, concentrated leadership and adopt instead a model of DL. The COVID-19 pandemic exposed healthcare systems globally to the greatest challenge of modern times and spotlighted the need for speedy decision-making, concern for staff and a call "to get serious about distributed leadership" (Cordoba et al., 2022, p. 45). Looking to the future, we hope that lessons were learnt following the pandemic and that these will help create space for progressing DL thinking and practice.

Interest in DL has been increasing steadily among researchers and practitioners since the start of the millennium (Bolden, 2011), but its theoretical roots can be traced back to 1250 BC (Oduro, 2004) making it one of the oldest leadership approaches. So what then is DL? DL is a widely discussed concept and there have been several attempts to define the term (Hasselgren et al., 2021), but Harris et al. (2007) suggest that these definitions vary. To complicate matters further, the term DL is often used interchangeably with shared leadership and democratic leadership (Spillane, 2005), which can result in mixed-up meanings and interpretations. Most conceptualizations of DL express it as practice that requires interactions between leaders, employees and their situation or context. Thus, DL is exemplified by interactions between individuals and their setting, routines and tools and emanates from activities of leadership rather than the role, routines and functions of an individual leader; important though these may be (Spillane, 2005). The aim in using a DL approach is not to generate additional leaders but to generate improved leadership (Harris, 2013).

With regard to DL, leadership practice must be the "starting point" and a distributed perspective considers leadership to be the outcome of interactions among leaders, employees or team members and their setting or environment. This, Spillane (2005) points out is a critical point given that leadership practice from a distributed viewpoint is not the outcome of a leader's knowledge and skill but rather the interactions between individuals and their setting. Interactions, rather than a given action are the essential ingredients to leadership practice. Often, debates on DL refer to several people assuming leadership which Spillane (2005, p. 144) refers to as the "leader plus view". This, however, represents an incomplete picture since leadership practice from the perspective of DL emanates from interactions among leaders, other employees, team members and their settings.

Why DL?

A reasonable question to ask at this point is, why DL? In 2019, the Health Foundation organized a seminar in the United Kingdom to discuss NHS inquiries (Powell, 2019). These inquiries occurred over several decades, included different care facilities and investigated a range of issues including allegations of abuse and ill treatment of patients. Despite the range of issues examined, the various inquiries led to some shared findings and recommendations. These include "organisation geographical isolation which inhibits innovation and learning, inadequate leadership and poor communication" (Powell, 2019, p. 180). Many healthcare institutions still operate using heroic, concentrated, hierarchical approaches to leadership, which can restrain and undervalue the contributions of health professionals not in leadership or management positions. In 2011, the King's Fund Commission reported that traditional heroic approaches to leadership (where leadership is confined to a few senior personnel) are not capable of meeting the demands of contemporary healthcare organizations and put forward an argument for a distributed approach to leadership (The King's Fund, 2011). To emphasize further the merit and importance of DL, it is necessary to note that DL is a useful approach to leadership in health and social care where several healthcare professionals and patients need to work together and across several professional disciplines (Braut et al., 2022). Furthermore, researchers Leask and Macleod (2023) reported that healthcare continues to face challenges that are increasingly difficult to resolve with a single solution and that hierarchical structures and singular approaches to leadership may not be suitable for resolving difficult problems. Consequently, there have been calls for leaders in these health systems to amend such structures and promote leadership as a distributed enterprise, thus nurturing greater collaboration and improving innovation (Leask and Macleod, 2023).

CRM: Recovery is now considered a process as opposed to an event, and this approach has been pioneered within mental health services. It is now believed that one can live a full and meaningful life while also living with an ongoing and chronic mental health challenge (Higgins and McGowan, 2014). It is accepted that recovery is no longer universally defined, but rather it is defined for and by the person who is in the recovery process (Comiskey, 2020). The Substance Abuse and Mental Services Administration provides a working definition, recovery as, "a dynamic change process through which individuals improve their health and wellness, live self-directed lives, and strive to reach their full potential" (SAMHSA, 2012). Within this definition of recovery, an individual may or may not achieve a state of abstinence from an illness or condition. According to SAMHSA, community is one of the key dimensions that support a person in recovery. The CRM is therefore both the setting and the support within which the process of recovery is experienced.

CRM has been applied within a range of settings. The United Nations Development Programme (UNDP) refers to CRM and builds upon wide-ranging partnerships with national and local governments, NGOs, civil society groups and importantly, communities. UNDP emphasizes the human and social aspects of recovery (UNDP, 2017). The Australian National Emergency Management System builds upon these partnerships and highlights six basic principles, these being understanding the context, recognizing the complexity, using community-led approaches, coordinating all approaches, communicating effectively and recognizing and building capacity. The application of these principles is stated in the Australian response to the COVID-19 pandemic (Australian Disaster Resilience Knowledge Hub, 2023) and has been observed globally. The application of these principles is essential not only for community recovery but also for personal, holistic recovery within a community setting.

The WHO provides guidance on applying person-centered and rights-based approaches to all stakeholders who wish to develop community-based mental health recovery services (WHO, 2023). This guide outlines the connections needed between community services such as housing, education, employment and social protection sectors. Specific recommendations and action steps are presented for developing community mental health services that respect human rights and focus on recovery. Throughout the guidance document, the importance of leadership within CRM is highlighted, as is evident from the following quote,

> Strong coordinated leadership from multiple sectors, with accountability processes and a means to allow coordination throughout the system are necessary to make the collaboration work – from the policy level through to practical implementation at the service level on the ground.
>
> *(WHO, 2023, p. 183)*

The community reinforcement approach (CRA) within the range of treatments for substance use and recovery also focuses on a wider holistic person-centered CRM (Recovery Research Institute, 2023). CRA aims to accomplish user-defined recovery by looking at a person's environment and by replacing negative situations with positive activities and behaviors. It uses social, recreational, familial and vocational reinforcers to assist in the recovery process. During treatment, the person learns practical skills to meet his or her goals including communication, problem solving and assertive drink and drug refusal. The CRA can also incorporate job-hunting skills and social or recreational counseling to identify protective activities. To conclude, the key attributes of CRM are person-centered, participative, holistic care and leadership across a range of services identified by the person in recovery. The model which inspired this chapter is that developed by nurses, clients and academics working with a DL approach in community addiction services. The result of this was the formation of the healthy addiction treatment (HAT) recovery model (Comiskey et al., 2019, 2021).

Thus far, this chapter has addressed its first aim, which is to summarize key tenets of PCC, DL and a CRM. Next, this chapter discusses its second aim by addressing the question below.

How Might DL, Together with a CRM, Support the Implementation of PCC into a Community Health Setting?

Addressing this question was challenging given the lack of research on the combined use of DL and a CRM for supporting PCC within a community health context. As outlined in the first paragraph of the introduction, we used extant literature to determine the existence of similarities between the three concepts and used these to suggest provisionally, the combined use of DL and a CRM to support the implementation of PCC. These similarities are categorized under three themes: definitions, key principles and prerequisites.

Definitions

Despite the importance of PCC (Burgers et al., 2021) and calls for its implementation within healthcare (WHO, 2005; Byrne et al., 2020) there is still no agreed definition of the concept (Fridberg et al., 2022) which can make implementation burdensome and summarizing results from several studies difficult (Fridberg et al., 2021). In an attempt to address this gap, Byrne et al. (2020) carried out a literature review to identify if a common definition of PCC exists. Their findings revealed three core themes, people, practice and power. Similarly, DL, has amassed a large amount of scholarly literature (Cherkowski and Brown, 2013, Irvine, 2021) and the topic has gained significant attention over the last two decades, mainly because traditional heroic, concentrated leadership is no longer considered fit for purpose (Irvine, 2021). Despite this and the fact that the term is widely used both in literature and in practice, there is still no universally agreed definition of DL (Harris et al., 2007, Irvine, 2021, Hickey et al., 2022). This lack of definitional clarity can result in mixed-up meanings and interpretations and potential difficulties for researchers (Harris, 2013), resulting in many focusing their research on examining the features of activities that meet the requirements of DL rather than trying to define the term (Irvine, 2021). It seems reasonable to suggest, therefore, that both PCC and DL lack unanimously agreed definitions.

Regarding recovery, Jaiswal et al. (2020) noted that different individuals could perceive recovery-focused care differently. For example, individuals with mental health problems use the term to describe a personal life-changing journey while health professionals describe recovery in terms of quantifiable outcomes. Such variations in meanings demonstrate the lack of clarity of a recovery model of care, and this in turn can lead to variations in delivery of care. Furthermore, these researchers point out that the three themes (relationships, participation and sense of self) that emerged from their scoping study should facilitate discussions with clients, support staff and policy makers regarding the need to support individual recovery and promote the use of a recovery model. Our conclusion therefore is that the concepts of PCC, DL and recovery all seem to lack universally agreed definitions.

Key Principles

In a systematic review of centeredness (including person centeredness, patient centeredness and family centeredness) in healthcare, Feldthusen et al. (2022, p. 888) reported three key themes following a synthesis of reviews. These include "attributes of centredness, translation from theory into practice and evaluation of effects of centredness". The first theme summarizes the components of centeredness and includes, being treated with dignity and respect (treated as a human being with rights), importance of autonomy, being heard (service user must be allowed to articulate their experiences and preferences) and participating in one's own care (service user and healthcare professionals sharing power and responsibility). The second theme consists of strategies for action and prerequisites. Strategies for action include interacting with service users {getting to know them}, sharing information and exchanging knowledge and lastly, acknowledging service users as team members. Prerequisites include organizational leadership, training and education, time and flexibility (important qualities for aiding centeredness or PCC) and finally guidelines and documentation (to aid PCC and increase awareness of service user needs).

Santana et al. (2018) reported that while many frameworks of PCC exist, guidance on implementing PCC is sparse. To tackle this gap, these researchers utilized literature on PCC to develop a framework then used Donabedian's model (Donabedian, 1988) to catalog PCC components. The Donabedian model is a framework for investigating health services and assessing quality and consists of three linked stages: structure, process and outcomes. According to Santana et al. (2018), several domains or prerequisites required for promoting PCC emerged from literature reviewed, and these are addressed later in this chapter. An alternative to the model used by Santana et al. (2018) is the Gothenburg model of person-centered care (GPCC). This model is the outcome of work carried out by a group of clinical and non-clinical personnel at the University of Gothenburg in Sweden and resulted in the establishment of the center for PCC (Ekman et al., 2011). The aim of the center was to conduct a thorough exploration of PCC from the perspective of the person receiving care, the health professional providing the care and the institution responsible for organizing and delivering the required care. To guarantee reliability in the delivery of PCC, the researchers at the center felt it necessary to create a sequence of actions (or routines) that would allow PCC to take place in clinical practice every day rather than occasionally when time permits. The terms used by the center to describe these actions or routines are *initiate*, *integrate* and *safeguard*. Initiating refers to setting up a partnership with patients and includes listening to their narratives or personal accounts of their illness. The second action or routine is integrating, which refers to the health professional working in partnership with patients and includes sharing information and decision-making. The third action or routine is termed safeguarding. This refers to protecting the partnership created by documenting the patient narrative and includes for example, recording patient values, their preferences, the coordination of their care (is it well coordinated) and that the patient-provider relationship is well maintained. These actions or routines described by Ekman et al. (2011) are not dissimilar to those reported by Santana et al. (2018) given that they are likely to result in supporting the dignity and respect of persons, providing opportunities to be heard and increasing autonomy and self-governance.

With regard to DL, Spillane (2005, p. 144) suggests that leadership practice is critical to DL and states, "distributed leadership is first and foremost about leadership practice rather than leaders or their roles, functions, routines, and structures". Traditionally in healthcare, heroic, concentrated leadership has predominated, but health systems are becoming increasingly complex and therefore require leadership that draws on expertise from several individuals (Beirne, 2021; Cordoba et al., 2022). DL encourages people to work in ways that combine the knowledge, skills and abilities of many to achieve goals and recognizes that expert, specialist knowledge can come from several individuals and that this paves the way for leadership to emerge from those within a team (Leach et al., 2021). Gunzel-Jensen et al. (2018) put forward three core requirements for DL. First, the emergence of leadership is a central attribute of a group or network of people interacting with each other. Second, greater openness with regard to leadership is important, and the focus here is on inclusivity rather than exclusivity when deciding who can participate in leadership activity. Third, leadership is distributed among several individuals, not just those in designated leadership positions. With regard to PCC, the WHO (2007) explains that PCC includes all of those involved in the system of care and that CRM depend upon participative holistic care (Recovery Research Institute, 2023). Thus, it is clear to see that the key unifying principle among DL, PCC and CRM is interactive and wide-ranging inclusive decision-making.

Prerequisites

Prerequisites or antecedents are important considerations for facilitating or enacting any innovation or change and therefore worthy of discussion. For example, communication that is honest and clear is a precursor to trust (Curtis and Seery, 2017) and therefore essential to all aspects of health related work. As illustrated below, some of the prerequisites are similar across the concepts of PCC, DL and a CRM and derived from relevant research studies.

In their systematic review, Feldthusen et al. (2022) reported several prerequisites for PCC including (a) organizational leadership, (b) education and training and (c) time and flexibility. Organizational leadership is important for implementing PCC and creating a collaborative, supportive environment, building relationships and partnerships with other services, and creating and sustaining an empowering work environment. Feldthusen and her colleagues (2022) suggest that education and training emerged as the most important factor for centeredness (which includes PCC) in healthcare and that this education should include empathy, compassion, communication and shared decision-making. With regard to time and flexibility, these researchers stated that time is necessary for listening and building relationships and that flexibility must be built into all areas of care (services, policies and practices).

In relation to DL, a range of prerequisites similar to those addressed for PCC, have emerged from extant literature and it is important that health professionals address these before implementing DL. Prerequisites include (a) empowering structures and teams, (b) learning and development, (c) individually perceived autonomy and (d) empathy. Empowering structures are an essential precursor to implementing DL. Such structures allow staff members to participate in several work groups, which can create opportunities for joint problem solving and better decision-making (Grenda and Hackman, 2014). Research by Jiang et al. (2016) suggest that empowered teams are likely to engage in knowledge sharing with colleagues and that sharing knowledge aids team performance. Another prerequisite similar to that required for PCC is Learning and development. Healthcare continues to experience major changes, and this requires new competencies, knowledge and skills, which are updateable through planned learning opportunities and specialized continuing professional development programs. For example, learning and development are required for maintaining patient safety, a view supported by Sherwood (2015). Organizations with flat structures (few tiers of management) offer opportunities for employees to collaborate and innovate. Another advantage of such structures is increased autonomy. Unterrainer et al. (2017) found that individual perceptions of autonomy are critical to DL and that autonomy offers employees the opportunity to take on leadership functions and roles. Empathy is indispensable in healthcare and evidence, Holt et al. (2017) suggest that being able to show empathy is essential to effective leadership. It is often said that for a caring profession, health professionals do not always show compassion or display empathy; to quote Zulueta (2016, p. 1) "In many countries, there is a deep concern that modern health care has lost its moral compass and is struggling to provide safe, timely, and compassionate care to its citizens". This supports the point raised by Feldthusen et al. (2022) that continued education and training in empathy is imperative for supporting PCC.

SAMHSA (2012) in their working definition of recovery provide four key dimensions that support a life in recovery. Health and purpose are two of these. Interestingly the remaining two are home and community. Within these four dimensions, they place the principles of person centeredness, holistic care supported by peers and allies, relationships and networks and the involvement of the individual, the family and the community strengths and responsibilities. These prerequisites for the CRM have many commonalities with PCC and DL.

This comparison between PCC, DL and a CRM reveals similarities such as an absence of universally agreed definitions, similar principles across the three concepts, and shared prerequisites that require consideration prior to implementation.

In concluding this section, it is apt for us to end with a quotation from a document by the WHO. The document in question is the WHO Global Strategy on People-centered and Integrated Health Services which states in section 10.2

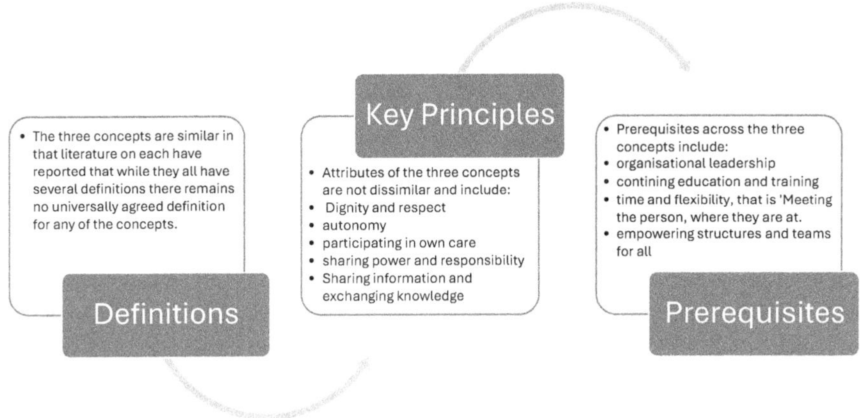

FIGURE 9.1 Similarities across definitions, key principles and prerequisites

Leadership for Change, that the delivery of people-centered health services will require a model of "distributed leadership that involves multiple actors working together collaboratively across organisational professional boundaries" (WHO, 2015, p. 35). This, in our view, certainly strengthens the argument for using DL and a CRM to support implementation of PCC into a community health setting. Note however, that research to establish compatibility and long-term utility of the combined use of DL and CRM for supporting the application of PCC is essential. Figure 9.1 below summarizes similarities among DL, CRM and PCC with regard to three key factors: definition, key principles and prerequisites.

Thus far, this chapter has summarized key aspects of PCC and drew attention to difficulties with its implementation. Additionally, it has summarized literature on DL and a CRM, alluded to the similarities between PCC, DL and a CRM, and on this basis has suggested the combined use of DL and a CRM for supporting PCC in the future. To encourage and support this, an example of a research study that combined a person-centered approach with a CRM follows. Testing DL was not included in the study's design; however, aspects of DL were utilized during parts of the study.

Example of a Research Study: Developing a Client-Centered, Nurse-Led Model of Care for Community Addiction Services (Comiskey et al., 2019, 2021)

Aim: To develop an evidence, person-centered community-based addiction treatment and recovery nursing model.

Background: The existing model was task orientated and reactive with caseloads equivalent to client registration lists.

Methods: A DL approach was taken by the Assistant Director of Nursing. Each of the nursing team members was asked to provide a summary of benefits and challenges of current nursing models. The academic team were asked to review the literature on nursing models and work with nurses and clients to assess needs. Clients articulated their needs in a series of one-to-one interviews and a wider group of clients provided quantitative data on their health and well-being. This wider group also contributed to decisions on what would be important to measure in the future. Trauma and adverse childhood experiences emerged as topics of importance to address.

Results: Client nursing needs were, managing methadone; expanding the nursing role; nurses as sources of psychological supports, service access and additional resources. Results informed the development of the HAT recovery model, a nurse-led, client needs and whole-clinic response. The model was finalized by consensus. The model refocused the community services on client's objective needs for their recovery, it addressed caseloads of nurses and measured impacts. The implementation of the model for clients and nurses involved the new measurements identified by the clients, it involved training in trauma informed service provision and a series of plan, do, study, act cycles with inputs from staff and clients as the model was rolled out and scaled up across the community nursing addiction services (Flanaghan, 2022)

Implications for nursing management: To date, there had been no nursing model for the community addiction services and nurses had no time for PCC. The proposed model addressed this. It provided an opportunity for DL across the stakeholders and for management to be guided by the experience of that leadership and subsequently streamline services, to allocate resources based on evidence of need from clients. It provided a PCC model for community-based, personally defined recovery led by the nursing services.

Future Considerations

In addition to the research example given above, an additional literature search to determine the compatibility between DL, a CRM and the GPCC produced no relevant research studies. However, based on the summary information presented in Table 9.1, is it not plausible to put forward a cautious suggestion that combining DL with a CRM might be a useful schema for the application of PCC using the GPCC model? While variables are not identical, there are similarities so is compatibility not conceivable? We leave such work to future researchers.

TABLE 9.1 Similarities between DL, CRM and GPCC

Distributed leadership (DL)	*Community recovery model (CRM)*	*The Gothenburg model of person-centered care (GPCC)*
What is it?	*What is it?*	*What is it?*
DL is not an action or set of actions carried out by one person. Rather, it is about a group activity and the ways in which individuals interact. It is based on the view that leadership involves several individuals within a team or organization. For some writers in the field (e.g. Gronn, 2002), this offers a different "unit of analysis"; where leadership is recognized as a holistic, interactive approach to leadership instead of the sum of individual efforts. Earlier sections of this chapter have indicated a call for healthcare to adopt a more distributed approach to leadership (West et al., 2015). Ahmed et al. (2015).	A CRM is first and foremost defined by the person in recovery. It is a process or journey taken by the person toward their recovery goal within a community setting. The community may involve family, peers, the healthcare and other professions and policy makers, each in an appropriate supportive role. The level of support will reflect the goal and the stage of recovery. The recovery goal may change during the process and the role of relevant members of the community will alter accordingly.	Authors such as Ekman et al. (2011, p. 249) claim that "PCC is the antithesis of reductionism" and that patients are people and should not be classified by their diagnosis only. Their strengths, plans and rights need to be considered too. This model of PCC advocates moving away from an approach where patients are viewed as passive receipts of care to one that includes their participation in decisions about their care. Despite the benefits of PCC (e.g. improved health outcomes and greater patient satisfaction), care continues to be mainly ritualistic (Ekman et al. (2011). PCC is considered important in healthcare given that it is a core value in maintaining high standards of care (WHO, 2005, 2015). Despite this however, the implementation of PCC remains challenging (Burgers et al., 2021).

(*Continued*)

TABLE 9.1 (Continued)

Distributed leadership (DL)	*Community recovery model (CRM)*	*The Gothenburg model of person-centered care (GPCC)*
Theory	*Theory*	*Theory*
Much of the literature recognizes activity theory as the theoretical origins for DL (Irvine, 2021, Bolden, 2011), but this is not universally acknowledged. In brief, activity theory is based on the view that activity is central; and "that doing precedes thinking … images, cognitive models" (Hashim and Jones, 2007, p. 1). According to Pau Yen Ho et al. (2016), actions by humans is acknowledged and understood within an activity system, and that this includes subjects (human doers) who have a desire to change an object (something that has to be done) into an outcome.	The community recovery model may reflect varying theories depending on the nature of the health challenge being addressed. However an appropriate overarching theory reflecting the person in recovery at the center with varying levels of support is Bronfenbrenner's (1994 and 2005) Ecological Systems Theory. This was originally developed for children but has expand to a bioecological theory given its universal applicability and recognition of the levels or systems within which we exist.	According Ekman et al. (2015) the theoretical foundation of the Gothenburg model of person-centered care is personalism. Philosophical personalism considers life sacred (Di Nardo et al., 2019) and views a human being as a whole person, with individuality and dignity. Pertinent features include self-possession which involves personal responsibility, self-governance (making decisions) and self-determination which is necessary to allow a person to determine their own destiny (Akrivou et al., 2023)
Key tenets	*Key tenets*	*Key tenets*
* DL is the collective property/output of a group or network of individuals interacting or working together. * DL is about expanding the boundaries of leadership. This means widening the number of leaders or those contributing to leadership. * DL implies that expertise emanates from many individuals not just those in senior positions (Bennett et al., 2003, Phillips et al., 2023).	Key dimensions include: Health Home Purpose Community Guiding principles include person driven, relational, supported and strengths based (SAMHSA, 2012).	Researchers at the Gothenburg Centre for Person-centered Care found that the key challenge was not convincing practitioners that PCC was important but rather to inform them that what they were doing was not actually PCC (were not considering the person before their diagnosis/disease). Consequently, the researchers developed three essential actions/routines that they believed would facilitate PCC. These were discussed earlier and include initiate, integrate and safeguard (Ekman et al., 2011).

Conclusion

In addition to presenting summaries of literature on PCC, DL and a CRM, we addressed key similarities between these concepts. Despite challenges with definitions, implementation and measurement of outcomes, it is clear to see that their strengths lie in their assertions of commonalities, interactions and most importantly, inclusivity. At a time of unprecedented challenges in international healthcare, where strategies recognize the need for proactive community health, now more than ever, these key tenants are essential for the foundations of the well-being of all our global citizens.

This chapter had two aims. Firstly, to summarize the main tenets of PCC, DL and a CRM. Secondly, to report similarities between these concepts and on this basis suggest tentatively the combined use of DL and a CRM to support the implementation of PCC into a community health setting. We hope we have managed to achieve this.

Acknowledgments

We wish to thank Dr. R. O'Connell for her assistance in critiquing this chapter.

References

Agledahl, K. M, Gulbrandsen, P., Forde, R., & Wifstad, A. (2011). Courteous but not curious: How doctors' politeness masks their existential neglect: A qualitative study of video-recorded patient consultations. *Journal of Medical Ethics, 37*, 650–654. https://doi.org/10.1136/jme.2010.041988.

Ahmed, N., Ahmed, F., Anis, H., Carr, P., Gauher S., & Rahman F. (2015). *An NHS leadership team for the future*. London: Reform Research Trust.

Akrivou, K., Bernacchio, C., Mele, D., & Scalzo, G. (2023) Editorial: Personalism and moral psychology: re-humanising economies and organisations. *Frontiers in Communication* https://doi10.3389/fcomm.2023.1182356

Áras Attracta Swinford Review Group. (2016). *What matters most.* Dublin: Áras Attracta Swinford Review Group, Health Service Executive.

Australian Disaster Resilience Knowledge Hub. (2023). *National principles for disaster recovery to COVID19.* Melbourne: Australian Institute for Disaster Resilience.

Beirne, M. (2021). Introducing the collection: A leadership book like no other! In E. A. Curtis, M. Beirne, J. G. Cullen, R. Northway, & S. Corrigan (Eds.), *Distributed leadership in nursing and healthcare: Theory, evidence and development* (pp. 1–16). London: Open University Press/McGraw Hill.

Bennett, N., Wise, C., Woods, P. A., & Harvey, J. A. (2003). Distributed leadership: A review of literature, National College for School Leadership. Available at: https://oro.open.ac.uk/8534/1/ (accessed 9 October 2024).

Berntsen, G. R., Yaron, S., Chetty, M., Canfield, C., Ako-Egbe, L., Phan, P., Curran, C., & Castro, I. (2021). Person-centered care (PCC): The people's perspective. *International Journal for Quality in Health Care, 33*(2), 23–26. https://doi.org/10.1093/intqhc/mzab052.

Bolden, R. (2011). Distributed leadership in organisations: A review of theory and research. *International Journal of Management Reviews, 13*(3), 251–269. https://doi.org/10.1111/j.1468-2370.2011.00306.x.

Braut, H., Oygarden, O., Storm, M., & Mikkelsen, A. (2022). General Practitioners' perceptions of distributed leadership in providing integrated care for elderly chronic multimorbid patients: A qualitative study. *BMC Health Services Research, 22*, 1085–1097. https://doi.org/10.1186/s12913-022-08460-x.

Britten, N., Moore, L., Lydah, l D., Naldemirci, O., Elam, M., & Wolf, A. (2016) Elaboration of the Gothenburg model of person-centred care. *Health Expectations, 20*, 407–418.

Bronfenbrenner, U. (1994). Ecological models of human development. In M. Gauvain, and M. Cole (Eds.), *International encyclopaedia of education* (pp. 37–43). New York: Freeman.

Bronfenbrenner, U. (2005). *Making human beings human: Bioecological perspectives on human development*. New York: Sage.

Burgers, J. S., van der Weijden, T., & Bischoff, E. W. M. A. (2021). Challenges of research on person-centred care in general practice: A scoping review. *Frontiers in Medicine, 8*, Article 669491. https://doi.org/10.3389/fmed.2021.669491.

Byrne, A. L., Baldwin, A., & Harvey, C. (2020). Whose centre is it anyway? Defining person-centred care in nursing: An integrative review. *PloS One, 15*(3), Article e0229923. https://doi.org/10.1371/journal.pone.0229923.

Cherkowski, S., & Brown, W. (2013). Towards distributed leadership as standards-based practice in British Columbia. *Canadian Journal of Education, 36*(3), 23–46.

Comiskey, C. (2020). *Addiction debates: Hot topics from policy to practice*. SAGE Swifts Series, SAGE, United Kingdom, ISBN: 9781526495761

Comiskey, C. M., Galligan, K., Flanagan, J., Deegan, J., Farnham, J., & Hall, A. (2019). Client's views on the importance of a nurse led approach and nurse prescribing in the development of the Healthy Addiction Treatment Recovery Model. *Journal of Addictions Nursing, 30*(3), 169–176.

Comiskey, C. M. Galligan, K., Flanagan, J., Deegan, J., Farnham, J., & Hall, A. (2021). The development and implementation of the healthy addiction treatment recovery model. *Journal of Addictions Nursing, 32*(1), E11–E20.

Cordoba, E. L., Shale, S., Evans, R. C., & Tracy, D. (2022). Time to get serious about distributed leadership: Lessons to learn for promoting leadership development for non-consultant career grade doctors in the UK. *BMJ Leader, 6*, 45–49. https://doi.org/10.1136/leader-2020-000395.

Curtis, E. A., Beirne, M., Cullen, J. G., Northway, R., & Corrigan, S. (2021). Epilogue: Where are we now and what is to be done? In E. A. Curtis, M. Beirne, J. G. Cullen, R. Northway, & S. Corrigan (Eds.), *Distributed leadership in nursing and healthcare: Theory, evidence and development* (pp. 256–263). London: Open University Press/McGraw Hill.

Curtis, E. A., & Seery, A. (2017) Trust and leadership. In E. A. Curtis and J. G. Cullen (Eds.), *Leadership and change for the health professional* (pp. 112–127). London: Open University Press.

Department of Health and Social Care (2024) Review into the operational effectiveness of the Care Quality Commission: full report. Available at: https://www.gov.uk/government/publications/review-into-the-operational-effectiveness-of-the-care-quality-commission-full-report/review-into-the-operational-effectiveness-of-the-care-quality-commission-full-report. Accessed on 16th November 2024.

De Zulueta, P. C. (2016) Developing compassionate leadership in health care: An integrative review. *Journal of Healthcare Leadership, 8*, 1–10.

Di Nardo, M., Ore, A. D., Testa, G., Annich, G., Piervincezi, E., Zampini, G., Bottari, G., Cecchetti, C., Amodeo, A., Lorussi, R., Del Sorbo, L., & Kirsch R. (2019) Principlism and personalism. Comparing two ethical models applied clinically in neonates undergoing extracorporeal membrane oxygenation support. *Frontiers in Paediatrics, 7*(312), 9. https://doi10.3389/fped.201900312

Donabedian, A. (1988). The quality of care: How can it be assessed? *The Journal of the American Medical Association, 260*(12), 1743–1748. https://doi.org/10.1001/jama.260.12.1743.

Ekman, I., Hedman, H., Swedberg, K., & Wallengren, C. (2015) Commentary: Swedish initiative on person centred care. *BMJ,* 350, 2. (Published 10th February 2015). https://doi.org/10.1136/bmj.h160

Ekman, I., Swedberg, K., Taft, C., Lindseth, A., Norberg, A., Brink, E., Carlsson, J., Dahlin-Ivanoff, S., Johansson, I-L., Kjellgren, K., Liden, E., Öhlén, J., Olsson, L-E., Rosén, H., Rydmark, M., & Sunnerhagen, K. S. (2011) Person-centred care – Ready for prime time. *European Journal of Cardiovascular Nursing, 10*, 248–251.

Estes, Z. (2003). A tale of two similarities: Comparison and integration in conceptual combination. *Cognitive Science, 27*, 911–921.

Feldthusen, C., Forsgren, E., Wallström, S., Andersson, V., Löfqvist, N., Sawatzky, R., Öhlén, J., & Ung, E. J. (2022). Centredness in health care: A systematic overview of reviews. *Health Expectations, 25*(3), 885–901. https://doi.org/10.1111/hex.13461.

Flanaghan, J. (2022). Embedding a new model of care in addiction nursing: How one team's journey influenced behaviours & practices across wider frontiers'. Presentation at NMPDU Dublin North Regional Nursing and Midwifery Conference, "The power of Nurses and Midwives to influence change" May 18th 2022. Retrieved from https://healthservice.hse.ie/filelibrary/onmsd/embedding-a-new-model-of-care-in-addiction-nursing-jean-flanagan.pdf on 16th October 2024.

Fridberg, H., Wallin, L., & Tistad, M. (2022) Operationalisation of person-centred care in a real-world setting: A case study with six embedded units. *BCM Health Services Research, 22*, 1160. https://doi.org/10.1186/s12913-022-08516-y

Gardiner, R. (2008). The transition from "informed patient" to "patient informed" care. *Study of Health Technology and Information, 137*(5), 241–256.

Giusti, A., Nkhoma, K., Petrus, R., Petersen, I., Gwyther, L., Farrant, L., Venkatapuram, S., & Harding, R. (2020). The empirical evidence underpinning the concept and practice of person-centred care for serious illness: A systematic review. *BMJ Global Health, 5*(12), Article e003330. https://doi.org/10.1136/bmjgh-2020-003330.

Grenda, J. P., & Hackman, D. G. (2014) Advantages and challenges of distributed leadership in middle-level schools. *National Association of Secondary School Principals (NASSP) Bulletin, 98*(1), 53–74.

Gronn, P. (2002) Distributed leadership as a unit of analysis. *Leadership Quarterly, 13*(4), 423–451.

Gunzel-Jensen, F., Jain, A. K., & Kjeldsen, A. M. (2018) Distributed leadership in health-care: The role of formal leadership styles and organisational efficacy. *Leadership, 14*(1), 110–133.

Harris, A. (2013). Distributed leadership: Friend or foe? *Educational Management Administration and Leadership, 41*(5), 545–554. https://doi.org/10.1177/1741143213497635.

Harris, A., Jones, M., & Ismail, N. (2022). Distributed leadership: Taking a retrospective and contemporary view of the evidence base. *School Leadership and Management, 42*(5), 438–456. https://doi.org/10.1080/13632434.2022.2109620.

Harris, A., Leithwood, K., Day, C., Sammons, P., & Hopkins, D. (2007). Distributed leadership and organisational change: Reviewing the evidence. *Journal of Educational Change, 8*(4), 337–347. https://doi.org/10.1007/s10833-007-9048-4.

Hasan, H., & Kazalauskas, A. (2014) Activity theory: Who is doing what, why and how. *Faculty of Businbess* – Papers (Archive). 403. Available at: https://ro.uow.edu.au/buspapers/403

Hashim, N. H., & Jones, M. L. (2007) Activity theory: A framework for qualitative analysis. https://ro.uow.edu.au/commpapers/408

Hasselgren, C., Dellve, L., & Gillberg, G. (2021). Conditions for distributed practices among managers in elder and disability organisations: A structural equation modeling approach. *International Journal of Nursing Studies Advances, 3,* Article 100049. https://doi.org/10.1016/j.ijnsa.2021.100049.

Hewison, A. (2020) Leading nursing beyond 2020: The challenge and the opportunity. *Journal of Nursing Management, 28*(4), 767–770. https://doi.org/10.1111/jonm.13022.

Hickey, N., Flaherty, A., & McNamara, P. M. (2022) Distributed leadership: A scoping review mapping current empirical research. *Societies, 12*(1), 1–20.

Higgins, A. (2008). *A recovery approach within the Irish mental health services, a framework for development,* Mental Health Commission, Ireland. Retrieved from https://recoverycontextinventory.com/images/resources/A_Recovery_Approach_within_the_Irish_Mental_Health_Services_2008.pdf on 16th October 2024.

Higgins, A., & McGowan, P. (2014). Recovery and the recovery ethos: Challenges and possibilities. In A. Higgins & S. McDaid (Eds.), *Mental health in Ireland: Policy, practice and law*, 61–78. Gill & Macmillan Ltd.

Holt, S., Marques, J., Hu, J., & Wood, A. (2017). Cultivating empathy: New perspectives on educating business leaders. *Journal of Values-Based Leadership, 10*(3), Article 3. https://doi.org/10.22543/0733.101.1173.

Institute of Medicine. (2001). *Crossing the quality chasm: A new health care system for the 21st century.* Washington, DC: National Academy Press.

Irvine, J. (2021). Distributed leadership in practice: A modified Delphi method study. *The Journal of Instructional Pedagogies*, *25*, Article 203270.

Jaiswal, A., Carnucgaek, K., Gupta, S., Siemens, T., Crowley, P., Carlsson, A., Unsworth, G., Landry, T., & Brown, N. (2020). Essential elements that contribute to the recovery of persons with severe mental illness: A systematic coping study. *Frontiers in Psychiatry, 11,* Article 586230.

Jiang, X., Flores, H. R., Leelawong, R., & Manz, C. C. (2016). The effect of team empowerment on team performance: A cross-cultural perspective on the mediating roles of knowledge sharing and intra-group conflict. *International Journal of Conflict Management, 27*(1), 62–87. https://doi.org/10.1108/IJCMA-07-2014-0048.

Leach, L., Hastomgs. B., Schwarz, G., Watson, B., Bouckenooghe, D., Seoand, L., & Hewett, D. (2021) Distributed leadership in healthcare: Leadership dyads and the promise of improved hospital outcomes. *Leadership in Health Services, 34*(4), ISSN: 1751–1879.

Leask, C. F., & Macleod, S. (2023) Exploring the implementation and evaluation of a distributed leadership model within a Scottish, integrated health and care context. *BMJ Leader, 7*, 285–290.

MAZARS LLP. (2015). *Independent review of deaths of people with a learning disability of mental health problems in contact with Southern Health NHS Foundation Trust 2011–2015.* London: NHS England.

Nkhoma, K. B., Cook, A., Giusti, A., Farrant, L., Petrus, R., Petersen, I., Gwyther, L., Venkatapuram, S., & Harding, R. (2022). A systematic review of impact of person-centred interventions for serious physical illness in terms of outcomes and costs. *BMJ Open, 12*(7), Article e054386. https://doi.org/10.1136/bmjopen-2021-054386.

Oduro, G. K. T. (2004, September 16–18). *'Distributed leadership' in schools: What English headteachers say about the 'pull' and 'push' factors* [Paper presentation]. British

Educational Research Association Annual Conference, University of Manchester, United Kingdom. https://www.google.com/url.

Pau Yen Ho, J., Chen D-T. V., & Ng, D. (2016) Distributed leadership through the lens of Activity Theory. *Educational Management Administration and Leadership, 44*(5), 814–836.

Phillips, D. R., Stewart-Fox, T., Phillips, S., Griffith, M., & Bhojedat, J. (2023) Distributed leadership in education: A systematic review of its role in fostering innovative practices and enhancing school performance. *International Journal of Science and Research, 12*(11), 4. Available at www.ijsr.net

Powell, M. (2019). Inquiries in the British National Health Service. *The Political Quarterly, 90*(2), 180–184. https://doi.org/10.1111/1467-923X.12696.

Quek, S. J., Thomson, L., Houghton, R., Bramley, L., Davis, S., & Cooper, J. (2021). Distributed leadership as a predictor of employee engagement, job satisfaction and turnover intention in UK nursing staff. *Journal of Nursing Management, 29*(6), 1544–1553. https://doi.org/10.1111/jonm.13321.

Recovery Research Institute. (2023). Community reinforcement approach (CRA). *Recovery Research Institute.* Retrieved 8th May 2023 from https://www.recoveryanswers.org/resource/community-reinforcement-approach-cra/.

SAMHSA (2012). SAMHSA's working definition of recovery. Retrieved from https://store.samhsa.gov/sites/default/files/pep12-recdef.pdf on 16th October 2024.

Santana, M. J., Manalili, K., Jolley, R. J., Zelinsky, S., Quan, H., & Lu, M. (2018). How to practice person-centred care: A conceptual framework. *Health Expectations, 21*(2), 429–440. https://doi.org/10.1111/hex.12640.

Sfantou, D. F., Laliotis, A., Patelarou, A. E., Sifaki-Pistolla, D., Matalliotakis, M., & Patelarou, E. (2017). Importance of leadership style towards quality of care measures in healthcare settings: A systematic review. *Healthcare, 5*(4), 73. https://doi.org/10.3390/healthcare5040073.

Sherwood, G. (2015). Perspectives: Nurses' expanding role in developing safety culture: Quality and safety education for nurses – competencies in action. *Journal of Research in Nursing, 23*(8), 734–740. https://dx. doi.org/10.1177/1744987115621142.

Spillane, J. P. (2005). Distributed leadership. *The Educational Forum, 69*(2), 143–150. https://doi.org/10.1080/00131720508984678.

The King's Fund. (2011). *The future of leadership and management in the NHS: No more heroes*. London: The King's Fund.

United Nations Development Programme (UNDP). (2017). *10 things UNDP does in disaster recovery.* New York: United Nations Development Programme.

Unterrainer, C., Jeppesen, H. J., & Jonsson, T. F. (2017). Distributed leadership agency and its relationship to individual autonomy and occupational self-efficacy: A two wave-mediation study in Denmark. *Humanistic Management Journal, 2*(1), 57–81. https://doi.org/10.1007/s41463-017-0023-9.

West, M., Armit, K., Loewenthal, L., Eckert, R., West, T., & Lee A. (2015). *Leadership and leadership development in health care: The evidence base*. London: The King's Fund.

World Health Organisation (WHO). (2005). *Preparing a health care workforce for the 21st century: The challenge of chronic conditions.* Geneva: World Health Organisation.

World Health Organisation (WHO). (2007). *People-centred health care: A policy framework.* Geneva: World Health Organisation.

World Health Organisation (WHO). (2015). *WHO global strategy on people-centred and health services: Interim report.* Geneva: World Health Organisation.

World Health Organisation (WHO). (2023). *Guidance on community mental health services: Promoting person-centred and rights-based approaches.* Geneva: World Health Organisation.

10

EARLY CHILDHOOD HOME VISITING – A COLLABORATIVE PERSON-CENTERED COMMUNITY APPROACH

Marion Byrne and Josephine Bleach

Introduction

Support programs have been used to assist the acquisition of parenting competencies, facilitating positive developmental practices, preventing and mitigating maltreatment and improving health outcomes (Mejdoubi, 2015; Eşkisu & Kapçı, 2021; Chan et al., 2021; Shanley et al., 2022; Brown et al., 2023). These programs focus on tailored support to individual families, identifying needs and linking with other services and resources. Despite some concerns regarding parental engagement (Whittaker & Cowley, 2012), such programs have generally demonstrated positive outcomes (Molloy et al., 2021; Brown et al., 2023). The delivery of programs can vary from individual sessions to group meetings or virtual modalities (Gagné et al., 2023; McKellar et al., 2023). They have also been targeted at underserved and at-risk communities, such as families experiencing homelessness (Sheller et al., 2018), ethnic groups (Osman et al., 2016; Andersson et al., 2024), equity-denied families (Komanchuk et al., 2024) or parents within the criminal justice system (Troy et al., 2018). It has been noted that people who lead parenting programs need to have certain competencies such as the ability to develop trusting relationships, good communication skills, openness and respect, being highly motivated and having knowledge to support the diverse issues parents require support in (Partain et al., 2019; Cohen et al., 2020). Moreover, parenting programs demonstrate positive impacts over time (Johnson et al., 2000; Gagné et al., 2023), although this depends on the quality of their implementation (Pinto et al., 2024). Within the programs, either paid workers or volunteers engage with families to map parenting supports to needs with a view to enhancing well-being. This approach concurs with community-centered approaches, particularly promoting families' control over their own lives, mobilizing social capital while promoting partnerships and leveraging community resources (Public Health England & NHS, 2015).

DOI: 10.4324/9781032662657-12

Parenting Programs in Ireland

In Ireland, the Community Mothers' Programme was established in 1983 in the former Eastern Health Board, offering a volunteer-led support system to families, particularly in disadvantaged areas. In 2019, the Community Mothers Programme was reviewed. Funding from the Sláintecare Integration Fund (a government fund to test and evaluate innovative models of care) and philanthropic donors led to the collaborative interagency development of an updated model, Community Families, which has also replaced the Area-Based Childhood (ABC) 0–2 Programme. The revised program aligns with key policy developments, including First 5: The Whole of Government Strategy for Babies, Young Children and Their Families (Department of Children, Equality, Disability, Integration and Youth [DCEDIY], 2018). Community Families deliberately puts parents and children first, empowering them through trusted relationships with their home visitor and the built-in flexibility to respond to all families and their unique needs and circumstances. A key aim is to empower families to develop confidence as they grow and build their local peer support networks, accessing supports and services within their local community. As such, Community Families leverages partnership approaches with families to empower parenting abilities and support children's health, development and well-being. Moreover, the program demonstrates how person and family-centered collaborations with communities can benefit all stakeholders. This chapter explores the co-production of an early years person-centered care support program, ABC 0–2 and subsequently the Community Families Programmes, in the context of evolving research, education, practice and policy at national and community level (see https://www.communityfamilies.ie/).

Background

The Community Mothers Programme was adapted from the Childhood Development Programme created by Dr Walter Barker of Bristol University in the United Kingdom (Johnson et al., 1993; 2000). The Bristol program highlighted that children in the participating families were more likely to have completed their primary and MMR immunizations, had better nutritional intake and received additional cognitive stimulation (Rowe et al., 1988). The children were also more likely to experience a more positive home learning environment, read books and visit the library regularly. With a strong evidence base, the Community Mothers Programme, at its peak, was delivered in 17 different communities across Ireland, providing support to 3,500 families each year (Brocklesby, 2019). In 2008, as the worldwide economic recession hit Ireland, there was a public service recruitment ban, and the public health nurses (PHNs) who coordinated the program on behalf of the health services executive Health Service Executive (HSE) were not replaced. This mainly impacted the greater Dublin area, while more rural areas, which were run by social services, now called Child and Family Services (Tusla), were impacted less. By 2013, program delivery was reduced to twelve communities, four managed by the HSE (three in Dublin and the fourth in Kerry) and eight managed by Tusla (all outside Dublin).

In 2014, the Irish Government, in partnership with Atlantic Philanthropies, launched the ABC Programme, which, through prevention and early intervention approaches, aimed to work in partnership with families, practitioners, communities, and national stakeholders to deliver better outcomes for children and families living in areas where poverty is most deeply entrenched. With the National College of Ireland (NCI) as the lead agency, a consortium of 48 organizations, who were already working collaboratively to address the deprivation within the area and improve outcomes for children, were awarded the contract to deliver the Dublin Docklands and East Inner City ABC Programme (ELI, 2015). As part of the application process, poor health outcomes (mental, physical, and general well-being) were identified as an issue within underserved families by the consortium. Additionally, challenges were recognized related to the lack of access to health information and advice on self-care, principally in relation to lifestyle, pregnancy, and childcare. These issues were particularly acute for parents with children from pre-birth to two years. Identifying a community-based need, PHNs in the area advocated for the (re)introduction of the Community Mothers Programme. At the time, there were licensing and centralized implementation support issues along with "programme fidelity drift", so this meant the national implementation support service for Community Mothers was not feasible. Working with local PHNs and the Clonmel Community Mothers Programme, who were delivering the program in South Tipperary, the ABC 0–2 Programme (which incorporated home visiting and parent support groups) was developed, with implementation commencing in September 2015. The home visiting team was recruited internally from experienced home visitors who undertook extensive training in early childhood development, nutrition and well-being. As noted previously, having facilitators with the requisite competencies is key to the program's quality, success and fidelity (Partain et al., 2019; Cohen et al., 2020).

Several contextual issues impacted the provision of and transformation in parenting support systems in Ireland; PHNs coordinating Community Mothers retired, HSE sites continued to close in Dublin, and the Tusla sites around the country experienced the impact of the country-wide recession. In addition, new research and emerging needs required the program to be standardized and updated. In 2019, a National Review of the Community Mothers Programme was conducted by the Katharine Howard Foundation (KHF) and the Community Foundation for Ireland. There was active participation of the HSE, Tusla and the remaining 12 Community Mothers sites, including the new ABC 0–2 Programme in the review (Brocklesby, 2019). A key recommendation was that a standardized national program model should be developed along with a strategy to ensure the sustainability and future development and governance of the updated program.

With funding from the Sláintecare Integration Fund and a private donor secured by NCI, the development of the standardized model and other key recommendations were progressed by the Tusla, HSE, KHF, NCI and the seven remaining sites from early 2020, leading to the creation of Community Families. In 2022, the National Community Families Oversight and Support Group, co-chaired by Tusla and the HSE, was established to support the transition of the original Community Mothers Programme sites, including the ABC 0–2 Programme, to Community Families and its continued roll-out, quality assurance and future development. A readiness assessment was completed in 2023 (Broderick, 2023) with the ABC 0–2 Programme fully transitioning to Community Families in 2024.

Principles, Aims and Objectives

The ABC 0–2 Programme was designed to meet the needs of children aged 0–2 years and their parents in the Dublin Docklands and East Inner City. Flexibility to respond to all families and their unique needs and circumstances was built into its initial design, thus reflecting the ethos of participation and the unique needs of families. Over the years, using a community action research approach (Bleach, 2016), the program evolved to adapt to emerging needs and changing contexts such as an increase in homelessness and waiting lists for key services, a local gangland feud and anti-refugee protests, as well as COVID-19. This demonstrates how communities have their own culture and the need for adaptability in applying bespoke approaches, modes of engagement and responses to individual needs. The three initial principles from which the aims and objectives have evolved were:

1 Person-centered care, which focused on partnerships, equity and mutuality of collaborations as key with the parent and child as the focus
2 Parents as the first and best educators of their children
3 Wrap-around interagency health and community signposting and referrals

The initial program aims were to:

- Support the special bond between parents and their children and recognize that this is at the core of subsequent child and family outcomes, from health and well-being to learning and succeeding in life.
- Improve children's lives by developing trusted relationships between experienced home visitors working in partnership with parents. This is done through home visiting and promoting the development of supportive community networks.

The initial objectives were to:

- Improve well-being, developmental and learning outcomes for children (0–2 years).
- Increase parental skills, knowledge, and engagement in all areas of their children's (0–2 years) development and learning.

- Ensure effective transitions for children (0–2 years) at key developmental stages and between home, hospital, early years, statutory and community services.
- Continue to improve the quality of the services (statutory, community and voluntary) provided to children (0–2 years) and their families.
- Enhance and develop the existing interagency collaboration within the area, including implementing the Meitheal Practice Model (see Cassidy et al., 2016).
- Enable children (0–2 years) and their families to experience a safe, secure, stable, caring, holistic, learning and restorative environment at home, in services (statutory, community and voluntary) and throughout the community.

Like the ABC 0–2 Programme, Community Families aspires to model strengths-based, non-judgmental relationships through all interactions, reflecting the person-centered philosophy of Rogers (1942) and Kitwood (1997). This focuses on a supportive, safe relationship with engagement, which leverages the strengths and positive attributes of the family to promote growth (Department of Health, 2017). This serves to increase the families' self-esteem and confidence in supporting their child's development. It is managed by home visitors or Community Mothers employed by the Health Service Executive, or community and voluntary organizations.

Developing the ABC 0–2 and Community Families Programme

This section examines the methodology used to develop both programs. The ABC 0–2 Programme was developed at the local level using community action research (Bleach, 2013, 2016), while the Community Families Programme was developed at the national level using a participatory co-production action learning approach (Pettican et al., 2022).

ABC 0–2 Programme

The development of the ABC 0–2 Programme consisted of several phases. Phase 1 encompassed an initial survey of need (Dartington Social Research Unit, 2006). The survey was completed by NCI before establishing the Early Learning Initiative (ELI), the lead agency of the Dublin Docklands and East Inner City ABC Programme. The survey findings demonstrated that while local parents had high educational aspirations for their children, they did not understand their pivotal role in realizing this and were not confident that they had the skills to support their children's learning. With support for parents as the primary educators of their children a priority, involving local people as co-constructors of programs (Bleach, 2013) and in the decision-making processes was perceived as key to educational change. As a result, a community action research (Bleach, 2016) approach was chosen to develop ELI's programs. This approach aligns with the principles of person-centered care at the community level, as it focuses on increasing community capacity (Dombroski et al., 2025). Acknowledging, respecting and utilizing the expertise and experience within the local families and communities is at the heart of the cyclical process, which revolves around stakeholders coming together to deliver high-quality services and share their learning. Over the past ten years, the process has evolved from a simplistic "plan, do, review" model (Lewin, 1946) into a developmental process of incremental change, informed by data and judgment that has led to the significant cumulative evolution of our theory, practice and programs (Patton, 1994). These changes are the result of a multitude of "dynamic conversations" (Schön, 1983) at each stage of the process through the systematic involvement of children, parents and front-line service delivery staff in all aspects of program planning, implementation and evaluation (Bleach, 2024). This mirrors the process described in Chapter 3 related to community profiling.

In phase 2 (September 2014), the ABC 0–2 years Working Group, consisting of representatives of the PHNs, social workers, maternity hospitals, family resource centers and the ParentChild+ Home Visiting team was established to develop the program with a coordinator employed in March 2015 (ELI, 2015). A retired PHN, who was involved with the Community Mothers Programme previously, was employed to support the coordinator in delivering the program, as well as training and supervising the home visitors. Home visitors were local women trained and employed by NCI to support parents in their own homes (Bleach, 2024). Building on previous experiences, learning visits were made to other Community Mothers Programmes in Dublin, while Tusla enabled the liaison with the rural Community Mothers sites in Clonmel, Nenagh, Athlone and Limerick, all of whom were willing to share their expertise and experience. The ABC 0–2 Home Visiting Programme began in September 2015 with 7 families, rising to 24 families later that year (ELI, 2016). Reflecting the growth of the program, in 2023–2024, 168 families were visited with 798 families attending group sessions, reflecting the growth in referrals, emerging needs, waiting lists for services and an increased culture of engagement by families.

In order to measure the effectiveness of a program, the ELI employs indicative evidence based on the following criteria: satisfaction rates, participation/attendance, aspirations and learning (Veerman & van Yperen, 2007). The results are compared to Irish national norms, the baseline data in the Evaluation Reports by the Children's Research Centre, Trinity College (Share et al., 2011), along with previous data collected through community action research processes. Gathered systematically, over several action research cycles, this data is used to provide indicative evidence of effectiveness and causality. This cumulative approach to knowledge generation (Blamey & Mackenzie, 2007) means that theory accumulates slowly within and across action research cycles rather than delivering "big bang" answers to questions of program effectiveness.

The tools used to evaluate the ABC 0–2 Home Visiting Programmes were:

- Attendance Records are kept of both intake and home visits.
- Progress Notes are completed by the home visitor after each visit.

- Participant Observations comprising comments made through informal feedback or interviews.
- Exit interviews are completed by parents and the home visitor when the program ends.
- Child and Parent Observations are completed by the home visitor within the first 2/3 visits and every 12 weeks thereafter. It tracks the well-being and development of the participating children and their parents as they progress through the program.

Community Families

In 2019, the ABC 0–2 Programme became involved with a National Review of the Community Mothers Programme, undertaken by Susan Brocklesby on behalf of the Katharine Howard Foundation and The Community Foundation for Ireland (Brocklesby, 2019). It recommended the development of an updated standardized national program. From early 2020, with support from the Sláintecare Integration Fund and NCI philanthropic donors, the Community Families Programme was developed using a participatory action learning approach and a collective iterative process. Structured reviews, consultative workshops, participant (including parents) interviews, observations and feedback were core methods for refining the program. The continuous engagement and sustained commitment of key national and local organizations, including the HSE, Tusla, KHF, NCI and 7 of the original Community Mothers sites, was central to successful co-production.

Content and Delivery

A universal, prevention-focused home visiting program, the ABC 0–2 Programme supports families to improve children's (from pre-birth to two years of age) well-being, developmental and learning outcomes while increasing parental skills, knowledge, and engagement. While the program's aims and objectives remain the same, the program content and delivery methods have evolved. Initially, the HSE *Caring for your Baby* booklet, which is distributed by the PHNs to all parents on the birth of their baby, was used by the home visitors to share knowledge and reinforce key health messages. In 2019, this was replaced with the more up-to-date My Child.ie website and booklet. With more knowledge of the impact of adverse childhood experiences and the increase in violence in the marginalized areas across the country, in particular Dublin's North-East Inner City (NEIC), there has been an increasing emphasis on infant and parental mental health and well-being, including the introduction of baby massage, restorative parenting, and trauma-informed practice. In 2018–2019, with an increase in the number of families living in homeless accommodation in the NEIC, a complementary *My Place to Play* program was developed in partnership with Tusla Partnership, Prevention and Family Support and the Children and Young People's Services Committee (CYPSC) (ELI, 2019). *My Place to Play* aims to enhance parent-baby interactions and children's physical (tummy time), emotional (sense of safety, well-being and belonging), cognitive and language development for infants living in homeless, emergency or overcrowded accommodation. For the general program, a home visitor is allocated to each family; the program takes place in the child's own home at a time that suits the parents/guardians. Visits last about an hour, with children up to three months receiving weekly visits. Depending on need, older children receive monthly visits. During the visit, the home visitor discusses how the parent and child are doing and what, if any, support is required. The HSE *My Child* Materials are used as a guide, with other materials provided as needed. Home visitors attend weekly supervision sessions with the program coordinator to reflect on their previous week's visits and plan the following week's visits. While visits with families are normally held face-to-face in person in the home, this provision has evolved over the years to accommodate diverse family circumstances. For example, where the current living situations are not suitable, visits are held in public places such as libraries and community centers. Moreover, the program adapted to contextual issues as with the introduction of COVID-19 restrictions in March 2020, virtual "home visits" via video/phone calls were introduced as well as socially distanced outdoor visits.

With interagency collaboration a key feature of the program, the home visiting team works in partnership with PHNs, Tusla Family Support Practitioners and other relevant professionals to provide continuity of care and reinforce key messages. Good relationships with social workers, homeless hubs and direct provision centers ensure that the most vulnerable families are supported. The increase in the diversity of the families engaging in the program has strengthened the existing interagency collaborations, referral pathways and signposting. The establishment of and our engagement in child and family, infant mental health, multi-disciplinary networks and partnerships with families help ensure that there is integrated wrap-around supports in place for children and families. Follow-on supports have been developed with most parents transferring into parent support groups, while others transfer into the more targeted ParentChild+ Home Visiting Programmes.

On average, 130 families receive 1,300 visits annually, with 1,083 in-home visits, 90 outdoor visits, and 63 video calls in 2022/2023 (ELI, 2023). Families may also exchange text messages with their home visitor between visits. Around 60% of referrals are from professionals, with the remainder recommendations from family members, friends or neighbors. In addition to home visits, families are encouraged to attend a wide range of community parent support groups and events with 600+ families involved each year. Participation in the program reflects the diversity of the catchment area with families from many different living and ethnic situations. This diversity is evidenced in the location of our home visits, which have taken place in many different living situations, e.g., apartments, flats complexes, direct provision and emergency accommodation.

This case study, compiled by the ELI ABC 0–2 team in 2024, reflects the complexity of delivery and referral networks for some families.

> A young mother and her 3-month-old baby living in emergency accommodation were referred to the programme by a Family Support Worker. Mam was very down and withdrawn at the start. Over time, the home visitor built the relationship with Mam as they discussed on a weekly basis how she and the baby were doing. Lots of encouragement and support were provided. Attending Meitheal (Irish interagency process) meetings helped the home visitor understand the family's situation and plan the content of visits around Mam and baby's needs e.g., providing a weaning pack and showing Mam how to make nutritious food for her baby with limited resources. The home visitor also encouraged Mam to take the baby to the groups ELI runs in the community and she even went with Mam to look for a creche place. Over time, Mam was able to get support for her mental health and in time the family got their own flat [apartment]. The home visitor continued to connect with Mam, supporting her to set up a play space for the baby in their new home. When the child was two years of age, the 0–2 Coordinator linked the family with the ELI's Parent Child+ Home Visiting programme.

Impact

Starting with seven families in 2015, over 600 families have engaged with the program to date. Feedback has been very positive. Of the 391 parents who completed evaluation forms, 99% ($N = 386$) found the program useful/beneficial and were happy to recommend it to a friend. Ninety-eight percent ($N = 385$) of parents reported learning new approaches and ideas from their home visitor and felt confident in using these. In reporting specifically on what they learnt from engaging in the program, parents noted practical tips around playing and interacting with their baby, including tummy time and sensory play, tips on supporting their child's development, and tips on caring for their baby, including sleep and nutrition.

Participant Observations

Comments (taken from ELI End of Year Reports) from participants over the years reflect the value and impact of the support to parents. The first three quotes reflect the changes in thinking and behavior of the parents, whereby they began to believe in themselves, manage their feelings and the stressors involved with having a new baby. They also learnt how to talk, interact and play differently with their baby.

> I learnt that it was great to trust my own instincts rather than following a rulebook. I learnt a lot about play and child development. I think the support offered was great. It was a very specific time to think about what is working or not.
>
> *[Parents, 2016]*

> How to keep calm, got to enjoy my child's different stages of his development. Got great breastfeeding advice, done lots of activities and floor time and when he was asleep, the home visitor was a great support for me. I was able to have great conversations with her and often got to offload to her about my motherly concerns and other things. I loved that the visits were baby, parent-led which resulted in a lovely, relaxed atmosphere during each session and made me feel confident in my own ability.
>
> *[Parents, 2018]*

> I've learnt how to speak to my baby in a tone that makes her respond. Also using the technique wait/respond/wait. I've noticed that when my home visitor comes by baby is very attentive to her- quiet and calm tone. So, I was able to adapt it and get the most of our time together with my baby.
>
> *[Parents, 2019]*

Social isolation was huge for many parents, so being supported by the home visitors to meet other parents was important for their mental health and well-being.

> This programme helped me to cope with the pressure as a new mam and supported me during my Maternity leave which actually impacts all mams mentally. It helped me to meet other mams and build a circle to share the challenges I am facing. And it is great way for my little one to engage with other babies in different kind of sessions.
>
> *[Parent, 2022]*

The trusted relationship where they felt listened to and valued with their home visitor was really appreciated by the parents. They found the information provided helpful, as was the opportunity to ask questions that were relevant to them in their situation.

> ELI program was our source of trust besides our PHN for setting us up as new parents who respect, care and develop her child's physical and cognitive development. We had the chance to work with our home visitor, she is a great listener, an engaging trainer, a curious mind who always guides, encourages, champions, and motivates us.
>
> *[Parent, 2021]*

> The home visitor was an amazing. We really bonded with her, and our baby loved her. She gave us so much tips as we were new parents and always complimented us every time and in every way she can. I hope we can continue the relationship/ bond that we have formed with her and our family. Thank you, ELI. This is a great initiative. Keep it up!
>
> *[Parent, 2023]*

Child and Parent Observation Tool

The Child and Parent Observation Tool was developed in 2018–2019 to track the well-being and development of the participating children and their parents as they progress through the ABC program. The 1st Observation is completed after the 4th visit; the 2nd Observation is completed after the 12th visit, and the remaining stages of observations are completed every 12 visits thereafter. Due to the universal nature of the program, whereby all new parents in the catchment area are eligible participants, those who remain on the program for longer periods tend to be those most at-risk, which influences the average scores as the more vulnerable families progress throughout the observation stages. Table 10.1, compiled by the ELI team, presents the average percentage scores over the period 2020–2023, when delivery was impacted by COVID-19 lockdowns, with virtual delivery and outdoor visits the norm in 2020–2021. By 2023, we had reverted to home visits with some virtual and outdoor visits.

As can be seen from the findings, there is a consistent need for social support for parents who live in isolation within the Inner City. Due to the process of gentrification, we have found that the influx of the young, educated workforce has resulted in a high number of first-time parents who are away from their own families and lacking a system of social supports. It is also concerning that 30% of the parents reported health issues themselves. The biggest impact was the growth in parents' knowledge and confidence throughout the program, along with their responsiveness to their baby's cues. While most children were healthy, developing

TABLE 10.1 Home visitor parent and child observations

	*Observation 1**	*Observation 2**	*Observation 3**	*Observation 4***
	***N* = 313**	***N* = 258**	***N* = 111**	***N* = 51**
* Universal Plus (Levels 1–3); ** Most vulnerable families (Levels 2–3)				
Parent observations by home visitor				
Social support	36%	36%	44%	35%
Isolated	30%	30%	25%	34%
Health	56%	65%	52%	65%
Warmth	93%	97%	99%	98%
Responsiveness	83%	92%	89%	95%
Knowledge	35%	46%	66%	76%
Confidence	56%	66%	66%	73%
Child observations by home visitor				
Responds to parent appropriately	81%	86%	85%	89%
Developing as expected	87%	89%	91%	83%
Healthy	91%	95%	89%	92%
Appropriate diet	90%	91%	87%	93%

as expected, responding to parents appropriately, and on a suitable diet when entering the program, the percentages, apart from developing as expected, remained consistent, despite the most vulnerable families remaining on the program after Observation 2. Similar to Finello et al. (2016) regarding other home visiting programs, the findings from ABC 0–2 Programme evaluations over the years appear to indicate that it has improved the lives of parents and children involved, creating all-around healthier and happier families. As the Community Families Programme is relatively new, its findings will be available in October 2025.

Discussion

Families with children in the ABC 0–2 parenting support program represent a diverse community, yet the application of this program was flexible enough to adapt to the contexts of the families' lives. In particular, the engagement, participation, and empowerment approaches demonstrate a mutual collaboration that respects the individuality and autonomy of the families receiving the service. Over the past ten years, there have been big changes in early childhood home visiting at both the local and national levels. When observing outcomes agreed in 2014 for the ABC 0–2 Programme, much has been achieved. Early identification of children's well-being, health, welfare and developmental needs enables more children to reach their developmental milestones with more support developed for those with additional needs. Parents' active engagement in supporting their children's well-being, development and learning ensures that they feel happier, more confident, informed and competent in their parenting role. Effective interagency partnerships have resulted in increased uptake in child health clinic attendances, better immunization rates and uptake of other well-being-related appointments. It has also enabled us to collaboratively address emerging challenges such as the 2016 violent gangland feud, COVID-19, the 2023 refugee crisis, along with significant increases in the number of children under two years in homeless and emergency accommodation and/or on waiting lists for disability services (Bleach, 2024).

Like other similar programs, the ABC 0–2 Home Visiting Programme was founded on the principle that parents are the key to positive change for their children (Sweet & Appelbaum, 2004). As it is usually delivered in the home, the program allows for a safe, natural environment in which home visitors can fully grasp the level of support needed by the family (Leirbakk et al., 2018) and foster the family's self-efficacy abilities. While there can be challenges with retaining and engaging families, particularly in diverse marginalized communities, focusing on relationships and parental experiences improves program quality and promotes success (Cho et al., 2017; Latimore et al., 2017). Taking parental feedback into consideration and ensuring home visitors have access to up-to-date, culturally informed (McMillin & Carbone, 2020) training and continuous professional development opportunities increases parental satisfaction (Latimore et al., 2017; Peacock et al., 2013) and engagement as partners in the process.

Employing local people as home visitors is also critical to the engagement and ownership by the local community (Bleach, 2024). Easily recognizable in their distinctive uniforms, the home visitors are the ambassadors for education and parent support on the street and in communities and provide an accessible point of contact, information, and referral for families. Moreover, reflecting the multitude of family diversity in communities, employing a home visitor who can speak the same language as the parents has increased the engagement of those parents.

This project is a good example of a future-oriented, policy-focused prevention and early intervention initiative, where practice, research and policy intersect in the collaborative strategic planning and transformation of an evidence-based early childhood home visiting program. It highlights the importance of dedicated champions, infrastructures, and resources at the national and local level to ensure sustained quality implementation, continued program efficacy and long-term positive outcomes for children and families. Capacity building through training, consultative workshops and communities of practice was important. Upskilling in scaling programs and emerging theories on child development, infant mental health and trauma-informed practice enabled us to innovate and incorporate these improvements into policy, programs and practice. Bringing national and local stakeholders together built relationships of trust and enabled us all to think differently, act differently, and relate to one another differently (Kemmis, 2009) in the best interests of children, parents and families.

At the national level, early childhood home visiting is now perceived as an essential local peer-led prevention and early intervention community lifeline for children and parents. It has been aligned with key Irish Government policies, including First 5, Sláintecare and Young Ireland, and incorporated into Tusla's Parenting Support Strategy and HSE's Women's and Infants, Health and Wellbeing initiatives, including Disability, Mental Health and Healthy Childhood Programmes. Through the First Five Strategy (DCEDIY, 2018), a national home visiting program office has been established in Tusla, and we are hopeful that a publicly funded national model will be agreed with Community Families scaled up across the country.

Conclusion

Change is a complex, analytical, political and cultural process of challenging and modifying the core beliefs, structure and strategy of a community (Pettigrew, 1987). This chapter has presented an example of a person-centered community-based family support initiative, where practice and policy are interconnected to develop an evidence-based early childhood home visiting program. Aligned with national policy, First Five, the journey from Community Mothers (1983) to the ABC 0–2 (2014) to Community Families (2024) highlights the importance of joint national and local partnerships, voices and ownership with all involved, professionals and parents, taking responsibility for the health and well-being of children. It also highlights the value and complexity of action research and learning, whereby programs adopt an individual-tailored approach, which enables self-efficacy and competencies in creating positive environments for children, at home and in their community.

References

Andersson, E., McIlduff, C., Turner, K. M. T., Carter, E., Hand, M., Thomas, S., Davies, J., Einfeld, S., & Elliott, E. J. (2024). Jandu Yani U (for all families): evaluating Indigenous Triple P, a community-tailored parenting support program in remote Aboriginal communities. *Australian Psychologist, 59*(3), 245–259. https://doi.org/10.1080/00050067.2023.2267159

Axford, N., & Whear, R. (2006). National College of Ireland early learning for children in North Docklands: Report of findings. In *Darlington Social Research Unit*. National College of Ireland. Retrieved from https://library.ncirl.ie/items/28372?query=Unit%29&resultsUri=items%3Fquery%3DUnit%2529%26offset%3D10

Blamey, A., & Mackenzie, M. (2007). Theories of change and realistic evaluation. *Evaluation, 13*(4), 439–455. https://doi.org/10.1177/1356389007082129

Bleach, J. (2013). Improving educational aspirations and outcomes through community action research. *Educational Action Research, 21*(2), 253–266. https://doi.org/10.1080/09650792.2013.789726

Bleach, J. (2017). Community action research in Ireland: improving educational outcomes through collaboration in the Dublin docklands. In: Rowell, L., Bruce, C., Shosh, J., Riel, M. (eds) *The Palgrave International Handbook of Action Research*. Palgrave Macmillan, New York. https://doi.org/10.1057/978-1-137-40523-4_11

Bleach, J. (2024). *Early Childhood Home Visiting- a Critical lifeline for families in Dublin's Inner City. - Jesuit Centre for Faith and Justice in Ireland.* Jesuit Centre for Faith and Justice in Ireland. Retrieved from https://www.jcfj.ie/article/early-childhood-home-visiting-a-critical-lifeline-for-families-in-dublins-inner-city/

Bleach, J., & Brocklesby, S. (2023). *"Early Childhood Home Visiting in Ireland"*. Education Matters Yearbook. Retrieved from https://irelandseducationyearbook.ie/downloads/IEYB2023/Irelands%20Yearbook%20of%20Education%202023%20-%20Early%20Childhood-7.pdf.

Brocklesby, S. (2019). *A National Review of the Community Mothers Programme.* Katherine Howard Foundation. Retrieved from https://www.khf.ie/community-mothers-programme/

Broderick, S. (2023). *Report on Readiness Assessment for Community Families* 2023. Unpublished Manuscript. National College of Ireland.

Brown, S., McConnell, L., Zelaya, A., Doran, M., & Swarr, V. (2023). Tailored nurse support program promoting positive parenting and family preservation. *Nursing Research, 72*(4), E164–E171. https://doi.org/10.1097/NNR.0000000000000662

Cassidy, A., Devaney, C., & McGregor, C. (2016) *Early Implementation of Meitheal and the Child and Family Support Networks: Lessons from the Field.* The UNESCO Child and Family Research Centre, The National University of Ireland, Galway.

Chan, S. W. Y., Rao, N., Cohrssen, C., & Richards, B. (2021). Predicting child outcomes in Bhutan: Contributions of parenting support and early childhood education programmes. *Children & Youth Services Review, 126*, N.PAG. https://doi.org/10.1016/j.childyouth.2021.106051

Cho, J., Terris, D. D., Glisson, R. E., Bae, D., & Brown, A. (2017). Beyond family demographics, community risk influences maternal engagement in home visiting. *Journal of Child and Family Studies, 26*(11), 3203–3213. https://doi.org/10.1007/s10826-017-0803–8

Cohen, F., Trauernicht, M., Francot, R., Broekhuizen, M., & Anders, Y. (2020). Professional competencies of practitioners in family and parenting support programmes. A German and Dutch case study. *Children & Youth Services Review, 116*, N.PAG. https://doi.org/10.1016/j.childyouth.2020.105202

Department of Health (2017). *Strengths-Based Social Work Practice with Adults.* DoH, London.

Department of Children, Equality, Disability, Integration and Youth. (2018). *First 5: A Whole-of-Government Strategy for Babies, Young Children and their Families* 2019–*2028.* Retrieved from https://www.gov.ie/en/publication/f7ca04-first-5-a-whole-of-government-strategy-for-babies-young-children-and/

Dombroski, K., Shiels, R., & Watkinson, H. (2025). Curating life in vacant spaces: Community action research and reversing the process of academic knowledge-making. *Gateways: International Journal of Community Research and Engagement, 18*(1), 1–17.

Early Learning Initiative (ELI). (2015). *End of Year Report 2014–15.* Unpublished Manuscript. National College of Ireland. Retrieved from https://www.ncirl.ie/Portals/0/Users/030/30/30/ELI%20End-of-Year%20Report%20%202014-15%20Summary.pdf

Early Learning Initiative (ELI) (2016). *End of Year Report 2015–16.* Unpublished Manuscript. National College of Ireland. Retrieved from https://www.ncirl.ie/Research/ELI-Research#6605594-reports

Early Learning Initiative (ELI) (2017). *End of Year Report 2016–17.* Unpublished Manuscript. National College of Ireland. Retrieved from https://www.ncirl.ie/Portals/0/Users/030/30/30/ELI%20Summary%20%20Annual%20Report%20%202016-17.pdf

Early Learning Initiative (ELI) (2023). *End of Year Report 2022–23.* Unpublished Manuscript. National College of Ireland. Retrieved from https://www.ncirl.ie/Portals/0/ELI/ELI%20Annual%20Reports/ELI%20End%20of%20Year%20Report%202022-23%20final.pdf

Eşkisu, M., & Kapçı, E. G. (2021). Efficacy of the parenting support program on child behavior problems. *Scandinavian Journal of Psychology, 62*(4), 449–459. https://doi.org/10.1111/sjop.12726

Finello, K. M., Terteryan, A., & Riewerts, R. J. (2016). Home visiting programs: what the primary care clinician should know. *Current Problems in Paediatric and Adolescent Health Care, 46*(4), 101–125. https://doi.org/10.1016/j.cppeds.2015.12.011

Gagné, M.-H., Brunson, L., Piché, G., Drapeau, S., Paradis, H., & Terrault, Z. (2023). Effectiveness of the Triple P program on parental stress and self-efficacy in the context of a community roll-out. *Journal of Child & Family Studies, 32*(10), 3090–3105. https://doi.org/10.1007/s10826-023-02663-4

Johnson, Z., Howell, F., & Molloy, B. (1993). Community mothers' programme: randomised controlled trial of non-professional intervention in parenting. *British Medical Journal, 306*(6890), 1449–1452. https://doi.org/10.1136/bmj.306.6890.1449

Johnson, Z., Molloy, B., Scallan, E., Fitzpatrick, P., Rooney, B., Keegan, T., & Byrne, P. (2000). Community mothers programme - seven-year follow-up of a randomized controlled trial of non-professional intervention in parenting. *Journal of Public Health Medicine, 22*(3), 337–342. https://doi.org/10.1093/pubmed/22.3.337

Kemmis, S. (2009). Action research as a practice-based practice. *Educational Action Research, 17*(3), 463–474. https://doi.org/10.1080/09650790903093284

Kitwood, T. (1997) *Dementia Reconsidered.* Open University Press, London.

Komanchuk, J., Letourneau, N., Duffett-Leger, L., Healy, P., Very, M., Huang, Z., Zheng, Z., & Cameron, J. L. (2024). Evaluation of the online first pathways program for equity-denied families: a randomized controlled trial. *Journal of Child & Family Studies, 33*(11), 3440–3454. https://doi.org/10.1007/s10826-024-02932-w

Latimore, A. D., Burrell, L., Crowne, S., Ojo, K., Cluxton-Keller, F., Gustin, S., Kruse, L., Hellman, D., Scott, L., Riordan, A., & Duggan, A. (2017). Exploring multilevel factors for family engagement in home visiting across two national models. *Prevention Science: The Official Journal of the Society for Prevention Research, 18*(5), 577–589. https://doi.org/10.1007/s11121-017-0767-3

Leirbakk, M. J., Torper, J., Engebretsen, E., Opsahl, J. N., Zeanah, P., & Magnus, J. H. (2018). Formative research in the development of a salutogenic early intervention home visiting program integrated in public child health service in a multiethnic population in Norway. *BMC Health Services Research, 18*(1), 741. https://doi.org/10.1186/s12913-018-3544–5

Lewin, K. (1946) Action research and minority problems. *Journal of Social Issues, 2*(4), 34–46.

McKellar, L., Eden, A., De Sousa Machado, T., Adelson, P., Stoodley, C., & Steen, M. (2023). #Parentlife: a feasibility study to explore a novel virtual early parenting programme. *MIDIRS Midwifery Digest, 33*(2), 177–182.

McMillin, S. E., & Carbone, J. T. (2020). A skillset and a stance: program planning for cultural competence and cultural humility in home visitation. *Evaluation and Program Planning, 81*, 101819. https://doi.org/10.1016/j.evalprogplan.2020.101819

Mejdoubi, J., van den Heijkant, S. C., van Leerdam, F. J., Heymans, M. W., Crijnen, A., & Hirasing, R. A. (2015). The effect of VoorZorg, the Dutch nurse-family partnership, on child maltreatment and development: a randomized controlled trial. *PLOS ONE, 10*, e0120182. https://doi.org/10.1371/journal.pone.0120182

Molloy, C., Beatson, R., Harrop, C., Perini, N., & Goldfeld, S. (2021). Systematic review: effects of sustained nurse home visiting programs for disadvantaged mothers and children. *Journal of Advanced Nursing, 77*, 147–161.

Osman, F., Klingberg-Allvin, M., Flacking, R., & Schön, U.-K. (2016). Parenthood in transition -- Somali-born parents' experiences of and needs for parenting support programmes. *BMC International Health & Human Rights, 16*, 1–11. https://doi.org/10.1186/s12914-016-0082-2

Partain, P. I., Kumbamu, A., Asiedu, G. B., Cristiani, V., Deling, M., Weis, C., & Lynch, B. (2019). Evaluation of community programs for early childhood development: parental perspectives and recommendations. *Maternal & Child Health Journal, 23*(1), 120–130. https://doi.org/10.1007/s10995-018-2601–3

Patton, M. Q. (1994). Developmental evaluation. *Evaluation Practice, 15*(3), 311–319. https://doi.org/10.1177/109821409401500312

Peacock, S., Konrad, S., Watson, E., Nickel, D., & Muhajarine, N. (2013). Effectiveness of home visiting programs on child outcomes: a systematic review. *BMC Public Health, 13*(1). https://doi.org/10.1186/1471–2458-13–17

Pettican, A., Goodman, B., Bryant, W., Beresford, P., Freeman, P., Gladwell, V., Kilbride, C., & Speed, E. (2022). Doing together: reflections on facilitating the co-production of participatory action research with marginalised populations. *Qualitative Research in Sport, Exercise and Health, 15*(2), 202–219. https://doi.org/10.1080/2159676X.2022.2146164

Pettigrew, A. M. (1987). Context and action in the transformation of the firm. *Journal of Management Sciences, 24*(6), 649–670.

Pinto, R., Canário, C., Leijten, P., Rodrigo, M. J., & Cruz, O. (2024). Implementation of parenting programs in real-world community settings: a scoping review. *Clinical Child & Family Psychological Review, 27*(1), 74–90. https://doi.org/10.1007/s10567-023-00465-0

Public Health England & NHS (2015). *A Guide to Community-Centred Approaches for Health and Wellbeing.* PHE, London.

Rogers, C. (1942). *Counseling and Psychotherapy: Newer Concepts in Practice*. Houghton Mifflin Company, New York.

Rowe, G., Sutcliffe, D., & Barker, W. (1988). *Community Health and the Child Development Programme.* University of Bristol, Bristol.

Schön, D. (1983). *The Reflective Practitioner. How Professionals Think in Action.* Temple Smith, London.

Shanley, J. R., Musyimi, C., Armistead, L. P., Mutiso, V., Hunsinger, M., & Ndetei, D. (2022). Supporting parents' abilities to care for their young children: initial testing of a newly adapted parenting program for delivery in Kenya. *International Journal of Child Health & Human Development, 15*(1), 53–62.

Share, M., McCarthy, S., & Greene, S. (2011). *Final Report, Baseline Evaluation of the Early Learning Initiative*. National College of Ireland. Retrieved from https://norma.ncirl.ie/1005/1/Evaluation_Final_Report.pdf

Sheller, S. L., Hudson, K. M., Bloch, J. R., Biddle, B., Krauthamer Ewing, E. S., & Slaughter-Acey, J. C. (2018). Family care curriculum: A parenting support program for families experiencing homelessness. *Maternal & Child Health Journal, 22*(9), 1247–1254. https://doi.org/10.1007/s10995-018-2561-7

Sweet, M. A., & Appelbaum, M. I. (2004). Is home visiting an effective strategy? A meta-analytic review of home visiting programs for families with young children. *Child Development, 75*(5), 1435–1456. https://doi.org/10.1111/j.1467–8624.2004.00750.x

Troy, V., McPherson, K. E., Emslie, C., & Gilchrist, E. (2018). The feasibility, appropriateness, meaningfulness, and effectiveness of parenting and family support programs delivered in the criminal justice system: a systematic review. *Journal of Child & Family Studies, 27*(6), 1732–1747. https://doi.org/10.1007/s10826-018-1034-3

Veerman, J. W., & van Yperen, T. A. (2007). Degrees of freedom and degrees of certainty: a developmental model for the establishment of evidence-based youth care. *Evaluation and Program Planning, 30*(2), 212–221. https://doi.org/10.1016/j.evalprogplan.2007.01.011

Whittaker, K. A., & Cowley, S. (2012). An effective programme is not enough: a review of factors associated with poor attendance and engagement with parenting support programmes. *Children & Society, 26*(2), 138–149. https://doi.org/10.1111/j.1099–0860.2010.00333.x

11

THIRD AGE

Celebrating Community

Anne Dempsey

Introduction

The principles of person-centered care are based on a non-hierarchical collaborative approach to enrich one's life. Centrally, this encompasses supporting individuals to maximize their potential and support their knowledge, skills and confidence (Health Foundation, 2016). As person-centered care has evolved, it has developed in five domains:

1 Policy development for transformation
2 Participatory strategies for public engagement
3 Healthcare integration and coordination strategies
4 Frameworks for practice
5 Process and outcome measurement (Phelan et al., 2020)

In recent years, these principles have transcended health and social care environments and have underpinned approaches in many community organizations. As described in Chapter 3, community-centered care pivots on identifying local needs and working with communities to identify and implement responses. This concurs with the Irish Government's (Government of Ireland, 2019) aim to foster a vibrant and active civil society with resilient communities. Predominantly working with an older population, Third Age is one such organization that has embraced the ethos of partnership, engagement and valuing everyone as an equal member of society while concurrently working with older people as a societal subgroup. This chapter applies a case study approach to community-centered care and examines how Third Age brings the model of person-centered care into the communities it serves by developing programs in which service users have an active say and can

DOI: 10.4324/9781032662657-13

influence service direction. In Third Age, each program and activity is created and developed in response to an identified community need.

Third Age

Established in 1988, Third Age is a community and voluntary organization working for, with and on behalf of older people. Third Age reaches out to thousands of people in Ireland each year with a range of socially useful programs at national, regional and local levels. A unique aspect of the organization's work is its volunteer ethos – trained older volunteers provide services for peers in a way that enhances the lives of giver and receiver alike. The work of Third Age also demonstrates the continuing potential and value of older people in responding to the diverse needs in their local communities.

The work of Third Age takes place against an aging demographic. Population projections point to a growth in demand for effective support for older people. The global estimates of demographic change suggest a rising older population (United Nations (UN), 2022a; World Health Organization (WHO), 2022). Similarly, in Ireland, the number of people aged 65 years and over is estimated to have risen by over 40% between 2013 and 2023, from 569,000 to 806,000, and is expected to double again to 1.6 million by 2051 (CSO, 2012, 2024). The most rapid growth rate is predicted in the over-85-years' age cohort. Internationally, we are seeing an increase in the number of older people living alone, many experiencing loneliness and social isolation (WHO, ITU, UN & Department of Economic & Social Affairs, 2021; Berlingieri et al., 2023). Loneliness describes a personal sense of being alone or a sense that one is not sufficiently wanted or needed. Social isolation includes an absence of social interactions, a lack of social support structures and poor engagement with friends or family (Ward et al., 2019).

Third Age takes a holistic approach to aging, focusing on services to help older people age better and providing them with responses to challenges and choices that influence mental and physical health. Ultimately, Third Age is focused on supporting people to embrace aging as an opportunity. In this regard, the organization works with the full spectrum of the older population, from active volunteers to more marginalized adults who require support mapped to individual need. Headquartered in Summerhill, County Meath, Ireland, Third Age provides local members with creative outlets and offers opportunities to take on new challenges through the development and delivery of activities and services within dedicated programs.

Three main programs are overseen by Third Age. The initial national program, SeniorLine, offers a national confidential listening service for older people. Lines are open every day of the year from 10 am to 10 pm with a Freephone number to discuss concerns or to seek conversation and support. A second national program, Fáilte Isteach[1] offers free language classes and integration support for migrants, international protection applicants and refugees. This program has grown and expanded to 3,500 trained tutors working in 296 communities nationwide. The third program, AgeWell, supports older people in County Meath, Ireland, to remain safe and healthy at home, promoting aging in place for as long as possible, providing early intervention if needed and helping to reduce the burden on acute emergency and long-term care.

Third Age founder Mary Nally retired as CEO in 2013 and Áine Brady, a former Teachta Dála (T.D. member of the Irish Parliament) and Minister for Older People and Health Promotion, was then appointed to the role. Under her guidance, the organization implemented a review of protocols, governance, management, reporting structures and responsibilities. This was supported by funding from The Atlantic Philanthropies, a private philanthropic foundation, to develop an Innovation Hub to screen and test new projects. The investment in innovation, quality assurance and governance allowed Third Age to pilot and evaluate potential new services in response to the age sector needs. This approach has informed service development in recent years.

Beginnings

In 1988, there were few activities or opportunities for older people in Summerhill village (County Meath, Ireland) – "there is nothing to do unless you like bingo" was one comment. Building on meeting local community needs, a local resident, Mary Nally, called a meeting to discuss how the quality of life could be improved for local older people and the Summerhill Active Retirement Association (S.A.R.A.) was born. The fledgling group had no premises and met informally for some years. In 1993, the European Year of Older People, the North-Eastern Health Board provided the Summerhill retirement group with a small, prefabricated building in the village and S.A.R.A. was registered as the Third Age Centre Ltd. Upon gaining charitable status in 2006, it became The Third Age Foundation CLG, trading as Third Age. The name is linked with the ages of life; the first is childhood and the second is young adulthood into middle age. It was recognized that human flourishing is key for all age groups, and Third Age is ideally a time for continued fruitfulness and productivity – a good fit for the mission and vision of Third Age.

Almost from the start, S.A.R.G. differed from the average retirement group. While there were the usual talks and activities common in such groups, a more community-focused approach prevailed. Residents from a long-stay community hospital in a nearby town, Trim, County Meath, were invited to join, as were Travelers[2] from a Training Centre in Navan, Co Meath. This integrated approach was innovative in breaking down barriers of age, disability and ethnicity within a local community. The principles of the organization, as originally established, underlined a robust and positive approach to growing older, which is still evident today. These principles helped, protected and fostered the rights of older people, supporting their voice, and encouraging them to remain active and interested in lifelong learning and community service. There was also the intention to dispel aging myths and stereotypes, and to promote physical and social well-being through an integrated community approach.

Within the initial activities of Third Age, a program was developed based on the needs and preferences of members. Activities included a weekly drama workshop, an exercise and activity program, a choral group, group holidays and socials. In 2006, the Department of the Taoiseach (Prime Minister in Ireland) provided funding for equipment and training, and weekly IT classes began. Older skills were celebrated with a focus on strengthening intergenerational solidarity. This involved an intergenerational knitting project, in which a small group of members traveled every Wednesday to nearby Dangan National School to teach the children to knit. However, the activity served a greater purpose, as between the "plain and the purl" of knitting, there were conversations about life experiences in the past and the present. Such interactions are recognized by the United Nations (2022b) as key to sustainable development, combating ageism and supporting environments where "nobody is left behind". In addition, other activities and supports sought to address issues of self-care, equality and equity. Third Age offered a Resource Centre, supporting members with applications for house adaptation grants and other entitlements, providing advocacy, regular talks from professionals and house calls, if needed. Third Age has also recognized the dynamic nature of community needs, leveraging social enterprise approaches to meet evolving and emerging contexts. Consequently, it was recognized that some services were of their time. For example, Third Age opened a small laundrette in response to a lack of local laundry services, while long waiting lists for local chiropody treatment prompted the opening of a monthly chiropody clinic in the Third Age center. The laundry service later closed as the need diminished over time. The community hospital residents grew too frail to attend activities, and the Traveler Training Centre closed. However, the provision of chiropody has flourished, and services have expanded with counseling, audiology, reflexology and a library exchange facility available to Third Age members. Today, the Summerhill center in County Meath has activities every day of the week – including chairobics, yoga, bingo, knitting, patchwork, line dancing and a social program of trips, holidays and outings.

Current Programs

SeniorLine

As activities consolidated, Third Age members began to talk about what they could give in response to community needs that would fit their skills. Around this time, Third Age heard of Filo d'Argento, an Italian telephone listening service for older people under the auspices of an association of retired trade union members. There was no such service in Ireland, so to ascertain its feasibility in the Irish setting, the Health Promotion Department of the North-Eastern Health Board conducted a series of seminars with 250 older people on addressing their needs. This maps to the approaches discussed in identifying community need in Chapter 3. The consultation identified several expressed needs. These were:

- The loneliness and social isolation experienced by many older people.
- The difficulty in accessing information on relevant services and entitlements.
- The need for the community to provide facilities, social outlets and support systems.
- The value for older people in proactively maintaining their own health.
- The role of the Health Board in responding to the needs identified.

It was agreed that the establishment of a telephone helpline could alleviate some of these challenges, and SeniorLine (originally Senior Help Line) opened in 1998 as a pilot telephone service for older people. Thirty-two volunteers signed up for training provided by Samaritans, Childline and the Health Board. Training covered listening and communication skills, with a non-judgmental, non-directive approach to callers. Referrals to other helpful services were also offered. Extra phone lines were installed in the Third Age Summerhill center, and a dedicated number was secured. The lines were open every Monday 10 am to 1 pm and Friday 7–10 pm and were manned by two volunteers. The service received 300 calls in the first year and was externally evaluated by St Patrick's College, Drumcondra, Dublin (Ireland) (now Dublin City University, St Patrick's Campus). The evaluation concluded that there was a clear need for the service to combat the loneliness experienced by many older adults. The peer-to-peer model was deemed effective, and the service was seen as cost-effective, offering great benefit to volunteers themselves (Morgan, 1998). This mirrors the important role of social prescribing as detailed in Chapter 15. The National University of Ireland, Galway, evaluated the service again in 2006. Findings concluded that the service had made a major contribution to targeting a response to the problem of loneliness and contributed to enhancing the health and well-being of older people at a relatively low cost while providing good value for money (O'Shea, 2006).

Over the next decade, SeniorLine recruited over 300 volunteers and opened 17 new centers, each managed by a volunteer coordinator, with office space provided variously by the Health Service Executive (reformed structure of the Health Boards), the local authority, parish organization or community centers. In 2013, it was decided to achieve economies of scale while maintaining service quality by centralizing the service in Dublin. The change was managed in cooperation with volunteers who had given many years of loyal service. During 2013–2016, SeniorLine completed the necessary rural closures, while recruiting, training and mentoring new volunteers to work in Dublin. This scaling down and simultaneous gearing up was achieved without loss of any rota hours, thanks largely to the generosity of all volunteers.

SeniorLine has had external recognition for its contribution to both the community and society. In 2019, SeniorLine was among 15 Irish projects chosen to share in the Google.org Dublin Impact Challenge. It was demonstrated that the project responded to loneliness identified by callers by offering peer-to-peer courses in digital skills and a drop-in center to isolated older people in Dublin's city center. In 2019, SeniorLine gained the Volunteer Ireland Invest in Volunteer Quality Mark Award. This involved external examination of policies, protocols and independent interviews with volunteers. In their citation, Volunteer Ireland highlighted the quality of SeniorLine volunteer training, and the care and commitment demonstrated by the service toward volunteers. In 2020, SeniorLine was shortlisted as one of five organizations selected by The Wheel for their Charity Impact Award, acknowledging the program's response to the loneliness suffered by many older people, particularly during COVID-19.

SeniorLine celebrated its 25th birthday in 2023. Over the years, the service has developed and gained expertise while remaining true to its original principles of hosting a peer listening and support service. The line is now open every day 10 am to 10 pm with a Freephone number and attracts 23,000–25,000 calls annually. The heart of SeniorLine remains committed to community service – being available to give time, empathy and non-judgmental attention to callers. People phone for many reasons. They may be anxious, unwell, in financial difficulty, experiencing family conflict, bereaved, suffering elder abuse or having thoughts of suicide.

Loneliness is implied or expressed in many calls (54% in 2023). Geographic isolation, illness, disability, bereavement, poverty, retirement, family emigration, shyness and being single are among the reasons identified. Longer lives are a cause for celebration, but the quality of that longer life may depend on family/community support and cohesion. The documented downside of longevity is the associated loneliness experienced by many older people at home. While older people today have a higher quality of life than in the past (McGarrigle & Ward, 2018), inequalities remain (Jolly, 2024). SeniorLine callers' stories illustrate the fact that many are disempowered from participating in society – through lack of income, ill health, disability and social or digital exclusion. In 2021, data on online usage indicated that almost half of those aged 75+ years had never accessed the Internet (CSO, 2022). In a society where much of life has moved online, this inability is a disadvantage in daily life. Many older people still live with the negative legacy of COVID-19, which deprived them of family, company, confidence and independence.

Supporting lonely people remains a core part of SeniorLine's work. The model of listening is to connect warmly with the caller, spend time understanding their concerns and encourage them to discuss their options. SeniorLine does not give advice but encourages the caller to self-reflect, which often helps the person to reframe a problem and see a new way forward. SeniorLine volunteers invite callers to phone again if needed and many keep in contact during times of crisis. Over half of callers contact the service very regularly, and SeniorLine has become an important part of their lives. Each volunteer also has a Directory of Services to which callers may be referred. These services offer relevant information and support in response to the caller's needs in areas of health, social contact and integrated care. SeniorLine promotes its service to general medical practitioners (GPs), public health nurses, hospital departments, libraries, pharmacies, community garda liaison officers, plus a wide range of community organizations and other non-government organizations (NGOs). Services are also highlighted through participation in Expos, Age Friendly and community events as well as participating in radio and print media. SeniorLine also provides presentations in person and online to groups working with a diverse range of older people and disseminates our publicity material widely to bodies such as active retirement groups, Meals on Wheels organizations, Men's Sheds and similar groups where older people come together.

Fáilte Isteach

The Third Age program Fáilte Isteach was also based on observed community needs. In October 2006, in the local supermarket in Summerhill, Co Meath, a young Argentinian mother was observed struggling to do her shopping because she couldn't translate the package labeling. Even a cursory survey of local migrant numbers demonstrated this was not an isolated experience. In common with many Irish towns and villages at the time, Summerhill and its environs were becoming home to new residents for whom English was not their first language. Many were experiencing daily difficulties due to this lack of fluency. Following discussions in Third Age, some members felt they had the time, interest and experience to offer a helpful intervention. On the basis of this, Third Age advertised free classes in conversational English. Twelve members signed up as volunteer tutors, outnumbering the seven students who arrived on that first Tuesday evening. However, this ratio soon changed and Fáilte Isteach developed rapidly following its national launch in 2008. It has been noted that language is key to enabling participation in communities (Pew Research Center, 2004; Krumm & Plutzar, 2004; World Economic Forum, 2017), a key component of community-centered care.

By mid-2024, the program had grown to 374 classes in 296 locations across 26 counties, with more than 3,500 volunteer tutors supporting the integration of 25,000 learners by delivering over 100,000 hours of free tuition annually. This expansion continues with new students enrolled, new tutors recruited and new classes regularly established. Fáilte Isteach is a community project involving predominantly older volunteers welcoming migrants, those seeking asylum and international protection applicants through conversational English classes, offered at beginner, intermediate and advanced levels. An informal approach to learning allows the most marginalized in society to engage and begin to integrate into life in Ireland. As well as improving language skills, classes can reduce loneliness and facilitate community integration.

Fáilte Isteach embraces a relaxed, unstructured learning environment. Tutors are encouraged to welcome participants through language, identify needs through conversation and focus primarily on fluency and confidence building.

The project has four aims:

- To provide the necessary language skills to migrants and international protection applicants in a student-centered and inclusive manner.
- To establish a network of Fáilte Isteach groups throughout Ireland.
- To involve older volunteer tutors and recognize their expertise and contribution.
- To promote greater integration and achieve a sense of community spirit by forging new friendships and facilitating learning among and about different cultures.

This person-centered project is tailored to suit the needs of migrants and to ease their transition to living in Ireland. Early topics deal with day-to-day needs: shopping, GP visits, children's homework and more. Classroom resources and support assist toward achieving active citizenship, form filling and CV creation. Class discussion helps students learn about their entitlements and employment, Irish political and cultural life and disseminates information from relevant state agencies. Fáilte Isteach salutes the potential of older volunteer tutors who make the project a reality and offer the opportunity for Irish people to reach out and welcome those in need. Tutors gain new skills, deepen their understanding of other cultures and a realization of the suffering and difficulties experienced by many in migration. The project is a testament to an Ireland full of people with compassion, altruism and a wish to care for others.

Over the past 20+ years, the Irish population has become increasingly diverse due to the arrival of a growing number of non-national immigrants. These include citizens from new European Union Member countries and beyond. These new arrivals are in search of a better life, often fleeing persecution in their own country, or displaced through famine, violence or racial/ethnic conflict. By 2011, there were 544,357 non-Irish nationals living and working in Ireland, representing 199 different nationalities (CSO, 2012). Eleven years later, this figure had risen to 632,000 (CSO, 2023a). Against this backdrop of diversity, Fáilte Isteach has developed and flourished, and as Ireland's migrant and refugee population grew, so too did the demand for Fáilte Isteach's services. The ability to speak the country's language is increasingly recognized as a vital skill for integration and advancement (Minuz et al., 2022). The project has grown organically. In the early days, any publicity invariably led to contact from communities throughout Ireland expressing interest in creating classes in their area. Third Age responded by encouraging the formation of a local group, traveling to meet each group to provide information on how to recruit students, and organize and run a class. A coordinator was appointed to each group, often a development worker from a local community organization or local partnership.

Over the years, Fáilte Isteach has built up working relationships with over 40 relevant organizations in the fields of education, justice, immigration, diversity and trauma support. The project also works with partners in libraries, schools, local authorities, parish centers, Local Area Development Companies and Direct

Provision Centers. Direct Provision is Government-provided accommodation to people seeking international protection. In 2017–2018, Fáilte Isteach began to work in Direct Provision Centers with those seeking asylum. These classes welcomed many who had come from war-torn situations in their own countries and needed specialized support and attention. By 2019, Fáilte Isteach was providing a comprehensive framework for new group establishment, ongoing training and support to all branches, tutors and coordinators. An in-house curriculum had been designed for the Irish context in consultation with tutors and coordinators. Extensive tutor teaching packs and student textbooks at all levels were created and distributed to support engagement. To further develop best practice, regional seminars were organized for groups to meet, address any concerns and explore emerging issues. These new issues included giving tutors an understanding of racism and conflict-induced trauma for particularly vulnerable migrants.

Similar to the SeniorLine, Fáilte Isteach has had external recognition. In 2012, Fáilte Isteach received a positive evaluation from the School of Education in Trinity College Dublin with helpful recommendations on further development, which were subsequently implemented. Awards for Fáilte Isteach include:

- 2010: Awarded the Arthur Guinness Fund for providing an innovative and creative solution to a social challenge.
- 2013: The Council of Europe awarded Fáilte Isteach the European Language Label, acknowledging the project's innovative approach to language teaching.
- 2015: Selected from 106 applications to win the European Economic and Social Committee Civil Society Prize.
- 2016: Award from the European Lifelong Learning Platform in recognition of outstanding initiative in building inclusive societies and making lifelong learning a reality within them.
- 2017: The Report on Language and Migration in Ireland paid special tribute to Fáilte Isteach in combining education with integration.
- 2018: Chosen by the Council of Europe to distribute a toolkit of 55 lessons for tutors developed by the Council of Linguistic Integration of Adult Migrants (LIAM). Fáilte Isteach also worked with Monaghan Integrated Development in developing a pilot program, Ways to Work, aimed to improve migrant employability.
- 2022: County Winner in the Community section of the National Lottery Good Causes Award.
- 2023: shortlisted for Age Friendly Ireland Award Health & Wellbeing category.

Fáilte Isteach was also invited by Trinity College Dublin and Dublin City University to join a research project on online learning support for adult migrants post-pandemic. The results include a unique digital resource linked to the language used locally in Ireland, exploring phrases, accents and colloquialisms.

The war in Ukraine and the subsequent arrival of Ukrainian refugees to Ireland in early 2022 demonstrated Third Age's ability to respond to emerging needs. The new arrivals created an increased need for language tuition. Fáilte Isteach responded by identifying new community leaders and coordinators, forming new partnerships, recruiting more volunteer tutors and providing more classes. The work of Fáilte Isteach was recognized by the Ukrainian Ambassador in Ireland, who visited one of the groups in Cahir, Co Tipperary, in 2022. Fáilte Isteach demonstrates the collaboration of and within communities. It continues to combine emotional and practical support to migrants, refugees and those seeking asylum in a caring student-centered way that is particularly helpful to all who have suffered the trauma of making a home in a new country.

AgeWell

The AgeWell program evolved from "Mothers to Mothers" (M2M), an educational support program for HIV-positive pregnant women launched in 2001 by a team of South African obstetricians and gynecologists. On witnessing its positive impact, team member Dr Mitch Besser decided to apply its principles to address the needs of an aging population. With colleagues, he developed the AgeWell App and model of care and piloted it in Cape Town in 2014. Doctor Besser, while working with a group in Limerick, became aware of the Third Age peer-to-peer approach and contacted the current CEO, Áine Brady, to discuss possible involvement in the program. Third Age immediately saw its potential as a fit with our existing philosophy. As well as providing direct services and support to older people at home, the AgeWell model would engage older people themselves as volunteers, where they could respond to the needs of older community residents and link them in as necessary to relevant services.

In 2017, Third Age began introducing the program to Health Service Executive Primary Care Teams, Community Services, Gardai (Irish police service) and others in County Meath who could nominate older people as beneficiaries, demonstrating community-integrated care service provision. A recruitment campaign and training program were developed for AgeWell companions, with training assistance from AgeWell Limerick. Recruitment began in winter 2017, training was held in early 2018, and Meath AgeWell was launched in March 2018. By summer 2018, AgeWell had eight companions visiting 45 older people, with the program soon expanding to Meath North & West. Over 589 clients have been supported by the program since its inception, and today, over 100 older people are visited each week.

Clients may typically be isolated, vulnerable, frail, housebound, marginalized, at risk, have poor mobility, experience age-related and other disabilities, including serious health conditions, and many have multi-morbidity. With the rising cost of living, some clients make difficult financial decisions each week. The clients' mean age is 83 years. Clients live in both urban and rural areas, with slightly more living in rural areas in County Meath.

The AgeWell model recruits and trains people aged 50+ years as AgeWell volunteer companions to provide social engagement through weekly home visits and phone calls. The companions utilize a phone-based 20-question Wellbeing App to capture health, well-being and related information about clients. The App has a series of questions and observations asked on a fortnightly basis and is designed to register any deterioration in a client's physical, emotional/psychological health and well-being. The App also monitors changes in mood, social contact, access to services and any new symptoms occurring, such as confusion, changes in mobility, falls, appetite, pain or hospitalization. The platform processes the information using referral algorithms to generate suggested actions to explore with clients and can promptly link individual clients to appropriate services as needed. This provides a tailored support service and acts as an early warning system for identifying and addressing evolving health, social and environmental problems before they escalate. AgeWell is an example of the role of modern technology in connecting older people with peer and community resources. AgeWell collaborates with Community Health Nurses, social workers, physiotherapists, occupational therapists, police, Meals on Wheels service, transport initiatives, active retirement associations and other relevant health, community and social services as required by clients. Like other Third Age programs, the service supports and encourages clients to avail of the assistance they need. The program also helps to reduce isolation and loneliness and connects older people to appropriate care providers and information services regarding entitlements and other resources.

Every older person has the right to a happy, healthy life at home for as long as possible, and AgeWell supports this right. The program responds to potential problems before issues grow into something more serious, impacting well-being. AgeWell fosters independence and assists people to maintain, manage and improve their health, thus adding to their agency and self-efficacy, which is a core principle in person-centered approaches. AgeWell's Care Coordination Team provides support to companions by assessing all reported issues and responding appropriately. Regular independent client assessments are an important aspect of AgeWell's success. Before entering the program, each client receives an initial (Baseline) assessment followed by ongoing quarterly (Midline) assessments. Client assessments use the following scales: WHO5 (well-being) (WHO, 1998), MOSS 8 (informational and Emotional Supports) (Moss, 2019) and the UCLA (Loneliness scale) (Russell, 1996). AgeWell also measures clients' self-rated health and physical activity levels. Ongoing program evaluations have demonstrated a consistent reduction in loneliness, improved social, emotional and informational support, increased well-being, physical activity and self-rated health.

The success of AgeWell has also been demonstrated in attracting grants, illustrating its utility in delivery and award achievements. In 2018, AgeWell received a grant from the Social Innovation Fund, one of six awardees chosen from over 90 applicants offering mentoring and business support for program development. In November 2022, AgeWell was reviewed by Phelan (2022). The report concluded that the efficiencies of AgeWell are evident in three areas: firstly, it provides community-based support services for older people, which interconnect with the formal health and social care system while networking with other community services to promote person-centered services. Secondly, its early intervention remit enables the optimization of health and reduces premature cognitive and functional loss. Thirdly, it is cost-effective. More recently, in March 2024, AgeWell won the annual European Economic and Social Committee's (EESC) 14th Civil Society Prize, awarded to non-profit projects supporting mental health. AgeWell was chosen from over 100 applications from 27 Member States. In May 2024, AgeWell won the Meath County Council Civil Achievement Award, and in November 2024, AgeWell won both the Meath Co Council Trim District Area and the Countrywide Pride of Place Awards for Community Wellbeing.

AgeWell is developing against an absence of services that provide both companionship and a regular review of key health and well-being factors. This deficit can lead to a care system that over-emphasizes acute, emergency care services over prevention and early intervention services. AgeWell is also a timely service in an aging Ireland where growing numbers of older people are living alone (CSO, 2023b). Our national health service is under increasing pressure, often with long waiting lists for homecare support. This deficit can become critical when older people are discharged from the hospital, and service gaps may increase risks and vulnerability to readmission or progression to long-term care. Consequently, in identifying such gaps, Third Age believes there needs to be a coordinated approach to the care and support of older people, and that community-based initiatives play an important role in this process. AgeWell offers a solution to the support needs of our older population by enabling them to live well and age better in place. Moreover, in line with inter-sector collaboration (Government of Ireland, 2019), the program has the potential to complement the healthcare system by becoming part of an integrated hospital discharge and home support program for vulnerable older patients. Consequently, Third Age's vision is to expand to additional locations so that new populations of older people may experience the health and well-being benefits that the AgeWell program provides.

COVID-19

One of the strengths of community-centered care is the ability to respond rapidly and appropriately to changes in context. In early March 2020, it became obvious that the pandemic restrictions would have a significant impact on the work of Third Age throughout the year and beyond. Third Age was determined to maintain its programs and responded by focusing on priorities, providing public health briefings to staff and developing a service strategy in collaboration with its board of directors, funders, staff members and volunteers. These adaptations took a whole-organization approach. Each manager assumed responsibility for assessing and reconfiguring their program to make it fit for purpose, while the senior management team moved online to plan and problem-solve. All programs were repurposed to ensure that clients could continue to receive support while balancing services within public health guidelines to minimize risks to clients and staff. As the year progressed, programs came under increased pressure from a frightened and distressed older public who needed extra services, reassurance and support. Third Age became the social glue, offering practical and emotional contact to a wide circle of service users.

SeniorLine closed its three city center offices, and volunteers transferred to working from home, with no break in service. New rotas were set up while extra technical support was given to facilitate an efficient home service, and new channels were established for the daily capture of caller data. SeniorLine successfully sought funding to supply volunteers with SeniorLine dedicated phones to facilitate the working-from-home service. Volunteers received regular updated information on safety, community services and health concerns, enabling them to answer COVID-19-related questions with confidence. Volunteers also participated in regular online meetings which offered informal training and social contact. Today, SeniorLine remains a working-from-home service, with face-to-face training and monthly Continuous Professional Development (CPD).

Fáilte Isteach classes were suspended in line with public health guidelines, and the service began to train volunteer tutors to deliver classes online. As 2020 progressed, a growing number of classes were transferred online with the least possible break in service. The online network became a means for disseminating critical public health guidelines and information from state agencies. By September 2020, 50% of classes had moved online, involving 500 volunteers and 1,100 students. In 2021, 75% of classes had moved online, and today, a blended approach of online and offline tuition had proved to be a successful formula.

At the start of the pandemic, AgeWell carried out a risk assessment concerning public health restrictions and developed a program to safeguard companions and clients. Companions were provided with Personal Protective Equipment and received specific training on conducting home visits safely. Companions remained in constant touch with clients by phone, socially distanced door visits or home visits as permissible. The Wellbeing App identified any COVID-19 symptoms and supported clients to seek early medical help. Staff provided monthly steering meetings and fortnightly CPD sessions to companions.

Summerhill local activities initially closed in compliance with government regulations and to protect staff and members. Third Age mobilized its efforts to continue to support local older people. Staff immediately drew up a rota to enable contact with each member throughout the year, including daily/weekly phone calls, letters, birthday, Easter and Christmas cards. Staff also liaised with local shops to coordinate the delivery to members of groceries, household supplies, fuel and medicines. Summerhill staff delivered support packs to members containing books, puzzles, non-perishable foodstuffs, confectionery and flower seeds. Members were encouraged to phone SeniorLine for company and support. The Summerhill center itself acted as a conduit for government information and extended the database to include local people referred for support by County Meath Community Police. Overall, Summerhill services were a lifeline to members living in the wider catchment area. As restrictions lifted and people began to meet again, staff invited members to outdoor gatherings in the center and a local garden center. In early 2021, when vaccinations became available, Summerhill staff liaised with the local GP to establish a vaccination clinic for members with a recovery space in the center after the procedure. During 2021, activities returned to the center, and appointments for chiropody, counseling and other services were scheduled carefully to follow safety protocols.

Alliances

Building connections and networks is key to achieving goals in community-centered care. Recognizing this, Third Age is a member of The Alliance of Age Sector Non-Government Organizations (The Alliance), representing the collective thinking of NGOs working in the age sector. The other members are Active Retirement Ireland, Age & Opportunity, Alone, the Alzheimer's Society of Ireland, the Irish Hospice Foundation and the Irish Senior Citizens Parliament. In 2022, the Alliance published a report "Telling It Like It Is", capturing the experiences of a broad diversity of older people living in Ireland through the pandemic. The report demonstrated how the events of 2020/2021 affected older people negatively. Older people died and were bereaved disproportionately, their independence and decision-making were reduced, many living in their own homes felt frightened into isolation and the pandemic exposed the precarious and often inequitable nature of home care provision. In 2023, the Alliance published its second report "Telling It Like It Is: Combatting Ageism". This report highlighted the nature and influence of ageism in Ireland, set out the reasons why Ireland needs to take meaningful action to counteract ageism and listed some recommendations toward this outcome. These collaborative actions demonstrate the macro actions of Third Age in addressing the older community's needs in Ireland. Recommendations included the establishment of a Government Commissioner for Aging & Older People, a government-led awareness campaign, media guidelines on appropriate language, imagery and messaging regarding older people, revising ageist policies and practices and developing relevant education/training. Following the 2023 launch, a campaign group representing The Alliance, TDs and Senators was established to leverage the political support gained by the report.

Conclusion

This chapter has charted the activities and engagements of an NGO that works with communities to identify needs and generate community-based responses. Through its three major programs, Third Age has worked within the older person population and societal needs to identify what matters to people and developed responsive programs, leveraging and empowering older people within peer and intergenerational exchanges. Such programs have been recognized for their community contributions and ability to integrate people and services. Moreover, Third Age as a case study for community-centered approaches, has demonstrated its ability to flexibly adapt to using technology to enhance health and to adapt to emerging situations, for example, the COVID-19 pandemic and to act collaboratively on a macro level to address issues related to quality of lives for older people in Ireland.

Notes

1 Fáilte Isteach is translated from the Irish language as "Welcome in".
2 Travellers are an indigenous Irish ethnic group with a distinct culture, shared history and identity.

References

Berlingieri, F., Colagrossi, M., & Mauri, C. (2023, May 30). *Loneliness and social connectedness: insights from a new EU-wide survey*. JRC Publications Repository. https://publications.jrc.ec.europa.eu/repository/handle/JRC133351

Central Statistics Office (2012). *Census* 2011 *Profile 6 migration & diversity – A profile of diversity in Ireland*. CSO, Dublin.

Central Statistics Office (2022). *Internet coverage and usage in Ireland*. CSO, Dublin.

Central Statistics Office (2023a). *Census* 2022 *profile 5 diversity, migration, ethnicity, Irish travellers & religion*. CSO, Dublin.

Central Statistics Office (2023b). *Household, families and childcare*. CSO, Dublin.

Central Statistics Office. (2024, January 26). *Press statement older persons information hub 2024- CSO - Central Statistics Office*. Www.cso.ie. https://www.cso.ie/en/csolatestnews/pressreleases/2024pressreleases/pressstatementolderpersonsinformationhub2024/

Government of Ireland (2019). *Sustainable, inclusive and empowered communities. Department of rural and community development supported by the cross-sectoral group on local and community development*. GoI, Dublin.

Health Foundation (2016). *Person-centred care made simple. What everyone should know about person-centred care*. Health Foundation, London.

Jolly, R. (2024). *Inequality and ageing*. Age International, London.

Krumm, H. J., & Plutzar, V. (2024). *Tailoring language provision and requirements to the needs and capacities of adult migrants*. Retrieved from https://rm.coe.int/16802fc1c8

McGarrigle, C. & Ward, M. (2018). Quality of Life and relationships. In *Wellbeing and health in Ireland's over 50s 2009–2016*. (Turner, N., Donoghue, O., & Kenny, R. A. eds.) TILDA, Dublin. pp.25–46.

Minuz, F., Kurvers, J., Schramm, K., Rocca, L., & Naeb, R. (2022). *Literacy and second language learning for the linguistic integration of adult migrants*. Council of Europe, Strasbourg.

Morgan, M. (1998). *An evaluation of a new service aimed at isolated and lonely older people*. North-Eastern Health Board, Kells.

Moss, S. (2019). *Moss-PAS (Check): A questionnaire to identify potential mental health problems in people with intellectual disabilities*. Pavilion Publishing & Media, Shoreham by Sea.

O'Shea, E. (2006). *The senior help line: Older people working for older people-an economic and social evaluation.* NUIG, Galway.

Pew Research Center (2004). *Assimilation and language.* Retrieved from https://www.pewresearch.org/race-and-ethnicity/2004/03/19/assimilation-and-language/

Phelan, A. (2022) *The AgeWell programme as a public health intervention.* TCD, Dublin.

Phelan, A., McCormack, B., Dewing, J., Brown, D., Cardiff, S., Cook, N. F., Dickson, C., Kmetec, S., Lorber, M., Magowan, R., McCance, T., Skovdahl, K., Stiglic, G., & Van Lieshout, F. (2020). Review of developments in person-centred healthcare. *International Practice Development Journal,* 10(3). https://doi.org/10.19043/ipdj.10Suppl2.003

Russell, D. (1996). UCLA loneliness Scale (V3): Reliability, validity and factor structure. *Journal of Personality Assessment,* 66(1), 20–40.

The Alliance (2021). *Telling is as it is.* Retrieved from https://alzheimer.ie/creating-change/awareness-raising/alliance-of-age-sector-ngos/

The Alliance (2023). *Telling it like it is: Combatting ageism.* Retrieved from https://www.thirdageireland.ie/about/telling-it-like-it-is-combatting-ageism

United Nations (2022a). *World population prospects, 2022.* U.N., New York.

United Nations (2022b). *International youth day 2022: Intergenerational solidarity: Creating a world for all ages.* Retrieved from https://www.un.org/development/desa/youth/news/2022/06/iyd2022-intergenerational-solidarity-creating-a-world-for-all-ages

Ward, M., Layte, R. & Kenny R. A. (2019). *Loneliness, social isolation, and their discordance among older adults findings from the Irish longitudinal study on ageing.* TILDA, TCD, Dublin.

World Economic Forum (2017). *Stop telling immigrants to assimilate and start helping them participate.* Retrieved from https://www.weforum.org/agenda/2017/01/stop-telling-immigrants-to-assimilate-and-start-helping-them-participate/

World Health Organization (1998). *Wellbeing measures in primary health care/the depcare project.* WHO Regional Office for Europe, Copenhagen.

World Health Organisation (2022). *Ageing and health.* Retrieved from https://www.who.int/news-room/fact-sheets/detail/ageing-and-health

World Health Organisation, ITU, United Nations, & the Department of Economic & Social Affairs (2021). *Social isolation and loneliness among older people.* WHO, Geneva.

12

CIVIC ACTION FOR REAL-WORLD IMPACT

Trinity College Dublin's Journey in Advancing Civic Engagement for Societal Impact

Jo-Hanna Ivers, Sarah Bowman and Michael Foley

Introduction

While universities have a tradition of fulfilling a civic function, this role is dependent upon the historical context within which the university operates and who has access to it. Factors such as time, cultural norms, political climate, available resources, subject expertise, internal and external governance and partnerships, identified societal needs and levels of accessibility and inclusion continue to influence how a university understands and acts upon its civic function (Pinheiro et al., 2012). Today, civic engagement is recognized as a core function of higher education in Ireland and is understood as essential for fostering a wide range of benefits, including active citizenship that addresses societal challenges (HEA, 2013). Moreover, connected, engaged and empowered communities supported mutual well-being within academic and civic partners.

The relationship with society has been expressed as a fundamental part of how the university should operate, often described as a third mission alongside education and research (Maassen et al., 2019). This third mission challenges the university to create mutually beneficial partnerships, encouraging both the university community and its key civic partners to recognize their social responsibility in advancing societal impact. This impact can effectively address some of society's greatest challenges, including inequities, social disparities and knowledge gaps. For example, prioritizing cross-sectoral, interdisciplinary collaborations and transparent, inclusive processes helps "open" the university and further embed an ethos of the university as a relevant, critical asset to society (Ursić et al, 2022).

The benefits from a civically engaged university for students, staff and external partners are substantial: deep subject matter expertise is formed alongside critical

DOI: 10.4324/9781032662657-14

skills in leadership, communication, teamwork and problem-solving (Goddard et al., 2016). A civically engaged university enhances research relevance by cultivating an appreciation of evidence-informed approaches and mobilizing practical applications of knowledge. In a post-truth society, where public opinion may be shaped more by emotions, personal beliefs and repeated assertions rather than objective facts and evidence, the rigor a university community brings to public dialogue and debate is central to combating misinformation and false knowledge (Roozenbeek et al., 2023). Civic engagement influences the institution's reputation, making it an appealing or unappealing place for both current and prospective students and staff (Watson et al., 2011). By cultivating civic engagement, the institution establishes itself as a socially responsible partner, capable of influencing local, national and international policy, through the rigor of scientific, evidence-based recommendations. What has emerged is a sense of the positive societal impact that universities can have at a local and global level (Connell, 2019) and how collaborations, engagement and societal impact can define the ways in which a university functions and matters (Mattsson et al., 2024).

This chapter explores how Trinity is developing its civic engagement mission with opportunities for engagement by the academic community and wider society. The initiatives presented map with the principles of person-centeredness and align with strengthening communities, offering opportunities for synergistic, mutually beneficial relationships and collaborations while leveraging both communities' resources to increase collaboration and benefit society (Public Health England and NHS Trust, 2015).

Civic Engagement in European and National Contexts

The policies of the European Union, as well as national policies in Ireland, support and highlight the connection between universities and society. Internationally, efforts such as the establishment of the UNESCO Chair in Community-based Research and Social Responsibility in Higher Education (Hall and Tandon, 2017) and the OECD document "Higher Education and Regions" (2007) show the desire to move universities in this direction.

At a regional level, the European Union supports universities in enabling societal engagement (Institute for the Development of Education, 2023). Initiatives such as the Europe 2020 Strategy (European Commission, 2010); the European Pillar of Social Rights (European Commission, 2017); the European Democracy Action Plan (European Commission, 2020e); the Erasmus+ Programme (European Commission, 2021a); the EU Youth Strategy 2019–2027 (European Commission, 2018); Horizon Europe (European Commission, 2021b); the European Research Area (European Commission, 2020a); the Digital Education Action Plan 2021–2027 (European Commission, 2020c); and the European Skills Agenda (European Commission, 2020d) demonstrate multifaceted approaches for promoting active citizenship, democratic participation and social inclusion. Furthermore, the European Commission's Strategic Framework for European Cooperation in Education and Training (2009) set the stage for member states to work together on improving education and training systems through mutual learning and sharing of good practices. This framework underscores the importance of lifelong learning and social inclusion, which are essential components of civic engagement.

The European Union's focus on digital transformation, as outlined in the 2030 Digital Compass (2020b), also complements these efforts by aiming to enhance digital skills and inclusion across all segments of the population, thereby fostering a more engaged and informed citizenry. The focus at the European level has been on encouraging active engagement, especially for young people and older adults, by participating in democratic processes and contributing to the work of public entities, including universities, in their countries and across Europe.

Within the Irish context, the National Strategy for Higher Education to 2030 (Department of Education and Skills, 2011) was the first national policy in Ireland that placed engagement as a central pillar alongside teaching and research. The policy focused on engagement through teaching and learning, contribution and outreach. The Higher Education Authority Act (2022) included a deeper emphasis on community engagement. It sought to "strengthen engagement with the education system and society generally" (p. 15); "promote well-being, active citizenship, community engagement, inclusion, full participation in society and health in the learner" (p. 45); "meet the skills needs of the economy and society"; and "meet the needs of individuals, business, enterprise, the community, local interests and others at a national level and a regional level" (p. 45). The Department of Education's Action Plan for Education, published annually, outlines specific targets and initiatives to enhance community engagement and active citizenship among students. The Technological Universities Act (2018) was another significant policy, emphasizing the role of technological universities in regional development and community engagement. Impact 2030: Ireland's Research and Innovation strategy (2022) positioned research and innovation at the heart of addressing Ireland's societal, economic and environmental challenges, featuring a mission-oriented National Grand Challenges Programme that encouraged interdisciplinarity and engagement in research processes and programs. This included a focus on actions to "improve how research and innovation impact is defined, driven and monitored" and the strategy also highlighted the need to foster an environment within the research and innovation community that supports its ambition to be an Island of Inclusion and Engagement (p. 2). Ireland's policy landscape for higher education places significant emphasis on civic engagement, recognizing it as integral to teaching, research and societal impact.

Trinity's Role in Civic Engagement: Historical and Cultural Contexts

Founded in 1592, Trinity College Dublin has a long-standing tradition of serving both the local and global communities with alumni such as Nobel Prize winners, author Samuel Beckett and physicist Ernest Walton and former UN High

Commissioner for Human Rights Mary Robinson. In its early years, the institution primarily focused on providing a classical education to a section of the Irish elite. As Irish society and education policy changed (O'Sullivan, 2005), so did Trinity's mission and approach to education. The university gradually expanded its curriculum to include a wider range of disciplines and began to place greater emphasis on research and public service.

Over the past 20 years, Trinity has seen a move to more structured approaches to civic engagement, as the university began to seek to leverage its resources and expertise for the public good (Cameron-Coen and Allwright, 2016). During that time, there has been a growing focus on the importance of inclusivity and diversity in higher education (HEA, 2004). This has led to initiatives aimed at increasing access to education for underrepresented groups, such as the Trinity Access Programmes (TAP) (Bray et al, 2022). By fostering a more inclusive environment, Trinity ensures that its civic engagement efforts reflect the diverse needs and perspectives of the broader community. Another cultural shift has been the increasing emphasis on interdisciplinary collaboration. Recognizing that complex societal challenges cannot be addressed through single-discipline approaches (OECD, 2020), Trinity has promoted interdisciplinary teaching, management and research (Trinity College Dublin, 2019a). This shift is evident in initiatives such as the Healthy Campus Manager, responsible for health promotion in the university, working under the Vice President for Biodiversity and Climate Action, or in the many interdisciplinary research projects that have emerged from Trinity (Payne et al., 2022).

Today, Trinity has a vibrant community of over 22,000 students and is based in the center of Dublin city, with satellite campuses in Ireland and abroad, as well as three teaching hospitals: St. James's Hospital, Tallaght University Hospital and the Trinity Dental Hospital. Additionally, it has established global partnerships with prestigious institutions, including UC San Francisco in California and Fudan University in Shanghai, as well as other key academic collaborators such as Columbia University in New York, the University of Cape Town and the University of Melbourne, as examples. Within Trinity's strategic planning documents, the university articulates a strong sense of civic responsibility and its commitment to positive societal impact. This is reflected in its Strategic Plan, which states that civic action is used to "courageously advance the cause of a pluralistic, just, and sustainable society" (Trinity College Dublin, 2019a, p. 8). Trinity's research strategy (Trinity College Dublin, 2019b) emphasizes the importance of engaged research and co-creation as integral to Trinity's research future. This commitment flows from its Research Charter (Trinity College Dublin, 2019c, p. 12), which includes the key commitment to "Engage profoundly with our publics".

Trinity's Global Relations Strategy (Trinity College Dublin, 2019d) fosters international collaboration and cultural exchange, while its Equality, Diversity, and Inclusion (EDI) Policy ensures a supportive environment for all students and staff, underpinning effective civic engagement. Trinity's Student Partnership Policy (Trinity College Dublin, 2019e) engages students as active partners in governance, empowering them to contribute to civic initiatives. The university's Sustainability Policy (Trinity College Dublin, 2019f) embeds environmental responsibility across operations, aligning with broader civic goals.

The Trinity Education Project (TEP) (Trinity College Dublin, 2019g) integrates civic engagement into the curriculum, fostering a sense of responsibility and active citizenship among students. Trinity's Research and Innovation Policy (Trinity College Dublin, 2019h) supports research addressing societal challenges and encourages collaborations with external organizations. The Civic Engagement and Social Innovation Fund (Trinity College Dublin, 2019i), now renamed the Civic Engagement for Societal Impact (CESI) Fund, provides financial support for projects with a societal impact, promoting innovative approaches to civic engagement.

This commitment to civic engagement is furthered by Trinity's participation in the EU-funded Horizon 2020 and Horizon Europe projects, which focus on social innovation and inclusive growth through engaged research activities (European Commission, 2021b).

Development of a New Direction for Civic Engagement

In terms of its structure, Trinity is organized into three Faculties: the Faculty of Health Sciences; the Faculty of Arts, Humanities and Social Sciences; and the Faculty of Science, Technology, Engineering and Mathematics. Each Faculty encompasses various schools that facilitate teaching, research and other activities. Historically, civic engagement at Trinity has often been housed at individual and School levels, with notable examples of impactful initiatives emerging organically. For instance, the Faculty of Health Sciences demonstrated its strong commitment to societal impact through its Research Impact Metrics, which highlight significant contributions to community health and well-being, also recognizing that time-engaged research efforts require accounting within performance metrics. While these efforts have been effective on a localized scale, there has been a growing recognition of the need for a more coordinated and university-wide approach to civic engagement. This shift aims to build on the existing strengths of individuals, schools and faculties, fostering a unified strategy that amplifies the university's overall impact on society and builds meaningful partnerships with communities. The University Board, Executives and Deans have clearly stated their intention to elevate civic engagement to a more central mission for the university, providing stronger support to encourage authentic and coordinated approaches to civic engagement activities. Recognizing that a lack of coordination was placing the university and its partners at risk of inefficiencies, duplicative efforts, missed opportunities and stakeholder fatigue, Professor Jo-Hanna Ivers was appointed Associate Dean of CESI, under the Provost's Directorate, in 2022. Under her leadership, the CESI action planning process was initiated to encourage conversations on the necessary supports for CESI to thrive. This inclusive process engaged the university community and resulted in a prioritized set of actions to be implemented between

2024 and 2026 (TCD, 2023). Through this Plan, Trinity aims to advance the societal impact from its civic engagement efforts by:

- Promoting public dialogue and debate, welcoming diverse voices and perspectives;
- Nurturing mutually beneficial partnerships and collaborations across various sectors;
- Engaging with policymakers to inform public policy debates and advocate for evidence-based decision-making;
- Contributing to the well-being of individuals and communities, supporting the achievement of civic engagement goals;
- Advancing responsible practices in its operations, exemplifying environmental stewardship and ethical behaviors;
- Supporting, celebrating and rewarding quality approaches to engagement and impact; and
- Recognizing participation as an essential component in addressing social inequalities and fostering social cohesion.

Articulated in Trinity's CESI Action Plan, civic engagement refers to the active involvement of students, faculty, staff and alumni in their communities to address societal issues, promote democratic values and foster positive social change. This commitment to civic responsibility and the cultivation of associated knowledge, skills and attitudes enriches the academic experience, delivers impactful research and scholarship and fosters collective action for the public good. The CESI Action Plan acknowledges the local efforts already in place to create a more civically engaged university with positive impact, while also acknowledging the resources and supports required to encourage a culture of partnership. It aims to ensure greater awareness of Trinity's civic engagement champions, activities and opportunities, as well as address institutional barriers to civic engagement that emerged during the engagement process. The goal is for Trinity to live its mission as a recognized leader in civic engagement and social responsibility, mobilizing knowledge for the public good. This CESI Action Plan lays the groundwork for Trinity to be a better neighbor, an engaged partner and a determined leader advancing Sustainable Development Goals. It focuses the Civic Engagement Office's efforts as the university prepares for its next strategic planning cycle and encourages delivery of research, teaching, learning and extracurricular initiatives that positively impact on its students, its partners, including communities, at a national level and internationally.

Initial Preparatory Work

Development of the CESI Action Plan was based upon a clear vision by Prof Ivers for what should be at the heart of Trinity's civic engagement:

- *Empowered Students*: Preparing students with the knowledge and skills to be able to address complex issues in society;

- *Recognized Faculty and Staff*: Nurturing a culture where faculty and staff are driving societal change;
- *Meaningful Collaborations and Partnerships*: Harnessing diverse networks to address societal needs;
- *Multifaceted Approaches*: Innovating with novel perspectives and methodologies;
- *Community Engaged Research and Scholarship*: Advancing research with external stakeholders in order to ensure implementation and impact;
- *Ethical Leadership for Societal Impact*: Championing ethical, inclusive and equitable practices to achieve societal impact; and
- *Civic Engagement as a Sustained Commitment*: Cultivating lifelong engagement and learning to stay with change projects as they evolve.

As a first step in the process, Prof Ivers brought together a CESI Action Plan Development Team (Project Team) who had been involved in civic engagement activities as professional staff across Trinity. Collectively, this group had experience of, among other things: co-developing national strategies around engaged research; developing national and international training programs for engaged research; developing Trinity's public and patient involvement in health research; supporting and promoting Trinity-based volunteering; developing engagement with Trinity's local communities; capturing Trinity's societal impact; and promoting innovation processes.

One issue that guided the initial planning was that the university would be developing a new strategic plan during the lifetime of the CESI Action Plan. The CESI Action Plan would need to enhance Trinity's civic engagement to inspire the future strategy, but would also need to be flexible enough to be coherent with that strategy as it emerged. A second issue was that there was no definitive capture of civic engagement across the university. This process would, therefore, be focused internally to better understand the civic engagement activities, relationships, processes and structures of the university so that once this assessment was complete, there would be clarity for how to co-develop with Trinity's external partners a future civic engagement strategy, fully integrated into the forthcoming strategic planning engagement efforts led by the Provost's Directorate.

Based on the above, it was also agreed that a group facilitation approach would be taken during the Deployment Phase to encourage conversations and to reach some level of consensus about what issues were shared among those within the university. While opportunities would exist for people to respond individually to what emerged from those facilitations, it was decided that discussion and consensus conversations rather than individual inputs or surveys of staff or students would yield a more useful picture of what people valued, as well as immediate challenges that could be addressed within the two-year action planning period.

The development of the CESI Action Plan had four stages:

- Discovery Phase (January–September 2022)
- Development Phase (September 2022)

- Deployment Phase (October 2022–December 2022)
- Design Phase (January 2023–November 2023).

Discovery Phase

Between January and September 2022, the Project Team embarked on a thorough exploration to understand the civic engagement and societal impact landscape. As stated above, the Project Team was chosen due to their pre-existing experience and contacts in relevant fields of civic engagement both within and beyond Trinity. This included comprehensive reviews of literature around civic engagement (e.g., McIlrath et al., 2023). This discovery phase involved conducting interviews with colleagues from various institutions, including University College Cork, University of Limerick, Dublin City University, Royal College of Surgeons, ReThink Ireland, Campus Engage and the Irish Universities Association. The aim was to gather insights and best practices that could inform Trinity's approach to civic engagement.

Development Phase

In September 2022, the Project Team formalized membership of the Rapid Response Group, established the plan development process and set the timeline and communication channels. This phase was crucial for organizing the structure and ensuring that all necessary stakeholders were involved and aligned with the plan's objectives. The Rapid Response Group was assembled with the primary objectives of providing strategic direction and oversight in formulating the CESI Action Plan, evaluating and documenting progress against existing civic engagement initiatives and identifying ongoing or scheduled efforts within Trinity. The group also provided valuable insights into civic engagement needs, supports and opportunities. They identified and recognized key networks, individuals and initiatives aligned with these goals and pinpointed opportunities to enhance the coordination of infrastructural investments. This effort aimed to support and embed engagement across research, teaching, learning and other activities. Furthermore, the group contributed to developing the Action Plan and recommended approaches to integrate civic engagement and innovation into Trinity's next Strategic Plan, Research Strategy and other relevant guidance documents.

Deployment Phase

Between October 2022 and December 2022, the engagement plan for developing the CESI Action Plan was executed. This phase involved facilitating six workshops to advance understanding of Trinity's current civic engagement activities, identifying opportunities for collaboration and developing innovative approaches to enhance engagement efforts. During this phase, the Project Team focused on integrating the feedback and insights gathered during the discovery phase. Key activities during the deployment phase included:

Facilitated Workshops: The purpose of these Conversation Cafés was to convene the wider community with an interest in civic engagement from across the university community. Each "café" provided an opportunity to discuss the enablers for and the barriers to civic engagement in the university. It also provided an opportunity to identify Trinity's civic engagement champions and the activities that people wished to see. Through the discussions, it allowed people to share their experiences and reach some sense of consensus on what would make a difference in the development of Trinity's civic engagement activity.

Evaluating Input: The final process generated 991 inputs in total. Of these, 199 were reported as barriers to civic engagement, 198 were identified as enablers, 328 were suggested activities which were already happening and due to happen and 266 champions were also identified. Out of this process, it was necessary to, initially, group together common themes. After that, however, there was a need to develop a way in which the 725 enablers/barriers/activities could be ranked. The Project Team created a rubric that would consider the level of readiness for each action, the level of impact that the action would have and the ways in which it would align with the values of Trinity. Initially, the inputs were sorted under the core thematic dimensions of civic engagement for universities which emerged in the Erasmus + funded project to develop a toolbox *Towards a European Framework for Community Engagement in Higher Education* (TEFCE) project (Farnell et al., 2020a, 2020b):

- **Teaching and Learning**: Includes undergraduate and graduate curriculum and degree opportunities, as well as professional development credentials;
- **Student Engagement**: Refers to engagement activities with primary, secondary, undergraduate and graduate students;
- **Research and Innovation**: Presents opportunities to advance engaged research and innovation with a focus on better engaging across Trinity's campuses and teaching hospitals;
- **Management, Policies, Infrastructure, Supports**: Refers to Trinity's infrastructure that ensures monitoring, resourcing and communicating of CESI activities to encourage quality practices and advance a supportive culture through strategic initiatives;
- **Societal Engagement, Partnerships, Openness**: Refers to the resources, programs and supports with and for community partners, with a focus on how to enhance partners' efforts and capture the impact of Trinity's societal engagement.

This initial categorization ensured that the actions in the final plan would form a multifaceted approach to developing civic engagement that spanned the operations of the university, rather than emphasizing one aspect such as "policies, infrastructure, supports". To honor the input received, the Project Team developed a transparent rubric to allow for a ranking of proposed actions. This rubric (Table 12.1) addresses the level of readiness to implement the action, the level of impact it would have and the extent to which the action aligned with the values that would support and promote future civic engagement.

TABLE 12.1 Trinity's CESI action plan prioritization rubric

Dimensions	*Criteria*
Level of readiness	Actionable
	Timeline aligns
	Funding required
	Human support required
	Facilities required
	Level of effort for CESI
Level of impact	Fulfills university obligation or commitment
	Highlights TCD experience and expertise
	Numbers reached
	Benefits external stakeholders and advances the public good
	Encourages diversity and inclusion
Alignment with values	Overcomes an institutional barrier
	Ensures CESI activities are recognized and valued
	Improves understanding on CESI good practices
	Delivers enabling structures and supports for quality CESI
	Leverages existing activities and events

This rubric was applied individually by several members of the Project Team. After each Team member had scored the actions, there followed a consensus meeting where Project Team members justified their scoring and, where scoring diverged, aimed to reach an agreed order for actions. The top 40 actions which emerged from the rubric were then extracted. From these 40 actions, a set of physical cards were created. The team then sorted the cards into those which were alike. Each grouping of cards was then articulated as an overarching task that the CESI Action Plan wished to achieve.

It was agreed that 40 tasks would not be achievable during the period of the CESI Action Plan, and so the tasks were ranked into three tiers:

Tier 1: those which would be a priority for the CESI Action Plan (24 actions).
Tier 2: those which would be possible back-up activities if the priorities were achieved (4 actions);
Tier 3: those which would probably be beyond the scope of the CESI Action Plan but would indicate the ambition moving beyond the Plan itself and relevant to the university's strategic planning efforts moving forward (12 actions).

Once this was complete, a first draft of the Plan was complete, and the process could progress to the final stage.

Design Phase

In March 2023, the Draft CESI Action Plan was advanced for review. The draft was presented to the Rapid Response Group and other key advisors for feedback.

Subsequently, it was made available for a Trinity-wide consultation through the Civic Engagement website with a link sent to any contacts who engaged with the development process. This process ensured that the final plan, launched in November 2023, reflected the collective input and aspirations of the Trinity community.

Emerging Actions for Civic Engagement

What emerged from the work was the desire for the university to identify, capture and celebrate the civic engagement work that already existed across the university. Those involved also sought support, resourcing, good examples and learning opportunities to build their capacity to deliver and sustain better civic engagement. There was also a desire to understand how policies and procedures could be restructured to support better civic engagement.

Each action was organized by its task, which emerged from this process. Tasks and related actions are outlined in Table 12.2 below.

TABLE 12.2 Trinity's CESI action plan Tier 1 Actions

Tasks	*Actions*
Raise awareness on activities, champions and opportunities	Advance the Civic Engagement for Societal Impact (CESI) calendar for a consistent in-person presence
	Develop the CESI website to increase visibility and raise awareness
	Create an image portfolio of Trinity's CESI activities
	Develop five CESI case studies per annum
	Host a student intern to develop a social media strategy to engage students
	Advance a CESI social media campaign, in collaboration with Trinity Communications Office, for a consistent online presence and to share Trinity's CESI stories
	Deliver the CESI biennial survey for the university and prepare a state-of-the-union report for the Provost's Office
	Deliver Trinity's CESI Annual Report
Build capacity to advance quality approaches to civic engagement	Host two engaged research/PPI workshops per annum
	Host one engaged research event per annum
	Host one visiting lecturer event per annum
	Host external speaker events and information exchanges (for the community and by the community) to include international leaders and innovators
	Create a library of CESI methods with good practices
	Host two engaged teaching and learning workshops per annum

(*Continued*)

TABLE 12.2 (*Continued*)

Tasks	*Actions*
Overcome institutional barriers	Develop a guidance document: trinity community-friendly spaces and terms of use Utilize RSS to advance the CESI database to recognize champions Develop a guidance document: how to capture Trinity's CESI activity Develop a guidance document: fair budgeting for CESI efforts
Provide resourcing for civic engagement and societal impact to thrive	Submit two funding proposals per annum Enable access to key assets for partners (e.g., grounds, venues)
Recognize, reward and value good practices	Host the annual CESI awards and ceremony
Support colleagues and existing activities to extend impact	Engage members of the public during key events Provide support for partners' events Engage students during their key events

Not wanting to lose the ambition of the consultation process, Tier 2 and 3 Actions were included in the CESI Action Plan, but it was noted that they were not likely to begin or be achieved within the action planning timeframe. With the CESI Action Plan in place, Trinity invested in the creation of a CESI unit within the Provost's Directorate, which would provide continuity for Trinity's previous Civic Engagement work. This investment included dedicated office space and the appointment of a Civic Engagement Manager who would oversee the implementation of the CESI Action Plan and provide motivation for the improvements in the scope and amount of civic engagement that involves Trinity, particularly in the areas of service learning, engaged research and volunteering.

How Trinity's Civic Engagement affects Teaching, Research and Volunteering

The 2024–2026 CESI Action Plan outlines ambitious goals for further advancing civic engagement. Through these strategic initiatives, Trinity aims to create an optimal environment for community-based initiatives, leveraging the collective expertise of its diverse community to address various societal challenges from environmental sustainability to social justice. Trinity's commitment to fostering public dialogue, nurturing partnerships and engaging with policymakers underscores its role to make a positive contribution globally.

Central to the promotion of the university's third mission of developing partnerships to tackle societal challenges is its integration into the other two missions of education and research. This is achieved through service learning in education, where hearing from and working with external partners creates a deeper and richer learning experience. It is also achieved through engaged research, where the research team is part of a wider convening of societal partners that can help to shape the purpose and the impact of the research. This third mission also, however, recognizes that a university, by its nature, also instigates activities due to the nature of being a university that do not fall into formal student education or formal research. These activities may be due to the university's accumulated expertise, its location and estate, its human capital and other factors. These activities may be as diverse as an appointment to the board of a public body, promoting STEM education efforts in schools, providing arts performances for public audiences, facilitating citizen science opportunities, mobilizing knowledge in collaboration with corporate and government entities and supporting a patient advocacy group. Integrating civic engagement into Trinity's curriculum, research and extracurricular activities creates a rich environment to collaborate on social issues. These activities can have a profound impact, fostering a sense of social responsibility among those participating and generating tangible benefits for the community. As such, they are integral to Trinity's mission.

Service Learning: Service learning at Trinity integrates meaningful community service with instruction and reflection, enriching the learning experience and teaching civic responsibility. This approach allows students to apply classroom knowledge to real-world problems, enhancing their understanding of course content while making a positive impact on the community. The CESI Action Plan promotes service learning through running workshops and visiting lecturer opportunities. It also promotes service learning through the Civic Engagement Awards and the case studies developed and shared.

Engaged Research: Engaged research involves collaborative efforts between students, faculty and external stakeholders to address key issues. This method not only produces relevant and actionable knowledge but also empowers stakeholders by involving them directly in the research process, which allows mutual goals to be achieved. The CESI Action Plan will support engaged research through workshops and events, and the establishment of a methods library to support researchers new to this work. Guidance on fair budgeting is a key focus and is central to stakeholder involvement in research.

Volunteer Opportunities: Volunteering among both students and staff has been a cornerstone of civic engagement at Trinity. The CESI Action Plan will support NGO partners and develop guidance on community-friendly spaces and ways in which partners can engage with the University. The CESI survey will also aim to capture the breadth of volunteering that takes place.

Optimal Environment for Civic Engagement

Creating an optimal campus environment for civic engagement initiatives requires well-defined processes, comprehensive programs and robust structures that enable students and staff to form mutually beneficial collaborations with civic partners. Essential elements include dedicated spaces for collaboration, resources for project development and support systems for partnership management. Training programs in community engagement, interdisciplinary research opportunities and platforms for sharing best practices further enhance the capacity for impactful civic involvement. A supportive institutional culture that values and rewards civic engagement efforts is crucial for sustaining these initiatives and achieving long-term societal impact.

As staff and students develop their opportunities to engage in service learning, engaged research and volunteering opportunities, it raises the question about where this work can lead.

Increasing the civic engagement taking place across and beyond Trinity changes the environment in which the work happens, which then promotes and encourages more civic engagement. It fosters a collaborative campus culture through inclusive practices, interdisciplinary approaches and support structures that encourage joint, ethical and fair efforts between students, staff and external partners. These initiatives address various societal challenges while considering how relationships are mutually beneficial to collaborators while leveraging the collective expertise of the Trinity community. An optimal environment includes the following focus areas, which the CESI Action Plan aligns with through specific actions:

Inclusive Practices: Convening diverse stakeholder groups to discover and to co-create ways to work together can open possibilities for more inclusive practices across the university. The habits and processes of recognizing disparities and encouraging diverse engagement among stakeholders can also lead to similar practices with students and potential colleagues. It also provides insights among stakeholders into the university and how it works, thereby encouraging deeper future involvement in other ways. The CESI Action Plan seeks to make key assets available to partners, to provide support to them and to encourage and celebrate inclusive practices. This includes providing support for partners' events, as well as workshops to encourage good practice, plus access to key university assets for partners. This increase in inclusive practices creates greater potential for peer research, where those within a culture or community are creating knowledge to tackle issues. It also shapes the profile of the university as one where diversity is valued, and external partners are likely to encounter someone who is like them. The CESI Action Plan includes external speaker events and information exchanges (for the community and by the community) to include international leaders and innovators and further open the university to external perspectives and meaningful engagement and collaboration.

Interdisciplinary Approaches: Increased civic engagement can often reveal to university staff the pre-existing relationships with other parts of the university or with academics from other institutions. Communities can serve as the starting point for interdisciplinary work among academics. Recognizing that academics may be exploring or resolving the same issue from different disciplines can facilitate collaboration. The CESI Action Plan supports engaged research and provides a library of best practices and methods to foster interdisciplinary work.

That increase in interdisciplinary work can, in turn, make it easier to build and share community connections across disciplines, while also encouraging innovative practices.

Support Structures: Civic engagement often helps to interrogate the structures and mechanisms that currently exist to support the work of the university. It can lead to new models, such as engaging "experts by experience" or creating volunteering relationships with people external to the university. The CESI Action Plan seeks to overcome institutional barriers to greater civic engagement by hosting an annual CESI awards ceremony, engaging members of the public during key events, engaging students during their key events and submitting funding proposals for civic engagement to thrive. As support structures develop and adapt to progress civic engagement, it makes engagement more likely and, by extension, more likely that people with undertake new forms of engagement. The integration of these inclusive practices, interdisciplinary approaches and support structures at Trinity College Dublin creates an environment that is conducive to the success of community-based initiatives. By fostering a collaborative campus culture through inclusive practices, interdisciplinary approaches and robust support structures (Strategy 2020–2025, 2021), Trinity College Dublin creates an optimal environment for community-based initiatives. These efforts harness the collective expertise of the Trinity community to collaboratively address pressing societal challenges, demonstrating the university's commitment to CESI. Through these initiatives, Trinity not only enhances the educational experience of its students and the professional development of its staff but also contributes significantly to the well-being of the broader community.

Future Endeavors and Strategic Plan

The work of the CESI Action Plan begins to shape how the university considers civic engagement and the kinds of partnerships it is building or enhancing with external stakeholders. It focuses on raising awareness, overcoming institutional barriers and providing resources to support impactful, equitable engagement. The further integration of civic engagement activities into the Research Support System, the creation of an accessible, central calendar of events on the CESI unit's website, a biennial survey on CESI and annual reporting efforts are key components of the CESI Action Plan. These initiatives allow for a structured and comprehensive approach to fostering civic engagement within the university community, ultimately allowing the university to understand who is and who is not being engaged.

Where this Plan leads in the short term is toward the next strategic plan for the university, offering a preliminary assessment and addressing critical needs for fairer, more equitable, more enjoyable and impactful engagement experiences. It seeks to shape Trinity's strategic statement and its articulated strategic direction, allowing for more valuable external conversations given the university's focus to understand activities, barriers and opportunities more fully. In the medium term, those new and enhanced relationships should begin to suggest new ways of working together with both internal and external communities. A more nuanced understanding of civic engagement activities, along with emphasis on continuous improvement for those involved, should enhance Trinity's reputation in civil and public service, with international agencies, and within the NGO landscape. In the longer term, enhanced civic engagement should change how the university is considered. Rather than be seen as removed from everyday life, Trinity can be seen as a site of personal lifelong enrichment. It can be seen as a source of practical partnerships, emphasizing respectful approaches and appropriate opportunities for all sectors of society. The university should be seen as a place trialing innovative, transdisciplinary and open solutions to societal challenges in areas such as health, poverty, environmental crises, food production, energy and technology.

Conclusion

Trinity's journey toward civic engagement demonstrates the operational and strategic requirements for a higher education institution to develop the optimal environment for civic engagement to flourish and drive societal impact. In doing so, the process involved engagement with communities to co-develop civil engagement. This chapter explored Trinity's foundations, the strategic initiatives undertaken, and the ongoing efforts to create an inclusive and collaborative campus culture that fosters community-based initiatives with the key aim of weaving civic and community engagement into the fabric of the university's life, enriching academic experiences while addressing pressing societal challenges. By examining the historical and cultural contexts that have shaped Trinity's approach to civic engagement, it is clear that the institution has evolved continually to meet contemporary societal needs. From its early years of focus on classical education to its current status as a leader in interdisciplinary and inclusive practices, Trinity has shown a steadfast commitment to public service and social responsibility, albeit in a less strategic and coordinated fashion.

Trinity's strategic approach to civic engagement provides a case study of a journey of a higher education institution to making meaningful differences in society. By positioning civic engagement as a core value, Trinity not only enriches academic experience but also contributes significantly to the well-being of the broader community through equitable engagement and collaboration. This ongoing evolution ensures that the Trinity remains at the forefront of civic engagement, fostering a culture of active citizenship and social responsibility that prepares students and staff to be compassionate and influential leaders in their communities and beyond.

References

Bray, A., Hannon, C., & Tangney, B. (2022). Large-scale, design-based research facilitating iterative change in Irish schools – The Trinity Access approach. *Irish Educational Studies, 43*(1), 103–123.

Cameron-Coen, S., & Allwright, S. (2016). From colonisation to collaboration: Challenges of repositioning Trinity College Dublin, the University of Dublin, within its community. In *The Civic University: The Policy and Leadership Challenges* (Goddard, J., Hazelkorn, E., Kempton, L., & Vallance, P. eds.). Edward Elgar Publishing, Cheltenham. pp. 160–179.

Connell, R. (2019). *The Good University: What Universities Actually Do and Why It's Time for Radical Change.* Zed Books, London.

Department of Education and Skills (2011) *National Strategy for Higher Education to 2030.* Government Publications Office, Dublin.

European Commission. (2009). *Strategic Framework for European Cooperation in Education and Training (ET 2020).* Publications Office of the European Union, Luxembourg.

European Commission. (2010). *Europe* 2020*: A Strategy for Smart, Sustainable and Inclusive Growth. COM(2010) 2020 Final.* European Commission, Brussels.

European Commission. (2018). *Communication from the Commission to the European Parliament, the European Council, the Council, the European Economic and Social Committee and the Committee of the Regions. Engaging, Connecting and Empowering Young People: A New EU Youth Strategy. COM/2019/269 Final.* European Commission, Brussels.

European Commission. (2020b). *2030 Digital Compass: The European Way for the Digital Decade.* Publications Office of the European Union, Luxembourg.

European Commission. (2020c). *Digital Education Action Plan (2021–2027): Resetting Education and Training for the Digital Age.* Publications Office of the European Union, Luxembourg.

European Commission. (2020d). *European Skills Agenda for Sustainable Competitiveness, Social Fairness and Resilience.* Publications Office of the European Union, Luxembourg.

European Commission. (2020e). *European Democracy Action Plan. Luxembourg.* Publications Office of the European Union, Luxembourg.

European Commission. (2021a). *Erasmus+ Programme Guide.* Publications Office of the European Union, Luxembourg.

European Commission, Directorate-General for Education, Youth, Sport and Culture, Farnell, T. (2020). *Community Engagement in Higher Education – Trends, Practices and Policies – Analytical Report.* Publications Office of the European Union, Luxembourg.

European Commission, Directorate-General for Research and Innovation. (2020a). *A New ERA for Research and Innovation: Staff Working Document.* Publications Office of the European Union, Luxembourg.

European Commission, Directorate-General for Research and Innovation. (2021b). *Horizon Europe, the EU Research and Innovation Programme (2021–27): For a Green, Healthy, Digital and Inclusive Europe.* Publications Office of the European Union, Luxembourg.

European Commission, Secretariat-General. (2017). *European Pillar of Social Rights.* Publications Office of the European Union, Luxembourg.

Farnell, T., Culum Ilic, B., Dusi, D., O'Brien, E., Šcukanec Schmidt, N., Veidemane, A., & Westerheijden, D. (2020a). *Building and Piloting the TEFCE Toolbox for Community Engagement in Higher Education.* Institute for the Development of Education, Zagreb.

Farnell, T., Veidemane, A., & Westerheijden, D. (2020b). *Assessing the Feasibility of Developing a Framework for Community Engagement in European Higher Education.* Institute for the Development of Education, Zagreb.

Goddard, J., Hazelkorn, E., Kempton, L., & Vallance, P. (2016). Introduction: Why the civic university. In *The Civic University: The Policy and Leadership Challenges.* (Goddard, L., Hazelkorn, E., Kempton, L., & Vallance, P., eds.) Edward Elgar Publishing, Cheltenham, pp. 3–15.

Hall, B., & Tandon, R. (2017). *Mobilizing Community and Academic Knowledge for Transformative Change: The Story of the UNESCO Chair in Community-based Research and Social Responsibility in Higher Education.* The Canadian Commission for UNESCO's IdeaLab, Ottawa.

HEA. (2004). *Report of the High-Level Group on University Equality Policies.* Higher Education Authority, Dublin.

HEA. (2013) *Towards a Performance Evaluation Framework: Profiling Irish Higher Education.* Higher Education Authority, Dublin.

Institute for the Development of Education. (2023). *Policy Recommendations for the Enhancement of Community Engagement in Higher Education: European-Level Policy Recommendations.* Institute for the Development of Education, Zagreb.

Maassen, P., Andreadakis, Z., Gulbrandsen, M., & Stensaker, B. (2019). *The Place of Universities in Society.* Körber-Stiftung, Hamburg.

Mattsson, P., Perez Vico, E., & Salö, L. (2024). Introduction: Universities and the matter of mattering. In *Making Universities Matter: Collaboration, Engagement, Impact* (Mattsson, P., Perez Vico, E. & Salö, L. eds.) Springer, Switzerland, 1–10.

McIlrath, L., Bowman, S., & Lima, G. (2023). *Policy Recommendations for the Enhancement of Community Engagement in Higher Education: National and System-Level Policy Recommendations for Ireland.* Institute for the Development of Education, Zabreb.

OECD. (2007). *Higher Education and Regions: Globally Competitive, Locally Engaged.* OECD Publications, Paris.

OECD. (2020). *Addressing Societal Challenges Using Transdisciplinary Research: DSTI/STP/GSF(2020)4/FINAL.* OECD Publications, Paris.

O'Sullivan, D. (2005). *Cultural Politics and Irish Education since the 1950s: Policy, Paradigms and Power.* Dublin, IPA.

Payne, E., Whelan, C., & Patten, E. (2022). *Improving Arts and Humanities Engagement in Ireland's Civic and Community Sphere: Experiences, Challenges and Opportunities for Researchers Based in HEIs.* Trinity College Dublin, Dublin.

Pinheiro, R., Benneworth, P., & Jones, G. A. (2012). *Beyond the Obvious: Tensions and Volitions Surrounding the Contributions of Universities to Regional Development and Innovation.* Paper presented to the 7th International Seminar on Regional Innovation Policies, Porto, Portugal, October 7–11, 2012.

Public Health England and NHS Trust. (2015). *A Guide to Community-Centred Approaches for Health and Wellbeing.* Public Health England, London.

Roozenbeek, J., Culloty, E., & Suiter, J. (2023). Countering misinformation: Evidence, knowledge gaps, and implications of current interventions. *European Psychologist, 28*(3), 189–205.

Trinity College Dublin. (2019a). *Strategic Plan 2020 — 2025: Community and Connection.* Trinity College Dublin, Dublin.

Trinity College Dublin. (2019b). *A Living Research Excellence Strategy.* Trinity College Dublin, Dublin.

Trinity College Dublin. (2019c). *Trinity Research Charter.* Trinity College Dublin, Dublin.

Trinity College Dublin. (2019d). *Global Relations Strategy.* Trinity College Dublin, Dublin.

Trinity College Dublin. (2019e). *Student Partnership Policy.* Trinity College Dublin, Dublin.

Trinity College Dublin. (2019f). *Sustainability Policy.* Trinity College Dublin, Dublin.

Trinity College Dublin. (2019g). *Trinity Education Project (TEP).* Trinity College Dublin, Dublin.

Trinity College Dublin. (2019h). *Research and Innovation Policy.* Trinity College Dublin, Dublin.

Trinity College Dublin. (2019i). *Civic Engagement and Social Innovation Fund.* Trinity College Dublin, Dublin.

Trinity College Dublin. (2023). *Civic Engagement for Societal Impact Action Plan 2024–2026.* Trinity College Dublin, Dublin. https://www.tcd.ie/civicengagement/assets/pdf/actionplan/CESIActionPlan2426.pdf

Ursic, L., Baldacchino, G., Bašic, E., Sainz, A. B., Buljan, I., Hampel, M., Kružic, I., Majic, M., Marušic, A., Thetiot, F., Tokalic, R. I., & Markic, L. V. (2022). Factors influencing interdisciplinary research and industry-academia collaborations at six European universities: A qualitative study. *Sustainability, 14*(15), 9306. https://doi.org/10.3390/su14159306

Watson, D., Hollister, R. M., Stroud, S. E., & Babcock, E. (2011). *The Engaged University: International Perspectives on Civic Engagement.* Routledge, New York.

PART 3

Research Applying Person-Centered Approaches to the Community

13

RE-IMAGINING CARE – THE AUSTRALIA CARES PROJECT[1]

Brendan McCormack and Kate Harrison-Brennan[2]

Context

There is a drive to redress the imbalance in care from an ethos that is medically dominated, disease orientated and often fragmented, to one that is relationship focused, collaborative and holistic. The challenges, however, in making the shift to a more holistic model of care are continually emphasized, and at one level, we can attribute this to the complexity of (health) care systems and the impact of a diverse range of strategy and policy imperatives (Roncarolo et al. 2017). This inevitably translates into challenges experienced at the practice level that include, for example: increased emphasis on targets, the impact of organizational culture on individuals and teams, the increase in treatment options and technological care, the requirement of professionals to be technically competent, the drive for effectiveness and efficiency and an unrelenting focus on the financial bottom line.

Despite these challenges, and especially since the COVID-19 pandemic, there is an increasing desire to reaffirm the importance of the essentials of care, such as dignity, respect, privacy and communication (McCance and McCormack 2023), which are considered important to the care experience. It is in this context that we find increasing attention given to approaches that place the human experience at the center of care delivery. There is a strong synergy between caring and person-centeredness, with both ultimately focused on the quality of relationships that enable a good care experience to be realized (McCance and McCormack 2023).

'Care' is a word that is widely connected with professional healthcare practice, especially in nursing practice, but certainly not exclusively so. The word "care" is generally thought to be a positive term, implying love and kindness. However, it is not always straightforward. "Care" can be triggering and jarring for people who have had traumatic experiences of care systems or those whose caring labor

DOI: 10.4324/9781032662657-16

is undervalued or unacknowledged. People with disability often prefer the terms support worker and family member to care worker or carer, seeing the word care as paternalistic and patronizing (cf Davis 2013). Many early childhood educators have also rejected the word care, preferring to emphasize the educational role they play in children's development (Kamerman 2000).

A starting definition of care comes from feminist theorists, Fisher and Tronto (1990):

> Care is a species activity that includes everything that we do to maintain, continue and repair our 'world' so that we can live in it as well as possible. That world includes our bodies, ourselves, and our environment, all of which we seek to interweave in a complex, life-sustaining web.

Care really matters, it is deeply personal, even intimate, and it's a feature of our closest relationships, where vulnerability and dependence play out. We give and receive care across the course of life, from birth to death. When care goes right, it builds agency, dignity and connection through the reciprocal relationships between those giving and receiving care (Persson et al. 2020; Jennings 2018). When it goes wrong, it's a deep breaking of trust. At its worst, care can be exploitative and abusive. Every week we see and hear reports of people deeply shocked at the care received by their aged parents; colleagues, friends and family members with disabilities; and children. It happens across all types of care, leading to repeated tragedies, injustices and public scandals, as inquiry after review after royal commission continues to expose (Royal Commission into Aged Care Quality and Safety 2021). We hear stories of exhaustion, understaffing and low morale told by nurses, early childhood educators, teachers, paramedics, aged care workers, disability carers and many others (McKinsay & Company 2022; Buchan and Cotton 2023; Buchan, Cotton and Shaffer 2023). The many symptoms of our broken cultures, systems and practices of care are matched by a bewildering number of proposed remedies. It's as if a whole industry and infrastructure has grown up around plugging gaps and mending existing systems.

We're uncomfortable with care. Too often, there's an undertone that characterizes care as an unfortunate inconvenience, too private and too "female" to be aired in public (Green and Lawson 2011). Dependence and vulnerability are not words that come easy to us – we prefer to avoid thinking about them until we are forced to. "God forbid it should be me. It's undignified". We've painted those needing care as the unfortunate others, stripping them of their full personhood. So, we don't talk about it, even less celebrate it, and we've failed to understand and share the rich stories of beautiful care, respectful care, dignified care and care that shows what it is like to really help someone to flourish as a person.

We've also accepted the shocking disconnect present when we expect wonderful care, whether from paid or unpaid family and friend carers, but we completely undervalue carers. We set up systems with individualized care, designed to enable people needing care to identify their goals and seek services, then we expect that to be supported by people who are invisible, disrespected, unsupported or paid very poorly. It is a gap we're somehow not seeing (Commonwealth of Australia 2024).

The language we use and stories we tell hide inequality. Care is deeply racialized and stigmatized. We hear narratives suggesting there are people who are "deserving" and "undeserving" of care. Often, those who are "undeserving" are also those who aren't from racial or ethnic majorities. Those who are "undeserving" are often those who need care the most. And, ironically, those who are "undeserving" are often those who step into caring roles that others don't want to do, allowing our society and economy to keep ticking. Because we've failed to understand and value it, we've reduced care to a series of transactions, we deal with it in siloes and we think short term. Systematized policy responses to care have converted this deeply personal, unpredictable and relationship-based activity into units of labor and tools that can be standardized, measured and controlled. We look at it sector by sector, area by area, service by service, narrowing our field of vision and obscuring the interconnections between care as it plays out in different spheres.

So, in the Australia Cares Project, we set out to do something different, to re-imagine care and to do that drawing on sets of relationships and tools not usually deployed in policymaking.

Overview of the Project

We shaped the Australia Cares project through five questions:

1. What if we posed bigger questions about the place of care in the community and our economy?
2. What if we inverted the policymaking model, enabling communities to set the agenda and give policy guidance?
3. What if we brought people with diverse perspectives together to tackle those questions?
4. What if we used the expertise and infrastructure of the University of Sydney to partner with communities?
5. What if we stepped back from the short timeframes of political cycles?

To frame these questions and consider the many challenges associated with care, we framed care through the lens of "healthfulness": cultivating "environments of care that promote health", including "healthful relationships" that support a person to flourish. Care is about person-centeredness, relationships, professional care, nursing care, care theories, care and support economies and support services. It includes care for older people, children, people with disability, people from racial or ethnic minorities, people when they are sick and self-care. Care for Country is central to this approach to care as we recognize, value and center our connection to land and each other in the life-sustaining web of relationships of which we are a part. Care in all its guises is a vehicle for creating flourishing persons, communities and populations. Flourishing happens when we are "held" through various experiences as we move through life. We flourish when we experience beneficial, growth that pushes us to be the best versions of ourselves. When we are helped to make the most of our naturally occurring potential to care by channeling it for good, we don't just flourish as persons, whole communities have the potential to become more resilient. The context in which we live our life also plays a key role and our potential to flourish is context dependent. Conditions such as a culture that nurtures positive relationships, consistency between individual goals, desire for achievement and community goals, development strategies that invest in people as persons and approaches to learning, development and engagement that nurture individual and community vitality and energy, are essential. So, no matter how actively driven we might be toward our own flourishing, the cultures in which we work and live have a significant impact on our ability to do so.

Reimagining care encourages us to reflect critically on our language so that how we speak about care itself is caring. This means choosing language that helps people, including ourselves, to feel supported to live our best lives.

Methodology

Our work in the project explored community-led policymaking through two initiatives:

- Care Labs
- People's Assemblies on Care

We linked these initiatives with Stories of Care to complement perspectives obtained through the Care Labs and People's Assemblies.

We valued different forms of knowledge and invited diverse expertise from people with knowledge from personal experience, community knowledge, knowledge as a practitioner, organizational knowledge and academic knowledge (see textbox below). We convened activities bringing together people of diverse age, gender, socio-economic background and life experience. We created spaces that would maximize the opportunity for collaborators to have a positive experience of being and working together. From the design of activities and preparation of materials to the details of how spaces were set up, we created safe and inclusive spaces for knowledge co-production. In all our activities, we invited people to participate not only in their professional capacity but also by contributing their personal and lived experiences. We enabled opportunity for shared contemplation, attended to the inner worlds of collaborators and their social contexts and enabled emotional engagement. We facilitated a dance between the use of creative individual and group methods – clay, poetry and metaphor, for example – matched with deep thinking, reflective discussions and systematic approaches through structured deliberative practices. While we worked with structured plans, we were flexible with how these unfolded based on the flow of engagement with and between collaborators. We were able to stay focused on what was important in the moment and facilitate the emergence of new insights in a systematic and thoughtful way.

Participant Details

- 9 Care Labs
- 38 Care Lab collaborators
- 40+ People's Assembly on Care collaborators

Care Labs

These were online collaborations to discern care principles and apply these in thematic policy areas: aged care in the home and community and disability support in early childhood education and care.

We convened a series of online workshops and invited a diverse mix of collaborators. Across four core workshops and four shorter sessions, 38 people from different geographical locations collaborated in this policymaking. Many of these people joined us for a final Care Lab in November at the Australian Parliament House in Canberra with public servants and political staffers.

We adapted the methodology of Theory U (Scharmer and Kaufer 2018) to inform the Care Labs, enabling meaningful engagement from all collaborators. Theory U is an awareness-based methodology for changing systems which challenges us to connect with our internal world – our beliefs, values, experiences and assumptions – to engage fully with the external world. Theory U combines principles derived from participatory action research, design thinking, mindfulness and civil society movements. We shaped the work of the Care Labs through the five collaborative commitments of Sharmer and Kaufer to provide us with a framework to guide our movement around the "U". Importantly, our intention was to use the labs to get to the bottom of the "U" – presenting – where we could all be content our collaborative explorations resulted in a shared understanding of care principles we could all "settle with".

As we invited our collaborators into this process, we clearly signaled we were seeking to enable a way of being and working together that was different from the common experience of online workshops in which collaborators can be passive recipients of dense material presented by "experts". For example, we sent a Care Lab pack ahead of the sessions with a guide, creative materials and a snack. The initial signaling continued in the style of facilitation and theoretically informed modes of interaction. We used personal artifacts, clay modeling and poetry as stories of care were shared. We developed poetry and collaborative "inflammatory essays" (Siegel 1985) to uncover care principles. Policy ideas were posited and tested using the Disney Creative Strategy method (Designorate 2015)

People's Assemblies on Care

We worked with two communities where the University of Sydney has a physical presence and campus: Westmead in Western Sydney and Broken Hill in far-west New South Wales to hold People's Assemblies on Care. These People's Assemblies were designed as a response to the weariness members of the Australian public felt at successive Royal Commissions doing post-mortems of policy failures in key policy areas related to care (e.g. Royal Commission into Aged Care Quality and Safety 2021). Inspired by a wave of deliberative democratic exercises that have sprung up around the world, we selected a deliberative method to create a microcosm of a local community, a "mini public". We designed activities that sought to enable a movement from precognitive to cognitive engagement with the topics and subject matter. We worked with design thinking methods (Dust 2020) to create participatory and deliberative activities for the Assemblies.

For each Assembly, 20 community members were recruited. In Broken Hill, we worked with a broadly representative cross-section of the Broken Hill population, adjusted to ensure an equal representation of females and males as well as a higher proportion of Aboriginal and Torres Strait Islands people than in the general Broken Hill community and people with experience of chronic illness. In Westmead, we focused selection on a cross-section of members of the community who have a South Asian background. This was informed by insights from the first stages of the project in which those we spoke with in government and communities highlighted the need for policy development that reflected the values and expectations of culturally and linguistically diverse communities. We specifically sought families living in multigenerational households.

The Assemblies were designed to run in two phases in each location. Phase one, a three-hour evening workshop, was an exercise in consultation and agenda setting which set up for phase two, an all-day workshop on a weekend to deliberate on policy solutions.

About Care and Caring

Across the project, people spoke about the gulf between their aspirations to live in a caring society and their lived experiences of care. Beyond the published reports on broken systems, which are numerous and compelling, we unearthed a sense of anger and frustration, and a deep sense of those being cared for and those doing the caring not being seen.

In sharing stories of care, we recognized that in caring and being cared for, we experience our shared personhood. Our collaborators shared rich personal experiences: beautiful stories of relationships and community shared between those being cared for and those caring. We were moved by stories of love, each intimate and individual but linking us with something shared and essentially human. We heard of the strong bonds within communities and families that enable care, and the personal and cultural significance of caring for family members. Care is central to identity and culture within many of the communities we worked with.

> The beauty of being a carer to someone we love, it's enormous … And when my father for example, said to me, oh, living here with you every day, it's a Sunday. Because he felt my love and care that that made me feel tall and strong, no matter how exhausted I was. And when my mum living with dementia she looked at me and she said, 'oh, God loves me, because he gave me you to look after me.'
>
> *(Care Labs collaborator)*

In contrast, stories were shared of the shocking lack of care and value given to those they love, whether it be as they age, seek disability support or come to Australia as migrants. We heard about a distressing level of "othering" of people with disabilities, the invisibility of those outside of our major cities and the challenges of navigating ever more complex systems.

We heard that while caring is certainly difficult at times, it is not intrinsically burdensome. Our collaborators shared rich stories of the joys of caring – of enabling others to flourish. It is our cultures, systems and practices of care that impose a burden, placing pressure on the relationships between carers and those they care for. We heard stories of carers losing paid work to make phone calls and attend appointments, losing the capacity to build social connections; and facing poverty and lack of rest during retirement. We heard of the difficulties of navigating care in remote communities and the transcultural issues and challenges that get in the way of effective care and support for extended family systems in culturally diverse communities. There was a strong sense of these costs being invisible, to be covered privately and preferably quietly by individuals and households.

> Who do they think is sitting around with all this free time to be everyone's power of attorney with the pain and the hardship of the hours on hold? I'm not even talking about providing the direct care – the indirect care carries an enormous cost where you have to take a day of unpaid leave to do your old mum's calls, but the rest of the economy doesn't respect that, and still, you have to work on their time. So, the gerontologist's office will not commit to calling you at a particular time. The hospital will not commit. Nobody will facilitate anyone else.
>
> *(Care Labs collaborator)*

We clearly heard the anger of carers – anger at the load, invisibility and costs imposed by complex systems that are not working. Systems that don't make it easy for carers to access benefits and seem to serve the bureaucracy as an entity rather than those who are navigating it. Family and friend carers shared stories of how they grieve the opportunities taken away by our systems, just as they celebrate the relationships and experiences gained through the human activity of caring.

> I had to do a survey on wellbeing the other day and it wanted me to say I am happy a percentage of time and sad a percentage of time, and they had to add up to 100 percent. I'm like, emotions don't work like that. I can be 80 percent happy and 70 percent distressed.
>
> *(Care Labs collaborator)*

We heard the anger of those being cared for, of being "othered" and made invisible. In our current systems and cultures, too often the rights of those caring are pitted against those they are caring for, as if we were playing a zero-sum game. Our collaborators have pushed back against that: rights to care and be cared for must be seen as complementary rather than being in opposition. My right to care with dignity and agency at its heart need not undermine your right to recognition and compensation. Your right to a voice and to build your skills as a carer must not be at the expense of my agency and dignity as I am cared for.

The failures of our care systems are experienced differently across communities. We heard stories of the failures in care provisioning and suitability for Aboriginal and Torres Strait Islander peoples, women, migrants and those living beyond metropolitan areas. We sensed a series of underlying questions: Are there those that deserve care and those that don't? Do those with money and assets after a lifetime of "contributing" deserve more than those who have disability and will always require intensive support? Do we accept poorer quality care for some, just thankful that it's not us?

We heard the frustration and distress from underserved populations who are unable to access care for a range of reasons, from chronic shortages of care workers and care services to services that do not respond to cultural needs or are inaccessible because of policy imperatives. We heard of the domino effect when workforce shortages in one industry or sector of care have impacts across whole communities of care. We heard of the importance of trust in relationships of care and the sometimes-devastating impacts when this is absent.

We discovered care cannot be considered without also taking account of housing, economic security, visa status and safety. In many of our conversations and in different contexts, the giving and receiving of care were linked to factors that might at first glance seem unrelated. The reality for so many is that these are inextricably linked, and any meaningful consideration of care requires that we enable these connections to be acknowledged, described and analyzed.

These stories are consistent with what we know to be many of the problems and challenges in care systems. For example, there is consistent evidence over many years of international research that shows the impact on relationships, physical health, mental health and financial security of informal carer roles and family carer roles when they are not recognized, acknowledged and properly supported (Commonwealth of Australia 2024). The stories we heard bring this evidence into sharp focus and to life through lived experience.

The lived experiences of our collaborators also show how poorly equipped our care systems are to address geographic and cultural diversity among the Australian population. Arising from deeply listening to these stories are some fundamental questions we need to address as a society, including: How do we overturn histories of neglect, marginalization and discrimination from care systems among some populations and communities? How do we rebuild trust in decision-makers at all levels to engage in active inclusion strategies? How do we suggest decision-makers need to understand the whole picture to develop collaborative and inclusive policies on care?

Our collaborators were clear: we must do better with care policy. It should be underpinned by an interconnected set of principles and lead to a fundamental redesign of our systems. We worked with the Care Lab collaborators to systematically analyze the data collected during the Labs to generate four principles of care that transcend people, contexts and specialties (Figure 13.1). These principles act as "action guides" for shaping ongoing developments in care and future work of the Sydney Policy Lab.

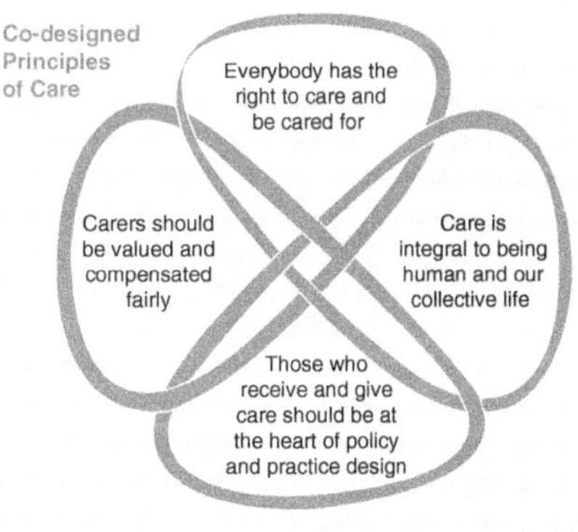

A cross-section of people collaborated in the Care Labs, including care givers and receivers, service providers and academics.

Their message was clear: We can do better.

Participants found Australia's current care system penalises and stigmatises people that are cared for and give care.

They felt care systems were often a burden that made these people invisible instead of helping them to flourish. Moreover, with the system focused on preserving itself, some people cannot find and afford quality care.

Together, participants co-designed four principles to address problems in the care system.

FIGURE 13.1 Co-designed principles of care

Policy Solutions

From the first phase of the People's Assemblies in Westmead and Broken Hill, driving questions for subsequent deliberation were developed. In Westmead, this focused on the care ecosystem and how transcultural issues and challenges get in the way of that ecosystem. While in Broken Hill, the driving question focused on care navigation and the complexities associated with finding one's way in, around and through the care system. Those gathered in the People's Assemblies on Care, supported by University of Sydney academics and professional staff, offered eight solutions to the challenges they identified (Table 13.1).

TABLE 13.1 Policy solutions identified

	Problem	*Solution*
1. Universal health care for all in Australia, regardless of visa	It's not guaranteed that if you're in Australia and in urgent need of health care you will receive that care. In emergency departments across the country, signs make clear that unless you have a Medicare card, you will have to pay for medical care received.	A humane approach to provision of medical assistance and care that provides a universal safety net for urgent and emergency care within Australia.
2. A new carer visa category	Parent Visas – contributory or non-contributory – are not meeting the needs of community members. The federal government 2023 Review of the Migration System highlighted that families are waiting for parent visas that never come (Parkinson et al. 2023). A growing migrant population has driven demand beyond places available. While recognizing that family structures and distributions of care across cultural groups differ, members of the migrant population experience acute and time-bound needs for care which are exacerbated when away from family members and others with whom they share long-term connections, language and culture.	Create a new carer visa category that has clear categories for qualification. For example, to provide care to a family member who has been diagnosed with terminal cancer, has been significantly injured in an accident or has been told by their doctor to be on bed rest during pregnancy. This could also enable caring for a very young child. The Sydney Policy Lab has addressed this issue with a "Carers Visa Policy Paper" that can be found here

(*Continued*)

TABLE 13.1 (*Continued*)

	Problem	*Solution*
3. Culturally integrated services network to uplift and facilitate cultural and religious needs in care provision	There are underserved populations whose various cultural and religious needs are not well understood by mainstream services. This means services are not accessed at all, services are accessed less than would otherwise be the case or public health messages are not received by members of the community because cultural and religious considerations and practices are not well understood or engaged with.	A network of care providers and volunteers who help uplift and facilitate specific community needs such as cultural meal delivery, end-of-life care, funeral service support, transport for community events; pre- and post-natal care, and health education on topics like the safety of co-sleeping with babies and infants.
4. One-stop shop to assist with retirement and later life planning for care	Ageing, for anyone, is like entering into another land. Ageing when you are a migrant compounds the sense of disorientation. Without signposts, it's hard to plan for the journey. In a world increasingly focused on digital solutions, this is no less the case when it comes to care services. However, so-called digital solutions bring layers of complexity and challenge that don't always result in meaningful outcomes for end users.	Create a one-stop shop that would help migrants – the Australian community, too – understand what might be ahead on the journey, choices they can make and how they and their loved ones can plan well for the future.
5. Community health education program	Carers of migrants who are also migrants themselves often find it challenging to navigate care services efficiently and effectively, and miss out on support and services.	Provide better education and information for the community, with the community and by the community. Work with existing community service providers to co-design education programs to improve care services and literacy of carers.

(*Continued*)

TABLE 13.1 (*Continued*)

	Problem	*Solution*
6. Families network forum for navigating and activating care	Navigating and then accessing care is difficult. It's hard to know which information to trust and to find care relevant to needs. We know care services are available, but we're lost trying to find them.	Create a digital resource curated and provided through trusted public apps to help individuals and the community navigate and access care relevant to them. Make it so that there is a seamless connection between the various actors who provide care and generate links with the physical places people go to access care.
7. Creative solutions to workforce shortages	The domino effect of workforce shortages in any one care sector generating a set of pressures on households and communities and contributing to workforce shortages not just in other care sectors, but across the local labor market.	Recognize that siloed thinking about interventions in one sector may exacerbate rather than solve broader workforce shortages. Learn from successes such as student placements that have led to ongoing work in community, and considered use of technology that enables care to be supported remotely. Developed solutions need to be holistic in nature, consider the whole care ecosystem and the relationships between individual components and embedded in established relationships with community organizations and service providers.
8. Care Navigators embedded in community	Shortage of services, as well as difficulties in navigating care systems, matched with long-standing fear and mistrust of formal systems, exacerbate barriers to accessing available care and support in a location.	Working in partnership with local communities, community leaders and people with lived experience, identify new ways to remove barriers to care through community asset mapping and co-creating solutions that draw on existing community assets and knowledges. Allocate resources to community-developed care navigation systems that are fit-for-place and commit to the development of new services that enhance access to care and services.

A Framework for Action

The Australia Cares project has demonstrated just what can be achieved when people are given the opportunity and support required to step back from systems and policy settings as they are and to imagine what could be. The problem definitions and solutions identified reflect what matters to a cross-section of people involved in care in Australia and two very different communities.

The policy recommendations we have made not only are highly desired by members of communities who have suffered from successive policy failures but also have the potential to be highly effective if refined and implemented with this same community leadership and university partnership. Governments at local, state and federal levels now have the opportunity – and need – to look beyond their near-term agendas in which they have sought to address the most urgent and pressing failures in current systems and policies related to care. These systems and policy settings have their origins in the 1950s, yet even measured by the values of decades past they have not succeeded.

Current harms, egregious policy and governance failures must, of course, be addressed, but it's time to transition to a new way of thinking about and doing care policy. It is time to move away from a dominance of neoliberal values that drive policymaking and delivery frameworks modeled on new public management to a greater emphasis on relationships and the relational economy that can drive innovative solutions for the future. A coherent, forward-looking framework for action is urgently needed to enable a person-centered approach to care that:

- is holistic, binding together care, well-being and health and therefore linked to other policy reform agendas
- listens to people throughout policymaking cycles
- builds a relational economy
- responds to community expectations
- is designed around the strengths and assets of specific cohorts and communities
- renews public institutions and invites partnerships
- spreads capital investment across the economy, especially to the forgotten parts

Summary

The Australia Cares project has demonstrated that a new framework for action is desirable, feasible and viable. As a community-led, multidisciplinary project, we have shown the potential for collaborations across sectors and between institutions to provide new solutions within such a framework. In the project itself, we have piloted various forms of community-led policy development. Drawing on what we've learned, these could now provide the basis for the way forward for care policy: community-led policies developed and implemented on an iterative basis. It remains the case that proactive approaches to seeking citizen-voice and participation are novel in policy making and there is a need for new methodologies such as that used in the Australia Cares project to be extended and expanded. We are committed to moving forward with communities across Australia on the Australia Cares project, and with this collaborative approach. Success will be when care policy enables communities across Australia to flourish in ways that are socially sustainable.

Notes

1 The full report of the Australia Cares Project can be found here Australia Cares Report.
2 We wish to acknowledge the co-authors of The Australia Cares Report – Marj O'Callaghan, Louise Beehag, Juliet Bennett, Christine El-Khoury and Max Hall, as well as the members of the Expert Advisory Group who guided the project processes. We also acknowledge the significant contributions of all the participants in the Care Labs and People's Assemblies on Care who gave so freely of their time, experience and care.

References

Buchan, J., & Catton, H. (2023). Recover to Rebuild: Investing in the Nursing Workforce for Health System Effectiveness. *International Council of Nurses*, *11*, 2023–03.

Buchan, J., Catton, H., & Shaffer, F. (2022). Sustain and Retain in 2022 and Beyond. *International Council of Nurses*, *71*, 1–71.

Commonwealth of Australia (Department of Social Services). (2024). The National Carers Strategy 2024–2034. https://www.dss.gov.au/supporting-carers/national-carer-strategy (accessed 19/12/2024).

Davis, L. J. (2013). Introduction: Normality, Power, and Culture. In L. Davis (ed.), *The Disability Studies Reader Fourth Edition*. New York: Routledge.

Designorate (2015). Disney's Creative Strategy: The Dreamer, The Realist and The Critic. https://www.designorate.com/disneys-creative-strategy/

Dust, F. (2020) *Making Conversation*. New York: Harper Collins.

Fisher, B., & Tronto, J. C. (1990) Toward a Feminist Theory of Care. In E. K. Abel & M. K. Nelson (eds.) *Circles of Care: Work and Identity in Women's Lives* (pp. 35–62). Albany: State University of New York Press.

Green, M., & Lawson, V. (2011). Recentring Care: Interrogating the Commodification of Care. *Social & Cultural Geography, 12*(6), 639–654. https://doi.org/10.1080/14649365.2011.601262

Jennings, B. (2018). Solidarity and Care as Relational Practices. *Bioethics, 32*(9), 553–561.

Kamerman, S. B. (2000). Early Childhood Education and Care: An Overview of Developments in the OECD Countries. *International Journal of Educational Research, 33*(1), 7–29. https://doi.org/10.1016/S0883-0355(99)00041-5

McCance, T., & McCormack, B. (2023). Developing Healthful Cultures through the Development of Person-Centred Practice. *International Journal of Orthopaedic and Trauma Nursing*. https://doi.org/10.1016/j.ijotn.2023.101055

McKinsay & Company (2022). Should I Stay, or Should I Go? Australia's Nurse Retention Dilemma. https://www.mckinsey.com/industries/healthcare/our-insights/should-i-stay-or-should-i-go-australias-nurse-retention-dilemma (accessed 19/12/2024).

Parkinson, M., Howe, J., & Azarias, J. (2023). *Review of the Migration System 2023*. Canberra: Commonwealth of Australia.

Persson, C., Benzein, E., & Morberg Jämterud, S. (2020). Dignity as an Intersubjective Phenomenon: Experiences of Dyads Living With Serious Illness. *Qualitative Health Research, 30*(13), 1989–2000. https://doi.org/10.1177/1049732320938343

Roncarolo, F., Boivin, A., Denis, J. L. Rejean, H., & Pascale, L. (2017). What Do We Know About the Needs and Challenges of Health Systems? A Scoping Review of the International Literature. *BMC Health Services Research, 17*, 636. https://doi.org/10.1186/s12913-017-2585-5

Royal Commission into Aged Care Quality and Safety. (2021). https://www.royalcommission.gov.au/aged-care/final-report (accessed 19/12/2024).

Scharmer, O., & Kaufer, K. (2018). *The Essentials of Theory U: Core Principles and Application.* Oakland, CA: Berrett-Koehler Publishers.

Siegel, J. (1985 December). Jenny Holzer's Language Games. *Arts Magazine, 4*, 64.

14

CO-DESIGNING INTEGRATED CARE TECHNOLOGY WITH OLDER PEOPLE AND THEIR SUPPORT NETWORK IN THE COMMUNITY

Insights from The ValueCare Project

Andrew Darley and Áine Carroll

Introduction

As populations age globally, ensuring the well-being of older adults has become a critical public health priority. We have reached a period when people are expected to live longer than at any other time in history. Healthcare advancements and access, living conditions and greater awareness of health behaviors have shaped how population-level life expectancies are at an all-time high, with an estimate that, by 2030, one-in-six Europeans will be aged over 60 years and, by 2040, one-in-four older people will be aged over 85 years (United Nations, 2017; World Health Organisation [WHO], 2022). While this projected demographic shift indicates societal progress in promoting healthy lifestyles and addressing environmental factors, it also increases the likelihood that more people will experience a chronic or complex health condition during their lifespan (Partridge et al., 2018). Older people are often faced with conditions and circumstances that can limit their ability to live as they wish.

To address this, healthy aging has become a key global strategy which focuses on "the process of developing and maintaining the functional ability that enables wellbeing in older age" (WHO, 2022). Healthy aging does not simply focus on promoting a person's physical health status, but is a multidimensional concept that encompasses psychological, social, environmental, cultural and spiritual components (Menassa et al., 2023). It embodies the proactive promotion of people's ability to learn, maintain relationships, make decisions and contribute to society throughout the lifespan (Beard et al., 2016). Healthy aging centers on creating the environments and opportunities that enable people to be and do what they value throughout their lives (WHO, 2021). To achieve this, the World Health Organization has urged entities to focus not on the increase in longevity, but rather on finding ways

DOI: 10.4324/9781032662657-17

to support the quality of the extra years, encouraging older people's activity, autonomy and sustained engagement in society (WHO, 2017).

For healthy aging initiatives to be successful, health and social care services must be structured and resourced in a way that facilitates a holistic care approach, supporting older people to achieve fulfilling lives. However, this can be a great challenge, as health systems are commonly structured in a way that fragments pertinent care services (Strange, 2009). This is particularly important for the care of older people, as they often have multiple conditions that require a multidisciplinary care approach. This siloed structure of health systems has been associated with poor medication management (Anderson, 2010), preventable hospital admissions (Nyweide et al., 2013) and increased mortality rates (Prior et al., 2023).

Integrated care is a movement which seeks to provide person-centered and coordinated care for people across their lifespan (Goodwin, 2016). In Ireland, a specific national clinical program has been implemented to deliver integrated care for older people, aiming to improve healthcare delivery and address the challenges of an aging population (Health Service Executive, 2017; Harnett et al., 2020). Digital health is a proposed solution to support both healthy aging (Neves et al., 2022; Helbostad et al., 2017) and integrated care (Shah et al., 2022). While technology may offer a valuable tool to support older people in their home environments and communities, technological innovations must be grounded in the values of the people they intend to support. This represents a core principle in person-centered care approaches, while concurrently creating partnerships with older people as a community, which reflects the ethos of this project. Participatory research methods, such as co-design, are becoming increasingly prevalent in designing and evaluating person-centered health and/or social care solutions, which directly involve people in developing the solution they seek to support (Donetto et al., 2015).

As older people represent an increasingly larger proportion of our population, health systems and local communities must respond, adapt and provide ways to meet the priorities and preferences of people as they age. Community well-being encompasses various aspects of life that contribute to the overall quality of life, including social, environmental and cultural (Phillips and Pittman, 2009). For older adults, community well-being is crucial as it can significantly impact their health, independence and life satisfaction (Schulz and Eden, 2016). Drawing on the exemplar of the European-funded research study, The ValueCare Project, this chapter outlines the underlying principles and methodology for co-designing an integrated care digital health technology to support the well-being of older people in their communities within the Irish context.

Integrated Care for Older People

Recognizing the increasing global population of older adults, health systems will need to adapt to meet the well-being needs of older people and reach them within their community settings. Older people commonly experience multiple or complex health conditions which require a holistic understanding and comprehensive care approach from multidisciplinary care providers (Banerjee et al., 2015). However, our health systems are not structured in a way that facilitates a comprehensive, coordinated care approach, aligning people's medical, psychological and social well-being needs to ensure they are addressed effectively. Interprofessional collaboration and teamwork are known to be inhibited by differences in organizational cultures, professional boundaries and communication barriers (Lingard et al., 2017; Suter et al., 2009). Lack of coordination between necessary health and social care services can result in suboptimal outcomes for older people that inhibit their quality of life, such as repeated hospital admissions, delays in receiving appropriate care and increased levels of anxiety and depression as they struggle with navigating complex healthcare pathways (Baxter et al., 2018; Rosenwohl-Mack et al., 2020). Health and social care services operating in isolation can make it challenging for older people and their supportive network to access the care providers who would most effectively support them in their needs.

Integrated care is valued as a critical approach to reforming and supporting health systems to cope with demographic aging (Lourenço et al., 2023). Integrated care seeks to address the known fragmentation and overlap that can occur within existing healthcare systems, which can impact people's well-being (Goodwin, 2016). While there is no universal definition of integrated care, the most commonly used definition (Armitage et al., 2009) comes from the World Health Organization (Waddington, 2008): "The Organisation and management of health services so that people get the care they need, when they need it, in ways that are user friendly, achieve the desired results and provide value for money". More specifically, integrated care for older people refers to a continuum of services that shifts health and social care toward a more person-centered and coordinated approach, thereby optimizing the intrinsic capacity (encompassing both physical and mental capabilities) and functional ability of older individuals (World Health Organisation, 2022). Evidence to date suggests that integrated care can have a positive impact on the well-being of older people, including improved management of chronic health conditions and complex needs, reduced hospital admissions and fewer emergency department visits (Goodwin et al., 2014; Kirst et al., 2017). By integrating relevant health and social care services into the livelihoods of older people and applying an interdisciplinary model of care, integrated care has the potential to provide comprehensive and holistic support tailored to the unique needs of older individuals, ultimately promoting healthy aging and well-being.

Integrated Care for Older People in Ireland

In the context of Ireland, it is projected that by 2041, one-in-four Irish people will be over the age of 65, necessitating the development of comprehensive and coordinated care strategies (Central Statistics Office, 2017). The Irish government and policymakers have placed substantial emphasis and investment in supporting older people's choices to live safely and independently in their own homes and community for as long as possible, commonly known as "ageing in place" (O'Sullivan et al., 2022). Supporting people to live in their homes and communities can enable "older people to maintain independence, autonomy, and connection to social support, including friends and family" (Wiles et al., 2011, p. 357). The national Irish health service, the Health Service Executive (HSE), developed and implemented strategic frameworks aimed at promoting integrated care including the National Clinical Programme for Older People (NCPOP) and the National Integrated Care Programme for Older Persons (NICPOP) (HSE, 2017), which seek to enhance and bridge existing gaps between primary, secondary and social care services.

The NICPOP in Ireland was established with the primary goal of supporting older people in their home setting. A key innovative feature of NICPOP is the establishment of pioneer community-centered integrated care hubs for older people (Barry et al., 2021). These integrated care hubs are situated within the HSE's Older Persons' and Chronic Disease Service model, which seeks to shift older person care to proactive and preventive settings, away from acute settings where older people are known to experience poorer health outcomes and morbidity. Integrated care hubs are geriatrician-led ambulatory specialist services for older people, functioning as outpatient day hospitals and staffed by a core multidisciplinary team that addresses common health challenges, such as falls, memory clinics, movement disorders and frailty (NCPOP, 2012).

The Integrated Care Program for Older Persons (ICPOP) Hubs are distinctive in their ability to undertake Comprehensive Geriatric Assessments (CGA), which are deemed the "gold standard" in assessing and managing the health and social well-being needs of older people, thereby avoiding fragmented care approaches in community settings (Turner, 2014). Upon completing the CGA, each older person receives a personalized, tailored care plan based on their identified needs and returns to their home in the community. These plans are centered on both the results that emerged in the context of the CGA and the co-production of care plans with the older person and their care supporters. In essence, the ICPOP Hubs are designed to expand and integrate health services, providing specialist support within older people's communities and promoting their well-being. This model of integrated care in Ireland provides specialist, multidisciplinary care that aims to support the well-being and independent living of older people, prevent acute health events and identify and address psychosocial challenges to living well in their own communities.

The Role of Digital Health in Integrated Care for Older People

The use of technology in the provision of health and social care, commonly referred to as digital health, presents an opportunity to reimagine how care is delivered and promote healthy behaviors among older people. Digital health technology has been recognized for its ability to place and empower people at the center of their care, improve health literacy and support informed decision-making regarding management or treatment plans (WHO, 2021). More specifically, digital health is regarded as a valuable tool in supporting older people in their self-management practices and well-being in their homes (Maeder et al., 2020; Tannou et al., 2022), as it is understood that the management of most health conditions relies on personal maintenance rather than clinical care. In Ireland, the value of digital technology is reflected in the "Stay Left, Shift Left" initiative, which seeks to support well-being in their home using proactive and preventative supports through digital mediums and ultimately avoid hospital or acute services (HSE Digital Transformation, 2020).

On a personal level, digital health technologies can enhance the service user's health engagement and self-management. Mobile health applications (apps) and wearable devices empower older adults to take an active role in their health by tracking their physical activity, medication adherence and other health-related behaviors (Kvedar et al., 2014). This increased engagement may lead to better health outcomes and a greater sense of autonomy among older patients (Ienca et al., 2021; Xie et al., 2022). Family caregivers benefit from digital health technologies through improved communication with healthcare providers and access to educational resources. Mobile apps and online platforms can offer guidance on caregiving tasks, reducing stress and enhancing the quality of care provided (Zhai et al., 2023; Darley et al., 2024).

Digital health technologies offer numerous advantages in the context of integrated care for older people. Technology can facilitate remote monitoring by healthcare providers to older people in their home setting, which can track health indicators, promote healthy behaviors and provide health and social care professionals with real-time data that can inform shared decision-making (Kampmeijer et al., 2016). In this way, digital health technologies can enable the effective sharing of well-being information amongst various healthcare professionals across disciplines. This interoperability ensures that all members of a healthcare team have access to well-being data, which can improve coordination of care and reduce potential errors or duplications (Bates et al., 2018). This process is particularly relevant for facilitating integrated care for older people, who often require the services of multiple specialists from various disciplines. By capturing this well-being information, integrated care professionals can create holistic care plans to support their well-being based on information directly reported or tracked by older persons. Recent evidence (Melchiorre et al., 2018) suggests that digital health technology has led to improved care integration and management practices. Therefore, it is likely that digital health may inform or become a key facet of integrated care models in the future (Shah et al., 2022).

Despite these benefits, several challenges exist to adopting digital health technology in integrated care for older adults. Evidence to date highlights how technological literacy, previous exposure and access to technology inhibit the adoption of technology among older people. These barriers are associated with socioeconomic factors, educational opportunities and physical and/or cognitive limitations related to aging (Friemel, 2016). Concerns about privacy and security have also been found to deter older people from engaging with technology to support their health

(Jockisch et al., 2022). Recognizing that digital health may be an appropriate vehicle for providing and enhancing integrated care, we need to understand at a local community level how to best support older people in a person-centered manner and create the conditions for authentic participation and involvement in their own care. While technological innovations may improve care coordination and accessibility, we must ensure that these advancements are created with the people they intend to support, thereby providing the greatest potential to enhance their well-being and enable them to live their lives in the best way they see fit.

Co-designing Digital Health with Older People

Patient and public involvement (PPI) has become a prevalent approach in rethinking how health and social care services are delivered, with the primary aim of ensuring they are person-centered. Co-design is a key research methodology within PPI, which emphasizes collaboration between people living with well-being challenges and their supportive care network to create solutions that meaningfully meet their needs. As such, the principles of co-design are oriented toward person-centered care, focusing on individual needs, partnerships and collaborations around care plans. Involving and collaborating with older people in the design process helps create solutions that avoid assumptions about what would be helpful. By directly working with key stakeholders, the project's direction can be aligned with targets that benefit the community of older people. Maintaining a multi-perspective approach increases the likelihood that the technology aligns with the priorities and preferences in care for older people, while also being clinically appropriate and feasible within the healthcare setting in which it is intended to be implemented. An evident synergy exists between integrated care and co-design research, as both aim to create person-centered care services that view people as partners and collaborators in their development (Lewis and Ehrenberg, 2020; Bate and Robert, 2007).

Several benefits have been identified regarding co-designing with older people in digital health technology. Involving older people in the design process ensures the resulting technology is tailored to their specific needs and requirements, which can lead to increased usability and adoption rates (Harrington et al., 2018). A sense of ownership has been identified among older adults through the co-design process, as they have played a key role in its creation, which in turn enhances user engagement and satisfaction (Harrington et al., 2018; Lyles et al., 2022; Tsekleves et al., 2016). The co-design process empowers older adults by valuing their input and experiences. This inclusion promotes social engagement and combats the isolation often experienced by older individuals (Vines et al., 2015).

Context of The ValueCare Project

While the shift toward integrated care is occurring in Ireland, there has been no evidence to date regarding the co-design of digital health to support integrated care for older people living in their community and home settings. The ValueCare Project is a European research project, funded by the Horizon 2020 Programme, which seeks to co-design and deliver integrated care to older people living with chronic health conditions across seven European integrated care contexts (Bally et al., 2022). The underlying objective aligns with the Quadruple Aim (Sikka et al., 2015), which aims to enhance the quality of life and well-being of older people, as well as that of their integrated care providers, and promote the sustainability of healthcare systems in Europe. While this project operates on a European scale, its research design and co-design methodology aim to support older people living with various health conditions at the local community level within partner countries.

In the context of the ValueCare pilot study in Ireland, the aim of the study is to develop digital health technology that supports older people living with mild to moderate frailty in the integrated care community settings of Cork and Kerry. Age-related frailty and cognitive decline are complex multidimensional conditions that significantly impact the ability of older adults to sustain functional capacity and independence. The vision for the co-designed technology is to align with the current Older Persons'/Chronic Disease Service Model and Integrated Care Model (i.e. Supports to Live At Home) (Harnett et al., 2020). Acknowledging that the Irish pilot of the project was conducted in collaboration with ICPOP, the study sought to achieve the Quadruple Aim and identify how digital health support could be effectively implemented into current integrated care clinical practice. The study was conducted with two pioneer integrated care hubs, representing both urban and rural populations and services in Ireland.

Co-Designing Digital Health Technology to Support Older Person Community Well-Being

The ValueCare Project methodology was guided by the principles of experience-based co-design (Bate & Robert, 2006). Experience-based co-design is a participatory approach used primarily in healthcare settings to improve services by actively involving service users, families and healthcare staff in the design process. This methodology emphasizes the collaborative nature of service improvement, where stakeholders share their experiences, identify areas needing change and co-create solutions (Donetto et al., 2015). By adopting a co-design methodology, the research team did not premeditate the functionality or content of the technology for the communities and their members (older people, family caregivers, health and social care professionals), which the project sought to support. It was fundamental to co-design the digital health technology in partnership with integrated care professionals and managers to ensure that the solution would be feasible and appropriate for the integrated care community-centered setting in Ireland. In addition to older people and their families, the health and social care professional fields represented in this process included geriatric consultants, physiotherapists, nurses, occupational therapists, dietitians, social workers, pharmacists, community support workers, age advocacy groups and individuals who work in social and cultural activities for older people.

Three overarching rounds of co-design were conducted. The first round focused on the priorities and preferences for well-being and support care. The second round focused on the feasibility, appropriateness and functionality of how technology could support these priorities and preferences. The third round involved testing a technology prototype to gather feedback before the pilot. While the first round featured single-stakeholder focus groups and interviews, the subsequent rounds involved groups with various stakeholders to ensure diverse representation of perspectives and a collective agreement on technology (Bate and Robert, 2007).

The ValueCare Wellness App

The outcome of the co-design process was the creation of a wellness mobile app for older adults and a web platform for integrated care professionals. This app is centered on a virtual coach that provides participants with a wellness plan and goal setting, following health guidelines for older people in Ireland, as well as the IC-POP Hub team's assessment. The web platform, or dashboard, enabled integrated care professionals and the research team to register and create personalized wellness plans for participants who attended the hub, based on their CGA. Using the dashboard, a tailored wellness plan could be created for each participant regarding the four key areas that emerged during the co-design process: physical activity, nutrition, medication adherence and social connectedness. This app can be used on a person's smartphone or tablet. The research team provided data-enabled tablet devices for those who did not have access or prior experience. All participants were offered either group or one-to-one training, depending on their preferences.

Each participant was provided with their unique login and password to access their personalized wellness plan in their app. The virtual coach technology enabled participants to track their wellness goals progress, access educational materials and receive weekly motivational feedback and reminders. This approach demonstrates both empowerment and participation in their own care management. The basis of the virtual coach was that a weekly goal would be set with participants in one or more well-being components, in which they received educational content (videos, written guidelines) and motivational reminders. At the end of each week, the app reviewed their progress and provided written advice on how to improve their adherence to meet their goals, where relevant. Participants were also given the option to nominate family carers to view a restricted version of the dashboard, allowing them to see their progress with their consent. This nominated family member or friend was able to view their well-being progress, which may prompt interaction if they noticed a lack in one or more well-being areas.

A key feature of the app was a multimedia educational library featuring a variety of videos, written materials and visual aids to support individuals in understanding their wellness goals. As participants reported their progress on their wellness plan, it could be reviewed by the integrated care team in the ICPOP and tailored to meet the needs of each participant. It became apparent during the later stages of the co-design process, when developing the prototype, that existing educational video content available online often employed scientific language that was too complicated or too lengthy for older adults to engage with in the app delivery format. The research team created evidence-based scripts and filmed short educational videos featuring integrated care professionals on topics such as the importance of staying physically active, understanding nutrition as we age and the value of maintaining social connections. Within the library and motivational prompts, participants were provided with information and contacts that promote community well-being, including listings and notifications regarding cultural and recreational activities, to encourage community participation.

The care pathway of the app was situated in the ICPOP Hubs, which were intended to provide enhanced integrated care and reinforce care goals that the participants established within the practice following their CGA. As standard practice meant that older people attending the hub receive care planning for six weeks once referred, the app was designed to extend this period of care and could be used by participants for up to 12 months. A key finding from the pilot study was that older people attending the hubs often had complex needs or preferred not to participate in the research. Therefore, the research team needed to broaden their recruitment approach beyond the scope of the integrated care hubs and engage with community-centered services and supports for older people that the technology could also serve. This necessitated the expansion of the pilot recruitment strategy to include a second intervention arm in the pilot study, targeting older adults with mild to moderate levels of frailty in the community. As such, it was critically important that the virtual coach was based on the existing guidelines for older people in the Irish healthcare context. To recruit participants in this way, the research team took several approaches to reach older people in the community, including active retirement groups, daycare centers, positive aging exercise classes, age-friendly newsletters and bulletins and social media. This approach ensured that we were reaching individuals who had received integrated care through the community clinical pathway, as well as older adults who identified as having well-being support needs and wished to participate in the project. This dual recruitment model, operating within clinical community hubs and outreach in the wider community, aims to meet the target of 240 older people within the large-scale pilot.

Reflections for Community-Centered Well-Being for Older People

The underlying principles and methodology of The ValueCare Project signal several essential factors that could inform future initiatives to support community-centered well-being for older people. At a fundamental level, to create and implement community-centered well-being for older people in a meaningful way, we must actively challenge the explicit and implicit ageist views that exist in society and are inherently non-person-centered. By othering older people as a distinct and separate group of people in our communities, especially when developing and evaluating health and well-being supports, we are facilitating a narrative of how “we” can support “them”, thus reinforcing a biomedical perspective rather than a more holistic biopsychosocial approach. Acknowledging the demographic shift outlined at the beginning of this chapter, if current estimates of life expectancies are to be realized, those currently working in healthcare, research, academia and policy are more likely than ever to live into older age. We must approach well-being support with the understanding that we are all individuals at different points in our lifespan and that we are future-proofing our health systems and communities to adapt to the needs of older individuals.

Ageism and othering significantly impact the well-being of older adults, including social exclusion or isolation, low self-esteem, increased risk of chronic diseases, mental health conditions and decreased life expectancy (Holt-Lunstad et al., 2015; Levy, 2009). Framing older adults as a distinct group perpetuates an ageist belief system that older people are a homogenous group defined by their age-related limitations rather than their diverse experiences and abilities. This, in turn, can implicitly create a barrier to their experience, which may inhibit person-centeredness when developing supports. Efforts must not only be made to support life expectancy and clinical outcomes but also to enhance life fulfillment based on the values and lived experiences of older people. In this way, older people as a community can be reframed as a heterogeneous, empowered population as rights-holders within an equitable health system and society. This reflects the central aspects of person-centered care and the driving force behind the co-design methodology of The ValueCare Project in Ireland. This co-design approach sought to ensure that the priorities and preferences of older people were listened to and responded to when designing the supportive technology. Internationally, there has been an increasing investment in developing digital support tools for people across the lifespan. The ValueCare App was created with the input of representative voices from the communities in which it was to be tested and aimed to support.

As this research is the first of its kind to co-design digital health for older people in Ireland, the methodology employed highlights several implications for future research in the field of community well-being, even beyond the scope of digital health. Collaboration from the outset with older people, family caregivers and health and social care professionals ensured that the technology aligned with current clinical practice while providing an enhanced integrated care pathway for older people. While challenges of engaging older people in co-design research have been identified (Harrington et al., 2018; Tsekleves et al., 2016), to ensure that older people within communities across the region of Cork and Kerry, the research team engaged in extensive stakeholder mapping, gatekeeper relationship building and knowledge sharing, technological literacy assessment, training and support to use digital platforms to take part in the co-design process and transparent and age-friendly study information and materials (Darley and Carroll, 2022).

Additionally, the co-design process highlighted to the research team that community well-being for older people should not be focused solely on health; it must also consider how people maintain their intrinsic capacity and derive meaning from life. It has been observed that there is an overemphasis on individuals and the healthcare system, whereby the community is commonly overlooked or is an afterthought when examining societal well-being (Russell, 2020). The co-design process emphasized the importance of social and cultural events to ensure community participation among older people, i.e., bringing people together for those who want it. During the co-design process, the importance of knowing what events and activities were happening in the community was commonly reported amongst all collaborating stakeholder groups. By focusing on the physical health of aging, we overlook the other supports or "community assets" (Russell, 2020, p. 3) that can support people in their daily lives and provide fulfillment. The co-designed technology within The Value-Care Project pilot in Ireland not only reflected the individual care needs of the person as they aged but also focused on promoting their engagement with the community and local social and cultural activities, which is a key facet of integration in Ireland. While digital health has predominantly focused on improving clinical health and social care outcomes, this project highlights its capacity to provide person-centered health and social care, as well as enhance overall well-being and connect people to others. The stakeholders in Cork and Kerry created an app that focused not only on clinical health outcomes but also on overall well-being and education in these areas, as well as community participation and engagement.

Acknowledging that community-centered initiatives are a key component of integrated care, this care approach presents a promising opportunity to not only improve the coordination of health and social care for older people using a person-centered approach but also connect individuals to their community for well-being support. Through an interdisciplinary approach, which is fundamental to integrated care, healthcare professionals have the opportunity not only to collaborate more effectively and understand the role of their peers' disciplines but also to create well-being goals that are co-created with those they are caring for, which are realistic and tailored to their preferences and care needs. Integrated care models that incorporate interprofessional collaboration have been linked to reduced hospital admissions, enhanced chronic disease management and improved mental health outcomes (WHO, 2016). Given that initiatives promoting shared learning and teamwork are essential for the future of integrated care (Lennox-Chhugani, 2023), the digital health technology developed in the project facilitated interprofessional collaboration and engagement with participants through the goal-setting process and transparent data flow for well-being progress reporting. A key component of this project has been learning about this new community-centered, integrated care clinical service on how to implement research to support evidence-based practice, as well as offering digital health as part of their care practice.

While digital health may not provide a solution to all well-being challenges or be the preferred or priority option among older people, it should be available as an option for those who wish to use it to support their well-being. This is particularly important with older people who may not have had experience or exposure to technology in their lifetime. Therefore, it is imperative to capture the experiences and attitudes of older people regarding their understanding of what technology is, what it can do and if they were to be supported in the future, what that support would look like. For any person, it would be challenging to imagine how they could be supported by a tool when they lack knowledge or experience of the tool itself. Equally, we must respect the preferences of older people who do not wish to be supported by technology and prefer traditional, in-person methods of health and social care with their professional team in the community. We are in an age in which society is learning how to partner with and provide support to people who are living longer, while simultaneously learning how technology can be utilized for health and well-being. At the heart of this project, the research team maintained the outlook that the project was not older person-centered but *human*-centered. If fortunate, every individual will have the opportunity to age in their community; therefore, we must identify meaningful ways to ensure people can achieve personal well-being across their lifespan, based on their values.

Conclusion

This chapter presents an insight into how the principles of person-centered care can be applied to facilitate community-centered well-being. With the vision of developing and piloting digital health technology to support older people, The ValueCare Project has set out to discover and engage with the priorities and preferences of care amongst older people in the community to inform the development of the technology. Furthermore, the research has captured the voices of older people's supportive networks in the development and implementation, including family caregivers, integrated care professionals and managers to ensure that the solution will be both effective in supporting the well-being of participants, as well as feasible and appropriate in the emerging integrated care context in Ireland. While the results of the evaluation regarding the impact of the technology on well-being outcomes are forthcoming, the co-design methodology employed to effectively create a tool to support community well-being in partnership with individuals we intend to support is presented in this chapter, which may inspire others working in older person care, digital health and other related fields. As the first study of its kind in the Irish context, The ValueCare Project lays the groundwork for inclusive collaboration with older people and their supportive networks, aiming to empower them to maintain their well-being within their community. This approach may also apply to other community contexts internationally. By emphasizing the importance of co-design and person-centered supports, this chapter aims to inspire further research and innovation in the fields of integrated care technology and community-centered well-being, ultimately leading to improved health outcomes for older people that meet their specific well-being needs, foster social connections, promote independent living and fulfillment.

References

Anderson, G. F. (2010). *Chronic care: Making the case for ongoing care*. Robert Wood Johnson Foundation, New Jersey.

Armitage, G. D., Suter, E., Oelke, N. D. & Adair, C. E. (2009). Health systems integration: State of the evidence. *International Journal of Integrated Care, 9*, e82. https://doi.org/10.5334/ijic.316

Bally, E. L., van Grieken, A., Ye, L, Ferrando, M., Fernández-Salido, M., Dix, R, Zanutto, O., Gallucci, M., Vasiljev, V., Carroll, A. & Darley, A. (2022). 'Value-based methodology for person-centred, integrated care supported by Information and Communication Technologies' (ValueCare) for older people in Europe: Study protocol for a pre-post controlled trial. *BMC Geriatrics, 22*(1), 1–2. https://doi.org/10.1186/s12877-022-03333-8

Banerjee, S., (2015). Multimorbidity—Older adults need health care that can count past one. *The Lancet*, *385*(9968), 587–589.

Barry, S., Fhallúin, M. N., Thomas, S., Harnett, P. J. & Burke, S. (2021). Implementing integrated care in practice–learning from mdts driving the integrated care programme for older persons in Ireland. *International Journal of Integrated Care*, *21*(1). https://doi.org/10.5334/ijic.4682

Bate, P. & Robert, G. (2006). Experience-based design: From redesigning the system around the patient to co-designing services with the patient. *BMJ Quality & Safety*, *15*(5), 307–310.

Bates, D. W. & Samal, L. (2018). Interoperability: What is it, how can we make it work for clinicians, and how should we measure it in the future? *Health Services Research*, *53*(5), 3270.

Baxter, R., O'Hara, J., Murray, J., Sheard, L., Cracknell, A., Foy, R., Wright, J. & Lawton, R. (2018). Partners at care transitions: Exploring healthcare professionals' perspectives of excellence at care transitions for older people. *BMJ Open*, *8*(9), e022468.

Beard, J. R., Officer, A. M. & Cassels, A. K. (2016). The world report on ageing and health. *The Gerontologist*, *56*(Suppl_2), S163–S166.

Central Statistics Office. (2017). *Population and labour force projections 2017–2046*. Central Statistics Office, Dublin.

Darley, A. & Carroll, Á. (2022). Conducting co-design with older people in a digital setting: Methodological reflections and recommendations. *International Journal of Integrated Care*, *22*(4). Retrieved from https://ijic.org/articles/10.5334/ijic.6546

Department of Health. (2021). *Sláintecare implementation strategy & action plan 2021–2023*. Department of Health, Dublin.

Donetto, S., Pierri, P., Tsianakas, V. & Robert, G. (2015). Experience-based co-design and healthcare improvement: Realizing participatory design in the public sector. *The Design Journal*, *18*(2), 227–248.

Friemel, T. N. (2016). The digital divide has grown old: Determinants of a digital divide among seniors. *New Media & Society*, *18*(2), 313–331.

Goodwin, N. (2016). Understanding integrated care. *International Journal of Integrated Care*, *16*(4). Retrieved from https://pmc.ncbi.nlm.nih.gov/articles/PMC5354214/

Goodwin, N., Dixon, A., Anderson, G. & Wodchis, W. (2014). *Providing integrated care for older people with complex needs: Lessons from seven international case studies.* The King's Fund, London.

Harnett, P. J., Kennelly, S. & Williams, P. (2020). A 10-step framework to implement integrated care for older persons. *Ageing International*, *45*(3), 288–304.

Harrington, C. N., Wilcox, L., Connelly, K., Rogers, W. & Sanford, J. (2018). May. Designing health and fitness apps with older adults: Examining the value of experience-based co-design. In *Proceedings of the 12th EAI International Conference on Pervasive Computing Technologies for Healthcare.* pp. 15–24.

Health Service Executive (HSE) Digital Transformation Office (2016). *Stay left shift left.* Retrieved from https://www.hsedigitaltransformation.ie/content/stay-left-shift-left

Health Service Executive (2017a). *National clinical programme for older people.* HSE, Dublin.

Health Service Executive (2017b). *Making a start in Integrated Care for Older Persons – A practical guide to the local implementation of Integrated Care Programmes for Older Persons.* HSE ICPOP, Dublin.

Helbostad, J. L., Vereijken, B., Becker, C., Todd, C., Taraldsen, K., Pijnappels, M., Aminian, K. & Mellone, S. (2017). Mobile health applications to promote active and healthy ageing. *Sensors*, *17*(3), 622.

Holt-Lunstad, J., Smith, T. B., Baker, M., Harris, T. & Stephenson, D. (2015). Loneliness and social isolation as risk factors for mortality: a meta-analytic review. *Perspectives on Psychological Science*, *10*(2), 227–237.

Ienca, M., Schneble, C., Kressig, R. W. & Wangmo, T. (2021). Digital health interventions for healthy ageing: a qualitative user evaluation and ethical assessment. *BMC Geriatrics*, *21*, 1–10.

Jokisch, M. R., Schmidt, L. I. & Doh, M. (2022). Acceptance of digital health services among older adults: Findings on perceived usefulness, self-efficacy, privacy concerns, ICT knowledge, and support seeking. *Frontiers in Public Health*, *10*, 1073756.

Kampmeijer, R., Pavlova, M., Tambor, M., Golinowska, S. & Groot, W. (2016). The use of e-health and m-health tools in health promotion and primary prevention among older adults: A systematic literature review. *BMC Health Services Research, 16*, 467–479.

Kirst, M., Im, J., Burns, T., Baker, G. R., Goldhar, J., O' Campo, P., Wojtak, A. & Wodchis, W.P. (2017). What works in implementation of integrated care programs for older adults with complex needs? A realist review. *International Journal for Quality in Health Care*, *29*(5), 612–624.

Kvedar, J., Coye, M. J. & Everett, W. (2014). Connected health: A review of technologies and strategies to improve patient care with telemedicine and telehealth. *Health Affairs*, *33*(2), 194–199.

Lennox-Chhugani, N. (2023). Inter-disciplinary work in the context of integrated care–a theoretical and methodological framework. *International Journal of Integrated Care*, *23*(2). https://ijic.org/articles/10.5334/ijic.7544

Levy, B. R., Zonderman, A. B., Slade, M. D. & Ferrucci, L. (2009). Age stereotypes held earlier in life predict cardiovascular events in later life. *Psychological Science*, *20*(3), 296–298.

Lewis, L. & Ehrenberg, N. (2020). *Realising the true value of integrated care: Beyond COVID-19.* Retrieved from https://integratedcarefoundation.org/wp-content/uploads/2020/05/IFIC3516-Covid-19-Thought-Leadership-Paper-A4-v7.pdf.

Lingard, L., Whyte, S., Regehr, G. & Gardezi, F. (2017). Counting silence: Complexities in the evaluation of team communication. In *Safer surgery: Analysing behaviour in the operating theatre*. (Finn, R. & Mitchell, L. eds.). CRC Press, Boca Raton, FL. pp. 283–299.

Lourenço, A., de Brito, M. F. & Gomes, B. (2023). The future of integrated care in aged individuals. In *Aging: From fundamental biology to societal impact.*. (Oliveira, P.J. & Malva, J.O. eds.). *Cambridge, Mass.* pp. 649–661

Lyles, C. R., Aguilera, A., Nguyen, O. & Sarkar, U. (2022). Bridging the digital health divide: how designers can create more inclusive digital. *California Healthcare Foundation*, 1–8. Retrieved from https://www.chcf.org/wp-content/uploads/2022/02/BridgingDigitalDivideDesigners.pdf

Maeder, A. (2020). Digital technology trends supporting assisted independent living of ageing population. *Studies in Health Technology & Informatics, 270*, 577–581. https://doi.org/10.3233/SHTI200226

Melchiorre, M. G., Papa, R., Rijken, M., van Ginneken, E., Hujala, A. & Barbabella, F. (2018). eHealth in integrated care programs for people with multimorbidity in Europe: Insights from the ICARE4EU project. *Health Policy*, *122*(1), 53–63.

Menassa, M., Stronks, K., Khatami, F., Díaz, Z. M. R., Espinola, O. P., Gamba, M., Itodo, O. A., Buttia, C., Wehrli, F., Minder, B. & Velarde, M. R. (2023). Concepts and definitions of healthy ageing: A systematic review and synthesis of theoretical models. *EClinicalMedicine*, *56*, 101821. https://doi.org/10.1016/j.eclinm.2022.101821

National Clinical Programme Older People (2012). *Specialist geriatric services model of care.* Health Service Executive, Dublin.

Neves, A. L. & Burgers, J. (2022). Digital technologies in primary care: Implications for patient care and future research. *European Journal of General Practice*, *28*(1), 203–208.

Nyweide, D. J., Anthony, D. L., Bynum, J. P., Strawderman, R. L., Weeks, W. B., Casalino, L. P. & Fisher, E. S. (2013). Continuity of care and the risk of preventable hospitalization in older adults. *Journal of the American Medical Association: Internal Medicine*, *173*(20), 1879–1885.

O'Sullivan, S., Buckley, M., Desmond, E., Bantry-White, E. & Cassarino, M. (2022). *Agency and ageing in place in rural Ireland.* UCC, Cork.

Partridge, L., Deelen, J. & Slagboom, P. E. (2018). Facing up to the global challenges of ageing. *Nature*, *561*(7721), 45–56.

Phillips, R. & Pittman, R. H. (2009). A framework for community and economic development. In *An introduction to community development.* (Phillips, R. & Pittman, R. H. eds). Routledge, New York. 3–19.

Prior, A., Vestergaard, C. H., Vedsted, P., Smith, S. M., Virgilsen, L. F., Rasmussen, L. A. & Fenger-Grøn, M. (2023). Healthcare fragmentation, multimorbidity, potentially inappropriate medication, and mortality: A Danish nationwide cohort study. *BMC Medicine*, *21*(1), 305.

Rosenwohl-Mack, A., Schumacher, K., Fang, M. L. & Fukuoka, Y. (2020). A new conceptual model of experiences of aging in place in the United States: Results of a systematic review and meta-ethnography of qualitative studies. *International Journal of Nursing Studies*, *103*, 103496.

Russell, C. (2020). We don't have a health problem, we have a village problem. *Community Medicine. 1*(1), 1–12.

Schulz, R., Eden, J., Engineering, & Medicine (2016). Programs and supports for family caregivers of older adults. In *Families caring for an aging. America*. (Schulz, R., Eden, J., eds). National academies Press, Washington. pp. 159–210.

Shah, A., Hussain-Shamsy, N., Strudwick, G., Sockalingam, S., Nolan, R. P. & Seto, E., (2022). Digital health interventions for depression and anxiety among people with chronic conditions: Scoping review. *Journal of Medical Internet Research, 24*(9), e38030.

Shah, B., Allen, J. L. Y., Chaudhury, H., O'Shaughnessy, J. & Tyrrell, C. S. (2022). The role of digital health in the future of integrated care. *Clinics in Integrated Care, 15*, 100131.

Sikka, R., Morath, J. M. & Leape, L. (2015). The quadruple aim: Care, health, cost and meaning in work. *BMJ Quality Safety, 24*(10), 608–10.

Smith, A. (2017). *Winter.* Hamish Hamilton, United Kingdom.

Stange, K. C. (2009). The problem of fragmentation and the need for integrative solutions. *The Annals of Family Medicine, 7*(2), 100–103.

Suter, E., Arndt, J., Arthur, N., Parboosingh, J., Taylor, E. & Deutschlander, S. (2009). Role understanding and effective communication as core competencies for collaborative practice. *Journal of Interprofessional Care, 23*(1), 41–51.

Tannou, T., Lihoreau, T., Gagnon-Roy, M., Grondin, M. & Bier, N. (2021). Effectiveness of smart living environments to support older adults to age in place in their community: An umbrella review protocol. *British Medical Journal Open, 12*(1), e054235. doi.org/10.1136/bmjopen-2021–05423

Tsekleves, E., Bingley, A. F., Luján Escalante, M. A. & Gradinar, A. (2020). Engaging people with dementia in designing playful and creative practices: Co-design or co-creation? *Dementia, 19*(3), 915–931.

Turner, G. & Clegg, A. (2014). Best practice guidelines for the management of frailty: A British Geriatrics Society, Age UK and Royal College of General Practitioners report. *Age & Ageing, 43*(6), 744–747.

United Nations (2017). *Population ageing and sustainable development.* Retrieved from https://www.un.org/en/development/desa/population/publications/pdf/popfacts/PopFacts_2017-1.pdf

Vines, J., Pritchard, G., Wright, P., Olivier, P. & Brittain, K. (2015). An age-old problem: Examining the discourses of ageing in HCI and strategies for future research. *ACM Transactions on Computer-Human Interaction (TOCHI), 22*(1), 1–27.

Waddington, C. & Egger, D. (2008). *Integrated health services—What and why.* World Health Organisation, Geneva.

WHO (2017). *Global strategy and action plan on ageing and health.* Retrieved from https://www.who.int/ageing/WHO-GSAP-2017.pdf?ua=1

Wiles, J. L., Leibing, A., Guberman, N., Reeve, J. & Allen, R. E. (2012). The meaning of "aging in place" to older people. *The Gerontologist, 52*(3), 357–366.

World Health Organisation (2016). *Framework on integrated, people-centred health services. Report by the Secretariat, 69th World Health Assembly.* WHO, Geneva.

World Health Organisation (2021). *Global strategy on digital health 2020–2025.* Retrieved from https://www.who.int/health-topics/digital-health#tab=tab_1

World Health Organisation (2022). *Ageing and health.* Retrieved from https://www.who.int/news-room/fact-sheets/detail/ageing-and-health

World Health Organisation (2021). *Decade of healthy ageing: baseline report.* World Health Organisation, Geneva.

Xie, L., Zhang, S., Xin, M., Zhu, M., Lu, W. & Mo, P. K. H. (2022). Electronic health literacy and health-related outcomes among older adults: A systematic review. *Preventive Medicine, 157*, 106997.

Zhai, S., Chu, F., Tan, M., Chi, N. C., Ward, T. & Yuwen, W. (2023). Digital health interventions to support family caregivers: An updated systematic review. *Digital Health, 9*, 20552076231171967.

15

AGE-FRIENDLY INDOOR AND OUTDOOR ENVIRONMENTS TO PROMOTE THE SENSE OF COMMUNITY

Joost van Hoof, Wilhelmina H. van Staalduinen, Zsuzsu Tavy, Rengin Aslanoğlu, Lucia Thielman, Hannah R. Marston, Grzegorz Chrobak, Małgorzata Świąder, Jan K. Kazak, Loredana Ivan and Jeroen Dikken

Introduction

Creating age-friendly indoor and outdoor environments is crucial for promoting community health, well-being and enhancing the quality of life for older adults (van Hoof et al., 2019; van Hoof and Marston, 2021). As populations continue to age globally, designing spaces that are accessible, safe and inclusive becomes increasingly important. Age-friendly environments (AFE) enable older adults to maintain their independence, stay active and engage with their communities, which in turn supports their physical, mental and social well-being. The notion of age-friendly cities and communities was laid down in the publication "Global Age-Friendly Cities: A Guide" (WHO, 2007), which has gained great traction in the past two decades. Over 1600 cities and communities worldwide have joined the World Health Organization's Global Network for Age-friendly Cities and Communities. The network was established in 2010 to connect cities, communities and organizations worldwide with the common vision of making their community a great place to grow old in (van Hoof et al., 2021a). The scope of age-friendly cities and communities includes both indoor and outdoor environments in the urban context, in which older people can thrive. The age-friendly movement focuses on community or neighborhood actions, with age-friendly solutions drawing on community or neighborhood features and characteristics. The fundamental notions of the age-friendly agenda align with McCormack and McCance's (2016) framework for person-centered care, which provides additional guidance on applying person-centered care principles at the community level. Originally developed for healthcare settings, this framework emphasizes the importance of valuing individual experiences, preferences and values. At the community level, this means creating environments that are not just safe and accessible but also resonate with the

DOI: 10.4324/9781032662657-18

personal and cultural identities of older adults. Applying person-centered care principles to community settings is essential for ensuring that the environments we create truly reflect the needs and preferences of older adults. The Gothenburg Model, developed in Sweden, also offers a framework for integrating person-centered care principles into community planning and development (Britten et al., 2017). This model emphasizes the importance of co-creation, where community members, especially those most affected by these environments, such as older adults, are actively involved in planning, designing and implementing community initiatives.

Age-friendly indoor environments are essential for the well-being of older adults, as they spend a very significant amount of time at home. Key elements include accessibility features such as ramps and wide doorways, safety modifications like grab bars and non-slip flooring and comfort considerations including adequate lighting and temperature control (Kazak et al., 2017). Architects, urban planning and supportive policies play a critical role in ensuring these modifications are accessible and affordable for all, including subsidies or grants for home modifications and incentives for developers to include age-friendly features in new housing projects. Additionally, outdoor environments play a vital role in community health by encouraging physical activity and social interaction. Age-friendly outdoor spaces should include well-maintained sidewalks, safe pedestrian crossings and accessible public transportation (Marston et al., 2022). For example, pedestrian crossings with longer signal times and audible signals can help older adults cross streets safely. Green spaces like parks and community gardens provide opportunities for exercise, relaxation and social engagement, which are crucial for mental and physical health. Features such as smooth walking paths, ample seating and shaded areas can make these spaces more inviting and usable for older adults (van Hoof et al., 2021a). Community centers offering programs tailored to older adults, such as fitness classes, arts and crafts workshops and social clubs, can further enhance social connections and reduce isolation. By creating environments that encourage older adults to remain active and engaged, communities can support healthier, more fulfilling lives for their aging populations. Moreover, investing in age-friendly infrastructure can lead to significant economic benefits, including reduced healthcare costs due to fewer injuries and illnesses, and job creation in sectors such as home modification, public transportation and community services. Considering cultural differences and tailoring approaches to meet the diverse needs of older adults, such as providing multilingual services and culturally relevant activities, are also essential for the effectiveness of these initiatives.

For policymakers, prioritizing the development of AFE is not only a public health imperative but also a strategic approach to addressing the demographic shifts occurring worldwide. Policymakers should advocate for and implement comprehensive age-friendly policies that encompass urban planning, housing, transportation and community services. This includes funding for home modifications, incentives for age-friendly business practices and investments in public infrastructure that supports active aging. Engaging older adults in the planning process ensures that their needs and preferences are directly addressed, leading to more effective and accepted solutions. Policymakers can promote cross-sector collaboration, bringing together government agencies, private sector partners and non-profit organizations to create integrated and sustainable age-friendly initiatives. By championing these efforts, policymakers can help build resilient, inclusive communities that support healthy aging and improve the quality of life for all citizens (Municipality of The Hague, 2020; Middlesbrough Age-friendly Charter, 2024).

AFE can foster intergenerational interaction, creating a more inclusive society facilitating a thriving environment for people of all ages and abilities. For example, well-designed public spaces can serve as common recreation grounds affording different generations to interact and strengthen community bonds. This holistic approach to community design benefits not only older adults but also the entire community by promoting a healthier, more cohesive and supportive environment. Additionally, the creation of AFE can stimulate local economies by attracting businesses and services that cater to an aging population.

In the context of partnership approaches fundamental to person-centeredness, older people and other stakeholders are increasingly asked to co-create, co-produce and co-design age-friendly solutions (James & Buffel, 2023). In such participatory sessions, participants are asked for their input, for instance, concerning the physical layout of the built environment, as well as in different intensities and levels of impact. As James and Buffel (2023) noted in their systematic review, co-research with older people offers improved understandings, more inclusive and responsive policy, practice and service design as well as opportunities for co-researchers to develop new skills. Similar notions were noted by Sanoff (2011), who posited that the participation of people in decision-making processes that are of concern to them can contribute to the legitimacy and democratic basis of the decisions that are being made. Older people's knowledge based on their personal experiences can be of value in shaping their social and built environment, including age-friendly indoor and outdoor environments (Buffel, 2019; van Hoof et al., 2021b; Tavy et al., 2022). The participation of older people in research and design projects is indeed at the core of the age-friendly agenda set out by the WHO, for instance, through the involvement of older people in the 5-year cycle of continuous improvement, as well as other programs launched by this organization. Such priorities reflect the inclusiveness and active participation of people in generating their preferences (McCormack & McCance, 2016) in the context of their lived environment. The World Health Organization (WHO: 11) Regional Office for Europe (2016) defined participation as:

> ...a process by which people are enabled to become actively and genuinely involved in defining issues of concern to them, in making decisions about factors that affect their lives, in formulating and implementing policies, in planning, developing and delivering services and in taking action to achieve change.

According to the WHO Regional Office for Europe (2016), the involvement and participation of older people in all decisions and processes is the single most important principle to facilitate the creation of AFE. Older people's experiences should be a starting point for the development of initiatives: "nothing about us without us!". Having said this, it is important to turn words into actions and look at meaningful methods for the participation of older people. One tool that can be used for the level of participation is the widely used ladder of citizen participation by Arnstein (1969) (see Figure 7.1), in which rungs of a ladder show the level of influence participants have. The higher on the ladder, the more power people have in determining the final outcomes of a process. Van Hoof et al. (2021) illustrated that it should not be a goal in itself to be as high on the ladder as possible. There is no ideal form of participation that is suitable for all situations; the level of participation deemed desirable by different stakeholders can depend on the goals, wishes and expertise of those involved.

The focus on participation of older people in shaping all aspects of their daily lives supplement the notions laid down by Phelan et al. (2020). In their work, Phelan and colleagues stated that in recent years, there has been a shift in orientation toward person-centeredness as part of a global move toward humanizing and centralizing the person within healthcare. Although AFE entail more than just healthcare – community support and health services are only one of the eight official age-friendly domains defined by the WHO – it is a crucial domain from which innovations can be taken as a source of inspiration for moving the age-friendly agenda forward. In this sense, it is again about putting older people and their needs and preferences central to the further development of AFE. Such approaches revolve not only about the older individuals themselves but also put the community of older people in the center, and indirectly all people who can benefit from our societies being more inclusive and accessible. In this sense, community-based approaches may promote community in terms of integration, democratic participation, equality and collaboration, to name a few.

In this chapter, we present three cases from projects located across Europe. These cases revolve around the participation of older people in designing, propagating and researching age-friendly indoor and outdoor environments in order to make their streets, neighborhoods, communities and cities more age-friendly. It is about putting the needs of older people and their wider communities first. The first case study is about collaborative project conducted in Poland, Romania and the Netherlands focusing on the design of a geoportal for researching the age-friendly context of a city through photoproduction by older people themselves. The second focuses on the European *Age-friendly Environments (AFE) Activists* project, which addressed the need for tailored training for adults aged 65 years and older who want to promote AFE in their cities and influence municipal agencies in their decision-making so that the infrastructure and services of the town or city are adapted to the diverse capacities, realities, needs and preferences of all residents of all ages. The third case is a study from the Netherlands focusing on participatory video approaches to investigate the age-friendliness of cities, in this case, the municipality of Delft. These three cases together showcase how older people can contribute to an age-friendly community in an active and meaningful manner.

Case 1: Participation and Geoportal Development

As urban environments become home to an ever-increasing number of older people, a distinct set of challenges emerges for this population. These challenges center around navigating their surroundings, accessing essential services and preserving their independence. This is akin to creating the conditions for human flourishing; a key priority in person-centered care (Ververda & Hauge, 2019). Understanding complex street layouts, ensuring walkable neighborhoods, utilizing public transportation effectively and locating appropriate rest areas have all become a challenge for many older people. Fortunately, a powerful set of tools known as geospatial technologies offers a promising solution to the challenges faced by older people in urban environments (Tupasela et al., 2023). These technologies encompass various applications, from urban planning to social collaboration (Kent & Specht, 2023). By providing data and tools that enhance mobility, access to services and social engagement, geospatial technologies have the potential to significantly improve the quality of life for older people and create more age-friendly urban environments (Angelidou, 2016). However, a major hindrance in creating truly age-friendly urban environments is the lack of a standardized, measurable approach to assessment (van Hoof et al., 2021a). This has limited progress in achieving the age-friendly agenda (Davern et al., 2020; Dikken et al., 2020). To bridge this gap, exploring qualitative methodologies that empower older adults as active participants becomes more important. These methods, such as photovoice which utilizes photography, and involved citizen science programs enable older people to become change agents by co-creating their ideal urban environments (Buffel, 2019; Gardiner et al., 2020; Marston, 2022; Ronzi et al., 2020). In this context, a user-friendly geodata data collection tool that allows the collection of photographs, comments and geographical locations that convey the issues that older people want to emphasize about the urban environments they live in, and a geoportal that presents this collected data, has been developed.

Based on older people's participation, a two-stage approach was used to co-create the geodata[1] collection tool (Aslanoğlu et al., 2024). Involving older people from two European sites (Wrocław (Poland, $n = 9$), and The Hague (the Netherlands, $n = 5$)), the initial design of the geodata collection tool was finalized. This co-created design was then adapted into KoBo Toolbox (which is an open-source and web-based geodata collection tool that can be used by smartphones or tablets) (Aslanoğlu et al., 2024).

In total, 76 older people participated in collecting geodata via KoBo Toolbox from Bucharest, Kraków, Wrocław and The Hague. They provided inputs from their urban environment using the World Health Organization's (2007) eight domains: outdoor spaces and buildings; transportation; housing; social participation; respect and social inclusion; civic participation and employment; communication and information; and community support and health services plus finance (Dikken et al., 2020). By using the aforementioned domains, participants pointed out the challenges related to age-friendliness and also which actions were needed to enhance urban environments. During the data collection, participants provided approximately 1100 inputs (in 4 months), where older people could take or upload photos, write comments (they were also asked to indicate if their comments were positive, neutral or negative) and add location data via the KoBo Toolbox.

Among the four cities from which the data were collected, Bucharest had the highest number of inputs. There were 713 data in total from 22 different participants. Each of the data sets contain nine domains along with photographs and comments. The participants from Bucharest provided more input (30%) on the WHO's *outdoor spaces and buildings* domain (Figure 15.1).

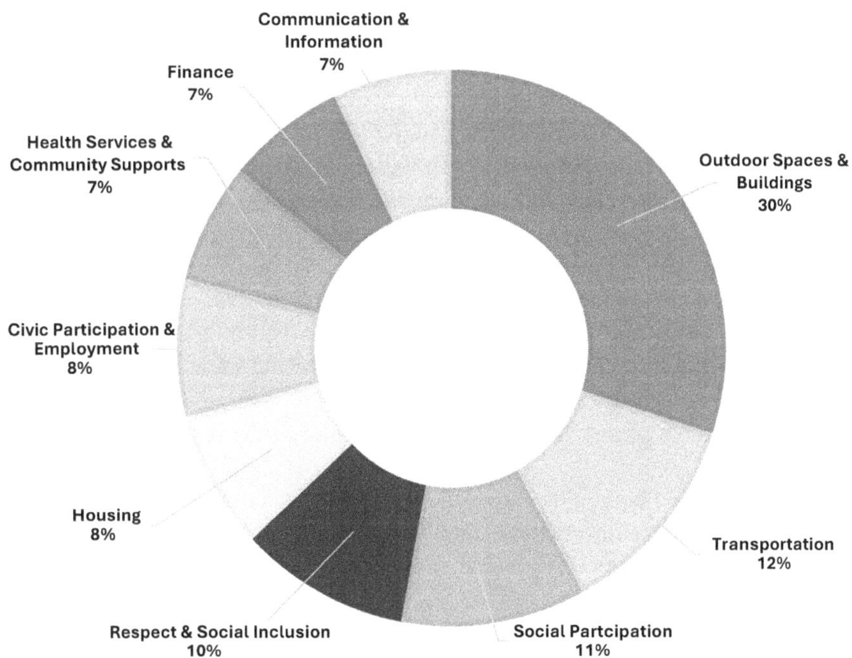

FIGURE 15.1 Percentage of the collected data from Bucharest by the nine age-friendly domains

The collected data was then analyzed and prepared to be used in the geoportal. Sentiment analysis (Stojanocski et al., 2016) was used to understand older people's opinions and identify areas of concern in urban environments, especially linked with the nine domains. The collected text data (i.e. comments) were categorized as positive (66.7%), neutral (0.5%) and negative (32.8%). Those additional layers of information provided a more comprehensive picture of the challenges and opportunities faced by older adults in urban environments. This analysis categorized participant comments into broad categories of positive, neutral or negative sentiment, which captures the finer details within the text. Considering this example categorized as negative: "I chose a negative example of graffiti painting on the façade wall panels [...] in Bucharest. It would be good if these young painters - talented by the way - display their graffiti drawings in specially arranged places", it is possible not only to collect the perspectives of the older people about their urban environments but also to see their suggestions for the improvement of those areas. This illustrates the possibility of specific and in-depth information being generated to enhance community-centered care. For example, the data extract identifies detailed information about a street in Sector 2 of Bucharest with the collaboration of older people. Through this comment, specific enhancements in the urban environment can be made. Another example can be provided from the domain *communication and information* which was categorized as neutral: "Accessibility of information and digitization of payments in our sector: I think that for some of our seniors this site is difficult to access". Although the overall comment was perceived as neutral, this comment highlights two different aspects of the older person's experience with digitized payments and that the participants themselves used the service, but others may find it difficult.

In relation to transportation, the positive sentiment analysis used for the comments from Bucharest identified the following quote:

> A commendable fact is that STB is equipped with modern trams (Imperial Metropolitan). These modern trams are equipped with air conditioning, have more seats, are roomy and have passenger access (easy boarding/disembarking, this being ensured through more doors situated on the old trams and are equipped with video screens that inform travellers about the route, the upcoming station as well as connections with other means of public transport.

These observations highlight successful initiatives that could be replicated in other parts of the city. This information can be used to inform future development projects, prioritizing the preservation of these positive aspects that contribute to a higher quality of life for older adults.

By investigating this data, alongside geospatial data, hotspot analysis and heat maps for the older participants were prepared (Figure 15.2). This underpinned the preparation of maps for positive and negative opinions, which can be appropriately named hot-spot places and hot spot anti-places (Świąder & Łukowiak, 2016). The hot spot analysis (Getis-Ord Gi*) represents the statistical analysis which

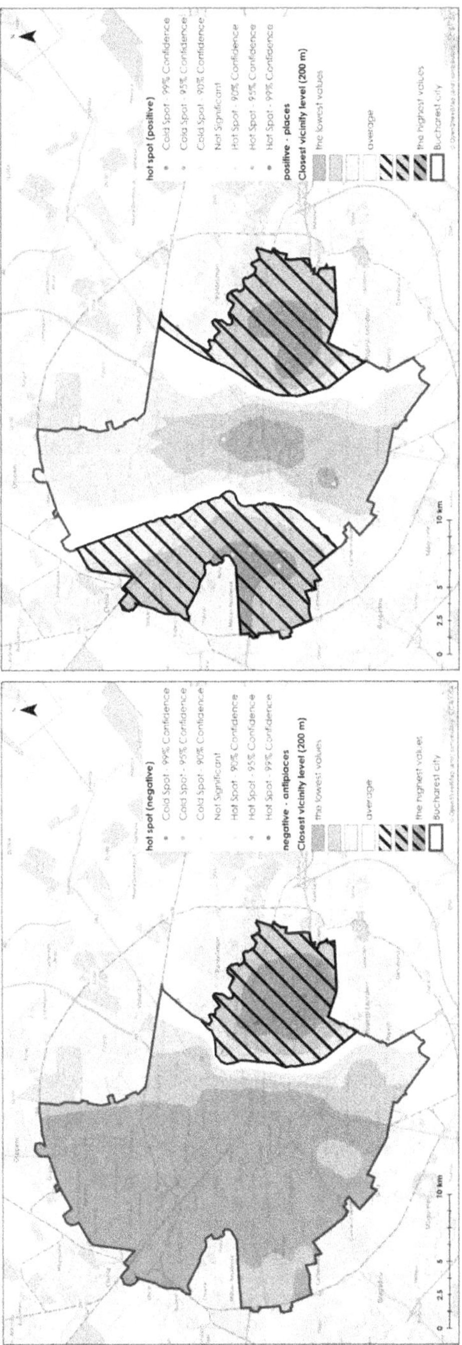

FIGURE 15.2 Heat maps prepared based on hotspot analyses for Bucharest (*N*= 658, left: negative, right: positive)

distinguishes the high and low-incidence locations. The result, defined as a "hot spot" is stated in terms of statistical certainty. There is a description of the heat-maps difference delimited based on hotspot, which is statistically significant, and other types – i.e., density analysis (classical density analysis), which show the heat areas of objects but not in a significant way. Therefore, unlike classical density analysis (an interpolated point data showing the density of occurrence), the final visualization – heat map – is less arbitrary (Dempsey, 2014). The heat maps created allowed for the identification of positive facilities that represent hot spot "places" or age-friendly areas. Conversely, facilities perceived negatively represent hot spot "anti-places" or areas that are potentially unfriendly to older adults.

The use of positive sentiment analysis allowed for delimitation of surfaces representing the highest occurrence of hot spot places, as well as anti-places. As a result, the hotspots with negative sentiment for "graffiti" can now be visualized on a map, providing city planners with a clear understanding of areas requiring improvements related to vandalism. This enables them to prioritize solutions with greater precision, targeting specific concerns in areas frequented by older adults.

The previously described sentiment analysis contributed significantly to the development of a comprehensive geoportal for age-friendly urban environments. This web-based platform serves as a central portal for the collected geodata, photographs and sentiment analysis results. By incorporating those data, the geoportal goes beyond just highlighting problematic areas. It also showcases positive aspects, such as "well-maintained parks" and "activities in senior centres" that contribute to a higher quality of life for older people. Overall, this allows for more targeted interventions, addressing specific concerns in areas frequented by older people. Therefore, city planners, policymakers and other stakeholders readily understand the spatial distribution of public concerns faced by older people within the urban environment. Moreover, some overlapping areas of places and anti-places could be identified, which could be a starting point for further analysis of urban space. Such results could mean that different social groups perceive the area differently which can be related, for example, to the accessibility of the area, in terms of physical (distance) or socio-economic (price/rates, status), social (problems of a particular group) and dimensions (Grant et al., 2010; Willberg et al., 2023). Consequently, such data also allow insights into promoting pre-conditions for person-centered communities in illustrating areas for improvement as well as examples of community cohesion.

In conclusion, this case collected detailed insights from Bucharest which have the strength to transform public perception into actionable knowledge. With this example, through the integration and collaboration of older people, policymakers and stakeholders will be able to make data-driven decisions that promote the creation of truly age-friendly cities that meet the specific needs of older adults.

Case 2: Age-Friendly Environments Activists

Case 2 focuses on the empowerment of older people to actively participate in society and to advocate their interests toward local or regional stakeholders, such as municipalities, ICT companies or housing organizations. The empowerment and training took place within the *Age-Friendly Environments Activists* project, which took place from 2018 to 2020.

The majority of environmental factors situated in our cities and communities were historically designed and developed in a different demographic context. The unprecedented increase in the aging population urges us to explore the fitness of our built environment, social environment, community and health support and modify those environments in a new demographic context and promote community-centeredness for all people. A promising strategy to deal with this issue is developing citizen competencies so that older adults take an active role in documenting features of their environment that can create barriers or enablers for active and healthy living and then voice them to policy and decision-makers to promote change.

The *Age-friendly Environments (AFE) Activists* project addressed the need for tailored training for adults aged 65 years and over who want to promote AFE in their cities and influence municipal agencies in their decision-making so that the infrastructure and services of the town or city are adapted to the diverse capacities, realities, needs and preferences of all residents of all ages. There were four main objectives of this project: (1) train, empower and support older people to get active for their cities/communities/neighborhoods, to bring forward their ideas and initiatives for AFE; (2) develop supportive, innovative and accessible training/learning modules and materials that are relevant to others (adult education providers, trainers, etc.); (3) raise awareness of the importance of AFE for active participation and civic engagement of older citizens; and (4) produce and disseminate sustainable outputs and outcomes and build strong networks for AFE and active participation of older citizens.

The objectives were achieved by a number of tasks, such as collecting, analyzing and showcasing inspiring grass-roots initiatives in different domains of AFE, as well as designing and testing a training program through cross-border cooperation and short-term study visits. This was followed by experiential and project-based learning enabling the older participants to initiate activities in the field of AFE. A transnational learning mobility was put in place to allow selected participants to gain first-hand experience of an AFE in The Hague and Udine (Italy), two cities which are members of the WHO's Global Network for Age-Friendly Cities and Communities. Furthermore, the project involved experts, public servants and different stakeholders in project activities.

Four outputs were delivered by the project partners:

1 A compendium of good practices of AFE containing exemplary grass-roots initiatives from European countries in different domains of AFE. The compendium was used as a training resource and as an awareness-raising tool for understanding activism and advocacy for and by older people and to gain inspiration to plan and implement small local projects.
2 AFE Advocacy training program can be used as a training resource for organizations/institutions interested in learning about AFE issues and including AFE

topics into their curricula and/or implementing AFE projects. A pilot training for *Age-friendly Environment Activists* was delivered by project partners in The Hague (the Netherlands), Hanau (Germany), Kaunas (Lithuania), Rome (Italy) and Vienna (Austria) between September 2019 and March 2020. The training program addressed information, advice and advocacy needs of older people to support them in making choices, making decisions, securing rights, acting in his or her interests as well as contributing to the life of the community and being fully engaged in society. A total of 75 older people participated in the training, consisting of approximately 75% females and 25% males. In addition to in-class training, the program included study tours to the age-friendly cities of The Hague and Udine for the selected participants to observe the local AFE initiatives and this experience facilitated the transfer of the knowledge gained to their peers.

3 AFE Advocacy Handbook containing the synopsis of good AFE practice examples: The handbook detailed the AFE advocacy training program, delivery methods, training tools and AFE advocacy projects implemented by AFE activists in partner countries.
4 The AFE Experience Handbook describes the educational approach of a study tour, the pathways of The Hague and Udine toward building a more inclusive society for people of all ages, the selected initiatives to be explored by the international team of AFE activists and the tools for observation, reflection and self-assessment. The Experience Handbook serves as an awareness-raising resource for older citizens, local authorities and municipal agencies, policy-makers, responsible businesses, philanthropists and innovators to understand the paradigm change. Thus, this aging perspective is shifting away from older age dependence to direct contribution and encouraging people to respond to the needs of aging citizens and engage them in participatory decision-making.

The target audiences of the project results are older adults aged 65 years and over, who want to remain active in their retirement phase by engaging in lifelong learning opportunities and becoming active members of civil society, adult education providers, local community and neighborhood groups, non-governmental organizations, associations of older people, local and national government agencies.

Case 3: Participatory Video for Studying the Age-Friendliness of Cities

The wider region of The Hague and Leiden in the Netherlands has nearly ten years of experience investigating the age-friendliness of outdoor environments and communities through participatory video (van Vliet et al., 2018; von Faber et al., 2020). Participatory video is an investigative method for co-producing age-friendly cities together with older adults. Participatory video research can be used to collect rich data about the age-friendliness of cities and the experiences, preferences and needs of older people living in these cities and neighborhoods (von Faber et al., 2020). In participatory video, community members are trained to create their own films to express their stories from their unique perspectives. This method can vary widely, from conducting brief video workshops in local communities to gather data on specific topics, to enabling participants to narrate, produce, share and own their stories through film. Despite these variations, most participatory video approaches aim to provide marginalized or underrepresented groups with a platform to depict their experiences through film (White, 2003). Additionally, the filmmaking process itself is often considered crucial, as it has the potential to transform and empower participants (White, 2003). This process includes developing skills, fostering interaction and bonding and reflecting on various topics or on one's identity or role within the community or society at large (White, 2003).

The methodology was introduced in the field of age-friendly cities in 2017 as part of the activities of The Hague Age-Friendly City (van Vliet et al., 2018). This method has since been used in various projects on age-friendly cities initiated by the project Regional Networks for the Social Welfare Domain The Hague & Leiden (*Werkplaats Sociaal Domein Den Haag en Leiden*), in collaboration with several municipalities in the Province of South Holland (Von Faber et al., 2020). The workshop hosted in this initiative contributed to the development of a regional network and the strengthening of the knowledge infrastructure around social issues.

The example shared here focuses on two of these participatory video projects that were conducted between 2020 and 2023 in Delft, a municipality in the Netherlands situated between The Hague and Rotterdam. In these two projects, a group of older adults (one group of six and a second group of seven participants) made a documentary about what is important to them looking at housing and aging in place. After the first project in Delft, the Municipality of Delft became a stakeholder and two social housing associations, and a local care organization was involved as well. The groups of older adults came together weekly for nine months with two researchers in project meetings of four hours at a community center or housing facility for older adults.

At the beginning of the project, only the issue of housing was chosen by the researchers and municipality, and the rest of the focused topics were open for older adults to decide. In the weekly sessions, the group came together to explore the topic by making a film together. They were trained to film using an iPad, as some participants had never used an iPad before. They learned how to conduct interviews and designed their questions based on what they thought was important or were curious to know from other older adults in their community. The older participants developed storyboards together, where they would choose what would be important to film and show. Participants held interviews with other older adults on video, and they chose to include housing initiatives to visit and film. The group analyzed the recorded interviews by watching them on a big screen together with the researchers and discussing what were important themes. This was an iterative process. The most important quotations, stories and images were chosen by the group to include in the editing phase. In the first project, the film was edited by the researcher due to COVID-19 restrictions at the time, after constructing the story together with the group. The second film was edited by older adults themselves, with the support of the researcher.

In the first project, the participants found it important to explore the housing market and be able to move to another home. They chose the topics of how older adults make the decision to move to a house that supports aging in place, the difficulties they experience when orienting on, and searching for, something new, and the possibilities available for them to relocate to suitable housing as they age (De Filmmakkers, 2021). The participants in the second project added to this the question of how to combine old and new friends once such a decision is made. Some of the most important topics to this second group were how to stay adventurous and active, how to stay connected and get people to be involved, how to look out for each other in a housing initiative or community and how the built environment of a housing initiative can support people to stay active and in contact within a community. For example, while visiting a housing initiative and interviewing older adults there, this group found that when the indoor spaces of a housing initiative were designed in an open way, with a shared kitchen and open areas where people could sit and see each other as they walk by, it encouraged community interaction. Participants emphasized the importance of having the choice to go out in the communal area or stay in their own place where they had everything they needed behind their own front door, thus having the ability to choose freely between social interaction within the community or the comfort of their own place and privacy. They also discovered that in such environments, people could support each other. One story this group included in the film was about a man who felt lonely and was supported by his neighbor. These themes can be seen in the two short Dutch documentaries "From door to door" (26 minutes) (De Filmmakkers, 2021) and "Ageing….and then what?" (33 minutes) (De Beeldschermers, 2024).

When the documentaries were ready, they were shown in the local theater during a festive event. Here, the results were also discussed in a panel with the alderman, a representative of a social housing initiative, and one of the older adults who produced the film. They discussed the significance of the results together, as well as with the people in the audience, who were all professionals who work in the field of housing, care or welfare and older adults themselves. In addition, the films were shown and discussed in community centers, housing initiatives and in meetings organized by the municipality with board members of housing, care and welfare organizations working together on the topic of aging in place.

The project demonstrated valuable results for participants, community strengthening, reflection and sparking discussions on aging and living environments. During the process of making a film together, participants (re)discovered talents and skills and engaged in new adventures, reflected on their everyday environment, highlighting the individual changes brought about by the project. Additionally, the project fostered new networks and cross-connections among participants.

The impact of the film as a product lies in the awareness it raises. Film is perceived as a valuable medium for representing experiences and communication of knowledge in an experiential way (MacDougall, 2006, 1998). When the film was viewed by other older adults in community centers, it prompted viewers to consider their own living options and how they want to age in meaningful ways. When shown to care and welfare professionals and students, municipal officials and architects, the films can provide insight into the lives and perspectives of older adults sparking meaningful discussions between professionals and older adults about future possibilities.

Increased awareness among participants and viewers also led to concrete actions: two participants moved to new homes, one participant registered in a new group housing initiative and new activities were initiated within their own community after reflecting within the group and "feeling inspired by people in the film". The municipality acted by establishing a connection with the each group shown in the video material, as they learnt about new informal networks in their municipality.

The project's impact extended to municipal and participatory engagement, with the groups of older adults continuing to show the films within the municipality and also participating in other meetings about aging in place. This initiative engaged a different group of older adults than usual reached by the municipality. Participation projects often struggle with diversity and representation, as participants may not adequately reflect the larger group (van Hoof, 2021b; van de Bovenkamp, 2013). These projects often demand specific skills, like articulating needs and speaking up in meetings, which can exclude certain groups and favor highly educated individuals (Vossen, 2010; PGO Support, 2019; van de Bovenkamp and Trappenburg, 2009). Participatory video opened up space for participants to share stories and experiences through different means, providing routes to participate in ways suitable for them.

Various important insights were gained through these participatory video projects. First of all, in creating contexts where older adults participate in meaningful ways, it is important to develop methods suited for older adults with different backgrounds. Second, participatory video can be a promising method in co-creating age-friendly cities together with older adults. Third, the process of making a film together through a participatory video format can foster reflection on themes related to aging in place and can bring positive changes for individuals and communities and strengthen participation. And fourth, the end-product (the film) can make an impact by increasing awareness of topics related to aging in place, among participants, older adults, policymakers and healthcare and social work professionals. These combined insights allow opportunities for strengthening community-centered care and promote active engagement of older people.

Afterthoughts

The previous sections have highlighted three projects from Europe in which older persons and their support networks were actively engaged in making their communities more age-friendly, with a particular focus on indoor and outdoor environments. These projects illustrated various degrees of participation, as described by Arnstein's ladder of citizen participation (Arnstein, 1969), where involvement ranged from consultation to partnership and even delegated power. Importantly, some projects have the potential to influence policymaking and even political decision-making, with outcomes that could be integrated into age-friendly action programs at the community or city level. By employing a diverse set of methodologies, these projects have shown that older people can significantly contribute to shaping their communities, enhancing the quality of life across several age-friendly domains, including social participation, respect and social inclusion, community support and health services and the design of outdoor spaces and buildings.

For example, in the geoportal development project, older adults from different cities were involved in co-creating tools that reflected their unique experiences and needs in urban environments. This participatory approach ensured that the tools developed were relevant and meaningful, aligning with McCormack and McCance's (2016) emphasis on shared decision-making and holistic care. Creating a person-centered community environment involves designing spaces that support autonomy and social participation. This was evident in the participatory video initiatives in the Netherlands. In this project, in the example of the Delft project, older adults were not just passive recipients of pre-defined services but active participants who documented their experiences and preferences regarding local housing and outdoor spaces. This aligns with the Gothenburg Model's (Britten et al., 2017) emphasis on inclusive engagement, ensuring that the voices of older adults are central in all stages of decision-making. The Gothenburg Model also advocates for shared decision-making, where older adults collaborate with planners and policymakers to develop solutions that cater to the diverse needs of the community.

Moreover, the Gothenburg Model emphasizes the sustainable implementation of community initiatives. Changes and developments should not only meet immediate needs but also be adaptable to future community shifts. In the Age-friendly Environments Activists project, older adults were trained to advocate for age-friendly changes that would not only benefit them now but also future generations, ensuring the sustainability of these initiatives. This long-term perspective supports person-centered care by ensuring that community environments remain responsive to the evolving needs of older adults, thereby promoting long-term health and well-being.

The integration of person-centered care principles into community settings is crucial for fostering environments that are supportive, inclusive and conducive to the well-being of all community members, particularly older adults. Both the Gothenburg Model and McCormack and McCance's framework provide valuable insights into achieving these goals through inclusive engagement, shared decision-making and sustainable implementation. By focusing on outcomes that enhance well-being and inclusion, communities can develop initiatives that not only improve the quality of life for older adults but also contribute to the overall health and vibrancy of the entire community.

In conclusion, the European projects discussed in this chapter serve as exemplars of how person-centered care principles can be effectively applied at the community level by prioritizing the needs and preferences of older adults and actively involving them in the planning and implementation of community initiatives. Future efforts should continue to build on these foundations, ensuring that the principles of person-centered care guide the development of environments that empower older adults and foster a sense of belonging and community for all.

Funding Acknowledgments

Case study 1 is a deliverable of the project City&Co: Older Adults Co-Creating a Sustainable Age-friendly City (JPI project number 99950200). This project was funded by the Taskforce for Applied Research (UTC.01.1), National Science Centre (UMO-2021/03/Y/HS6/00213) and Executive Agency for Higher Education, Research, Development and Innovation Funding (UEFISCDI) (Contract nr: 298 / 2022), as part of ERA-NET Cofund Urban Transformation Capacities (ENUTC), co-funded by the European Union's Horizon 2020 research and innovation program under Grant Agreement No. 101003758. Case study 2: Call 2018 Erasmus+, round 1, Key Action 2 Strategic Partnership Project. Cooperation for innovation and the exchange of good practices. KA220 – Cooperation partnerships in adult education. Age-friendly Environment Activists, Grant Number 2018-1-LT01-KA204–046947. Case study 3 is a joint deliverable of the Project Den Haag Filmt (*The Hague Films*), funded by Stichting RCOAK – Roomsch Catholijk Oude Armen Kantoor (grant reference 2019.279) and Werkplaats Sociaal Domein Den Haag & Leiden (*Regional Networks for the Social Welfare Domain The Hague & Leiden*), funded by the Ministry of Health, Welfare and Sport of the Netherlands (grant reference 330119).

Note

1 Geodata data, also known as geospatial data or geographic data, refer to information tied to a specific location on Earth. This location can be determined based on coordinates (latitude and longitude) or spatial relationships with other features.

References

Angelidou, M. (2016). Four European smart city strategies. *International Journal of Social Science Studies*, 4, 18–30. https://doi.org/10.11114/ijsss.v4i4.1364

Arnstein, S. R. (1969). A ladder of citizen participation. *Journal of the American Institute of Planners*, 35, 216–224. https://doi.org/10.1080/01944366908977225

Aslanoglu, R., Chrobak, G., van Hoof, J., Perek-Bialas, J. M., Ivan, L., Tavy, Z. K. C. T., Maj, M. & Kazak, J. K. (2024). A roadmap for the design of a public participation Geographic Information System to support urban ageing. *Geomatics and Environmental Engineering,* 18(5), 113–134. https://doi.org/10.7494/geom.2024.18.5.113

Britten, N., Moore, L., Lydahl, D., Naldemirci, O., Elam, M. & Wolf, A. (2017). Elaboration of the Gothenburg model of person-centred care. *Health Expectations,* 20, 407–418.

Buffel, T. (2019). Older coresearchers exploring age-friendly communities: An "insider" perspective on the benefits and challenges of peer-research. *The Gerontologist,* 59, 538–548.

Davern, M., Winterton, R., Brasher, K. & Woolcock, G. (2020). How can the lived environment support healthy ageing? A spatial indicators framework for the assessment of age-friendly communities. *International Journal of Environmental Research & Public Health,* 17, 7685.

De Beeldschermers (May 8th, 2024). *Ouder worden...en dan?* [Video]. Retrieved from YouTube. https://www.youtube.com/watch?v=fBdDrUIhkWI

De Filmmakkers (September 28th, 2021). *Van deur tot deur* [Video]. Retrieved from YouTube. https://www.youtube.com/watch?v=9eBl30Kty7E

Dempsey, C. (2014). What is the difference between a heat map and a hot spot map? *Geography Realm.* Retrieved from https://www.geographyrealm.com/difference-heat-map-hot-spot-map/

Dikken, J., van den Hoven, R. F. M., van Staalduinen, W. H., Hulsebosch-Janssen, L. M. T. & van Hoof, J. (2020). How older people experience the age-friendliness of their city: Development of the age-friendly cities and communities questionnaire. *International Journal of Environmental Research & Public Health,* 17, 6867.

Gardiner, P., Goldman Rosas, L., Rodriguez Espinosa, P., Winter, S. J., Sheats, J., Salvo, N, Aguilar-Farias, D., Stathi, A., Akira Hino, A. & Porter, M. M. (2020). On behalf of the Our Voice Global Citizen Science Research Network: Employing participatory citizen science methods to promote age-friendly environments Worldwide. *International Journal of Environmental Research & Public Health,* 17, 1541.

Grant, T. L., Edwards, N., Sveistrup, H., Andrew, C. & Egan, M. (2010). Inequitable walking conditions among older people: Examining the interrelationship of neighbourhood socio-economic status and urban form using a comparative case study. *BMC Public Health*, 10, 677.

James, H. & Buffel, T. (2023). Co-research with older people: A systematic literature review. *Ageing & Society*, 43, 2930–2956. https://doi.org/10.1017/S0144686X21002014.

Kazak, J. K., van Hoof, J., Swiader, M. & Szewranski, S. (2017). Real estate for the ageing society - The perspective of a new market. *Real Estate Management and Valuation,* 25, 13–24.

Kent, A. J. & Specht, D. (Eds.). (2023). *The Routledge Handbook of Geospatial Technologies and Society.* Taylor & Francis, New York.

MacDougall, D. (Ed.). (1998). *Transcultural Cinema.* Princeton University Press, Princeton.

MacDougall, D. (Ed.). (2006). *The Corporeal Image: Film, Ethnography, and the Senses.* Princeton University Press, Princeton.

Marston, H. R., Shore, L., Stoops. L. & Turner. R. S. (2022). *Transgenerational Technology and Interactions for the 21st Century: Perspectives and Narratives.* Emerald Publishing, Bingley.

McCormack, B. & McCance, T. (Eds.). (2016). *Person-Centred Practice in Nursing and Health Care: Theory and Practice.* (2nd ed). Wiley Blackwell, Chichester.

Middlesbrough (2024). *Middlesbrough Age-Friendly Charter. Middlesbrough, United Kingdom.* Retrieved from https://www.middlesbrough.gov.uk/adult-social-care/age-friendly-middlesbrough/age-friendly-middlesbrough-charter/

Municipality of The Hague (2020). *Seniorvriendelijk Den Haag. Actieprogramma 2020–2022.* The Hague: *Municipality of The Hague.* Retrieved from https://denhaag.raadsinformatie.nl/document/9555773/1/RIS307178_bijlage

PGO Support (2019). *De participatieladder voor wetenschappelijk onderzoek.* Retrieved from https://participatiekompas.nl/de-participatieladder-voor-wetenschappelijk-onderzoek

Phelan, A., McCormack, B., Dewing, J., Brown, D., Cardiff, S., Cook, N. F., Dickson, C. A. W., Kmetec, S., Lorber, M., Magowan, R., McCance, T., Skovdahl, K., Štiglic, G. & van Lieshout, F. (2020). Review of developments in person-centred healthcare. *International Practice Development Journal,* 10(Suppl), 1–29.

Ronzi, S., Orton, L., Buckner, S., Bruce, N. & Pope, D. (2020). How is respect and social inclusion conceptualised by older adults in an aspiring age-friendly city? A photovoice study in the North-West of England. *International Journal of Environmental Research & Public Health,* 17, 9246.

Sanoff, H. (2011). Multiple views of participatory design. *Focus,* 8, 11–21.

Stojanovski, D., Chorbev, I., Dimitrovski, I. & Madjarov, G. (2016). Social networks VGI: Twitter sentiment analysis of social hotspots. In *European Handbook of Crowdsourced Geographic Information.* (Capineri, C., Haklay, M., Huang, H., Antoniou, V., Kettunen, J., Ostermann, F. & Purves, R. eds.). Ubiquity Press, London, 223–236.

Swiader, M. & Lukowiak, M. (2016). Spoleczna waloryzacja przestrzeni zyciowej na przykladzie miasta Wolów (Polska, województwo dolnoslaskie) [eng. The social valorization of life space for Wolów city (Lower Silesia, Poland)] *Problemy Rozwoju Miast,* 3, 13–22.

Tavy, Z. K. C. T., van Bochove, M. E., Dikken, J., von Faber, M., Rusinovic, K. M., van der Pas, S. & van Hoof, J. (2022). The participation of older people in the development of group housing in the Netherlands: A study on the involvement of residents from organisational and end-user perspectives. *Buildings,* 12, 367.

Tupasela, A., Devis Clavijo, J., Salokannel, M. & Fink, C. (2023). Older people and the smart city: Developing inclusive practices to protect and serve a vulnerable population. *Internet Policy Review,* 12, 1–21.

van de Bovenkamp, H. M. & Trappenburg, M. J. (2009). Reconsidering patient participation in guideline development. *Health Care Analysis,* 17, 198–216.

van de Bovenkamp, H., Vollaard, H., Trappenburg, M. & Grit, K. (2013). Voice and choice by delegation. *Journal of Health Politics, Policy and Law,* 38, 57–87.

van Hoof, J. & Marston, H. R. (2021). Age-friendly cities and communities: State of the art and future perspectives. *International Journal of Environmental Research & Public Health,* 18, 1644.

van Hoof, J., Marston, H. R., Brittain, K. R. & Barrie, H. R. (2019). Creating age-friendly communities: Housing and technology. *Healthcare,* 7, 130.

van Hoof, J., Marston, H. R., Kazak, J. K. & Buffel, T. (2021a). Ten questions concerning age-friendly cities & communities and the built environment. *Building and Environment,* 199, 107922.

van Hoof, J., Rusinovic, K. M., Tavy, Z. K. C. T., van den Hoven, R. F. M., Dikken, J., van der Pas, S., Kruize, H., de Bruin, S. R., van Bochove, M. (2021b). The participation of older people in the concept and design phases of housing in The Netherlands: A theoretical overview. *Healthcare,* 9, 301.

van Vliet, J., Ligthart, M., Boon, M. & van der Pas, S. (2018). Leeftijdsvriendelijke stad in beeld: Documentaires maken met ouderen. *Geron,* 20, 56–59.

Ververda, J. & Hauge, S. (2019). Implementing active care through (cultural) activities of daily living: A person-centred approach to achieve flourishing. *Nursing Open,* 6, 583–590.

von Faber, M., Tavy, Z. & van der Pas, S. (2020). Engaging older people in age-friendly cities through participatory video design. *International Journal of Environmental Research & Public Health,* 17, 8977.

Vossen, C., Slager, M., Wilbrink, N. & Roetman, A. (2010). *Handboek participatie voor ouderen in zorg- en welzijnsprojecten.* CSO, Utrecht.

White, S. A. (2003). Participatory video: A process that transforms the self and the other. In *Participatory Video: Images that Transform and Empower* (White, S. A. ed.). Sage Publications, London. pp. 63–101.

Willberg, E., Fink, C. &Toivonen, T. (2023). The 15-minute city for all? Measuring individual and temporal variations in walking accessibility. *Journal of Transport Geography,* 106, 103521.

World Health Organization (2007). *Global Age-Friendly Cities: A Guide.* World Health Organization, Geneva.

World Health Organization Regional Office for Europe (2016). *Creating Age-Friendly Environments in Europe. A Tool for Local Policy-Makers and Planners.* WHO Regional Office for Europe, Copenhagen.

16

APPROACHES IN EDUCATION FOR PERSON-CENTERED AND COMMUNITY-CENTERED CARE

Amanda Phelan, Deirdre O'Donnell and Gobnait Byrne

Introduction

In the last number of years, there has been a deepening interest in innovation in third-level education and the promotion of student-orientated learning (Khalaf & Mohammed, 2018). As discussed in previous chapters in this book, communities are diverse, transcending geographical boundaries and include educational settings. Educational environments engender a sense of belonging, affiliation and a shared history (Chavis & Lee, 2015). This is demonstrated within artifacts such as school uniforms, crests or logos, college merchandize and institutional-related sporting activities. For former students, this connection to communities is frequently perpetuated through alumni relations and can be evidenced through activities such as continued following of sports teams or benefactor donations to former affiliated educational institutions. Within the system of third-level institutions itself, students are perceived as adults, where self-concept is consolidated in becoming a self-directed, autonomous learner wherein the adult learner experience translates to student maturation and is intricately linked to experience (Knowles, 1970), agency and creation (van der Walt, 2019). In a mini-systematic review of trends in educational programs and curriculum evaluation models undertaken by Nouraey et al. (2020), 63 papers were examined. Findings focused on theoretical bases and empirical foundations and concluded that the contextual arrangements, the purpose of the course and the expected learning outcomes underpinned curriculum models and program evaluation. Historically, learning has been within a power imbalance, where educators applied didactic methods to teaching, learning and assessment. The student passively received knowledge and skills while evaluation was dominated by traditional modes of assessment such as examination and assignments. Within a person-centered approach to education, the student is constituted as an active co-learner, who journeys

DOI: 10.4324/9781032662657-19

through an educational experience that includes mutuality in learning with educators, self-awareness and self-development. This chapter provides the background to the process and outcome of a European Union (EU) Erasmus-funded project with six countries which involved the co-development of a framework applying person-centered approaches to healthcare programs in third-level institutions using the McKinsey 7S (Waterman, 1980; Waterman et al., 1980) business model approach.

Curricula Transformation

Within healthcare service delivery, many organizational and policy agendas explicitly focus on person-centered care as a foundational philosophy (Health Service Executive, 2013; Health Foundation, 2016; Phelan et al., 2020; Australian Commission on Safety and Quality in Healthcare, 2022). In addition, health and social care curricula for various professionals include content that discusses the theory of person-centered care as a culture of service delivery and implementation in clinical practice. However, there remains a paradox. If we expect students to practice in a person-centered way, imbued with democratic partnerships, and safe spaces for whole-person learning and co-creation, should we not reflect this culture in the educational system (academic and clinical) in the context of student facilitation and engagement, organizational coherence, effective staff teams, appropriate skill mix and within program delivery and experience? Accordingly, curricula must intentionally enable and be experienced as person-centered, permeated with an orientation toward staff and students' learning and development, regardless of the physical site (McCormack et al., 2024). In other words, educators must address any theory-practice gap (Monaghan, 2015; Greenway et al., 2019) ensuring congruence across the formal academic setting and within all clinical areas that foster student placements. Moreover, curricula need to acknowledge and respond to domains that can often be overlooked. For example, in medical education, Torralba et al. (2020) discuss the need for psychological safety in learning environments and the need to recognize and be responsive to the hidden curriculum which encompasses the norms, behaviors and values within the culture of the environment. Equally, Clarke et al. (2015) note the need for organizational and system support within pedagogical transformations while the Office for Economic Co-operation and Development (OECD, 2019) points to the need for students to be supported to gain transformational competencies.

McArdle and Luiking (2022) suggest that applying a person-centered curriculum framework (PcCF) can potentially enhance cultures of care by having students experience person-centeredness embedded in their learning. Yet, an authentic focus on learning underpinned by person-centered principles can be lacking (O'Donnell et al., 2020). Thus, to transform program delivery, an Erasmus+ project focused on the development of a PcCF from 2019 to 2022.

For this project, two foundational anchors were stated:

Anchor 1 developed an agreed definition of what constitutes a shared curriculum. It is defined as:

> A Shared Curriculum Framework (SCF) is a complex system comprising facilitators of shared learning in community, and whose actions contribute to a common goal of supporting the design, delivery and evaluation of person-centred healthcare education [globally]. The use of a SCF creates consistency across education programmes, generates foundations for research and development, and supports the creation of pedagogical tools (teaching, learning, and evaluation) that align with the underpinning principles of the framework.

Anchor 2 looked at shared values within the curriculum's operationalization based on:

> A person-centred culture enables effective engagement based on the formation and fostering of healthful relationships between all persons. It has explicit values of respect for persons' self-determination, mutual respect and understanding. It creates the conditions for all persons to engage in continuous development and self/group/community/societal transformation.

One of the outputs of the project was to apply the McKinsey 7S (Peters & Waterman, 1982; McKinsey & Company, 2008) model as a lens to develop a PcCF that could be used by health and social care educators (academic and clinical) internationally (McCormack et al., 2022; O'Donnell et al., 2022; Cook et al., 2022; McCormack et al., 2024). Developed in the late 1970s, the McKinsey 7S model was promoted as "useful in diagnosing the causes of organizational malaise and in formulating programs for improvement" (Waterman, 1982: 68). Channon and Caldart (2015) indicate that this model transcends the classic simplistic assumption that structure follows strategy by incorporating five additional elements, namely, systems, style, staff, skills and shared values. The McKinsey 7S model has been developed and used as an analytical tool within organizational systems to examine their effectiveness and employee satisfaction and to improve success through implementing changes to strengthen teams and maximize operational efficacy and productivity (Bryan, 2008; Gechkova & Kaleeva, 2020). Examples of its diverse application include corporate succession (Putri et al., 2021), library data management (Lui, 2020), business start-ups (Putra et al., 2019; Mamun et al., 2020), hotels' effectiveness as organization (Odeh, 2021), dementia care in acute hospitals (Scerri et al., 2020) and digital transformation (Demir & Kocaoglu, 2019). Overwhelmingly, the McKinsey 7S model has been used to examine organizational systems, particularly within a commercial domain. Consequently, its application in the context of framing educational curricula is novel.

The McKinsey 7S has seven components as detailed in Figure 16.1. Each component is interlinked and important in analyzing and positioning the organization.

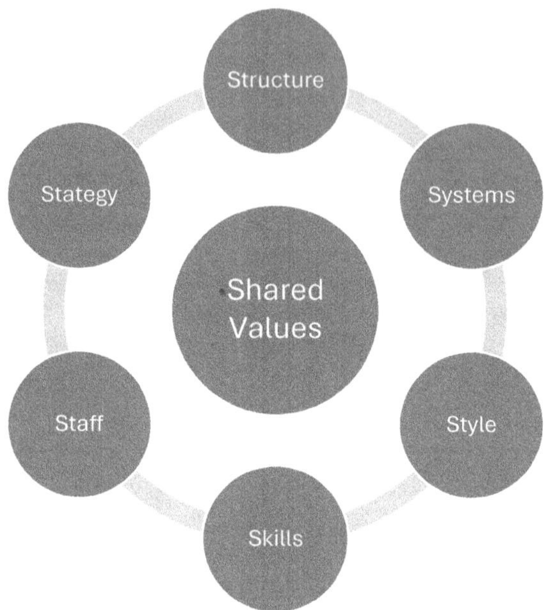

FIGURE 16.1 The components of the 7S model

Strategy, structure and systems are considered "hard" components as they are relatively concrete and easy to define and can be explicitly influenced by managers. The "soft" components (staff, style, skills) are less tangible and are influenced by the organizational culture (Gechkova & Kaleeva, 2020). Shared values are placed in the center as they bridge both "hard" and "soft" elements.

The elements of each S are demonstrated in Table 16.1, integrating descriptions from the work of Channon and Caldart (2015). This also presents a translation of the 7Ss to the context of the educational curriculum.

To achieve the full potential within the organization, all the Ss are presented in a non-hierarchical way to represent the need to have an equal focus on developing and fostering all domains.

Developing a PcCF

A team of educationalists, led by Professor Brendan McCormack from six different countries (Queen Margaret University, Edinburgh Scotland; Trinity College Dublin, Republic of Ireland; Ulster University, Northern Ireland; University of Applied Sciences, Utrecht, the Netherlands; University of Maribor, Slovenia: University of South-Eastern Norway, Norway), received funding from European Commission Erasmus + program to develop a PcCF for healthcare practitioners in Europe. The team agreed that the 7S framework provided a unique lens to develop a PcCF in the context of healthcare professionals' education (McCormack, 2022).

TABLE 16.1 The McKinsey 7S model and its translation to the context of educational curriculum

	Meaning	*Meaning in the context of educational curriculum*
Strategy	A set of actions the organization has in place to direct its response to the external environment. These provide the unique selling point and competitive advantage of the organization	Whole curriculum framework Identifies the unique selling point of the program and what makes it unique and attractive
Structure	Configuration of the organization. Incudes level of decentralization of decision-making, linkages between sections and ability to focus on components which are central to evolution and adaptability of the organization.	Structure of curriculum (modules/units/courses) to achieve intentions Institutional structure for curriculum
Systems	Ways which make the organization work-both formal and informal.	Teaching, learning and assessment methods used to achieve stated curriculum outcomes
Style	The type of leadership in the organization (micro-management versus detachment), risk-taking, market orientation and response pattern	Style of leadership used to deliver the curriculum.
Staff	Employees of the company. Transcends foci such as salaries and appraisals, morale, motivation and behavior. The model argues for a supportive environment which fosters young talent and career pathways.	General capabilities of the team delivering the curriculum. The make-up of the team and its "fit" with the curriculum intentions.
Skills	Capability evaluation of staff and mapping to changing environment	Knowledge, expertise, expertise and competencies of the academic team delivering the curriculum.
Shared values	A core element of the model. Key beliefs and objectives shared by the entire organization. Termed superordinate goals in the initial iteration of the model. Critical to the success of other components	Core values of the school/faculty/department and how these are made explicit in the curriculum.

This encompassed several project-related sequential methodological stages which are described below (see Figure 16.2).

Key to the development of the curriculum framework was the active involvement of all stakeholders in its development and direction. This reflects the principles of self-determination, autonomy, participation and collaboration to inductively

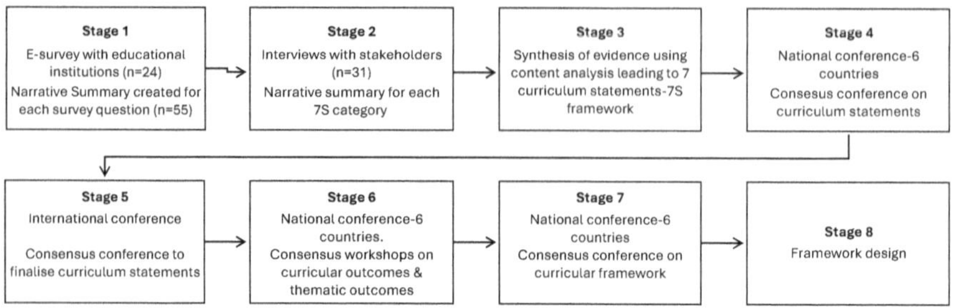

FIGURE 16.2 Overview of methodological stages (O'Donnell et al., 2022: 3)

empower participants to co-create the curriculum (Phelan et al., 2020). Stage 1 involved the development of an online survey, consisting of 35 open questions on the different components of the 7S framework. These questions focused on the existing curricula and participants were asked to comment on, for example, the stated values of the course team and how these values influenced curriculum delivery in their home institution. This questionnaire was distributed to healthcare educational leaders in different universities in Europe. The majority of participants ($n = 24$) were from three disciplines (nursing, medicine, occupational therapy) and responses were submitted from ten different countries (Australia, Germany, Malta, Northern Ireland, Norway, Republic of Ireland, Scotland, Slovenia, Sweden and the Netherlands) (O'Donnell et al., 2022). The project team analyzed the responses to the questions in teams and produced a narrative summary for each question.

The second stage comprised interviews with key stakeholders to further navigate the concept of person-centered care in healthcare professionals' education. Thirty-one online interviews were convened with students, educators and regulators from six different countries (Northern Ireland, Norway, Republic of Ireland, Scotland, Slovenia and the Netherlands). All interviews were recorded and varied in length from 20 to 70 minutes. Interviews were transcribed and findings mapped to the 7S Framework (O'Donnell et al., 2022). Following this, the third stage of the project involved the research team further analyzing the data from the online survey and interviews with key stakeholders to refine curriculum statements for the first draft of the PcCF. This process also included the development of draft outcome statements related to the implementation of a PcCF. To further validate the project outputs, stages four to seven included hosting both national conferences in the six collaborating countries and international conferences. During the national conferences, the draft statements were presented to key stakeholders in healthcare education. Participants were asked to review these statements to develop consensus on the PcCF statements. As a result of this consultation, the PcCF was revised. Subsequently, an international online conference was held in May 2021 where the second draft of PcCF was presented leading to further discussion and refinement of the statements.

Following the finalization of the PcCF statements within each of McKinsey's 7Ss, two further rounds of national conferences were held with the focus on ascertaining attendees' views on how this PcCF could be implemented in their programs. The outcomes of these discussions resulted in the development of thematic actions for each of 7S in the PcCF to support the implementation of the framework. Finally, the project team mapped the PcCF with the philosophical, methodological, learning environment's principles underpinning person-centered healthcare education (Dickson et al., 2020). Table 16.2 outlines the statement for one of the 7S (staff), the thematic actions and the mapping statements to the PcCF and learning principles.

Following the development of the PCCF, the team developed an essential guide to developing person-centered cultures in healthcare education and practice (McCormack, 2024). This guide has a chapter for each of the 7Ss and within each

TABLE 16.2 Example of McKinsey's 7S component related to staff, thematic actions and mapping statements within the PcCF (O'Donnell et al., 2022)

Staff	*Thematic actions: working toward statement*	*Mapping statements to the person-centered curriculum framework and principles*
All persons involved with the curriculum need to embody the values of person-centeredness through an explicit commitment to the facilitation of learning. Team capabilities need to be built on individual professional expertise that embraces the knowledge, skill and expertise to facilitate critical, reflexive, collaborative learning.	Build the complement of capabilities of the team to embody a culture of person-centeredness to enable delivery of a person-centered curriculum • Create sustainable opportunities for the academic team/education partners to develop their knowledge, skill, expertise and facilitation in critical, reflexive, collaborative learning and mentorship • Ensure job role specifications reflect the capabilities of the team needed to deliver a person-centered curriculum	Framework: Lifeworld Philosophical dimension: Co-constructed and Relational Methodological principle: • Curriculum encourages connectivity with self, other persons and contexts. • A co-constructionist approach to curriculum design and implementation where the curriculum is flexible and adaptive to the learner Learning environment: • Educators show courage, humility and vulnerability in the facilitation of learning • Critical questioning is embedded in learning processes

TABLE 16.3 Some activities focused on developing staff skills in facilitating a person-centered curriculum (adapted from Dunleavy et al., 2024).

Description of activity	*Aim of activity*
Person-centered simulation and reflection • Role play in simulated scenarios that highlight person-centered values	To develop a deeper understanding of person-centered values and practice them in real-life situations
Person-centered skill masters workshop	Enhance staff team's skills for delivering a person-centered curriculum
Identification of staff capabilities	Identify the staff capabilities and match talent with roles to foster team flourishing
Review of current induction program	Review current induction program to ascertain if it meets the needs of new staff and identify how to modify it to align to person-centered philosophy and curriculum.
"Flourish-O-Meter" evaluating staff and team development	To encourage staff to work together to evaluate progress and outcomes in the development of a person-centered culture and curriculum.

chapter, there are suggested activities to aid understanding. Dunleavey et al. (2024) identified some activities (see Table 16.3) focused on the staff component of the PcCF. These activities serve to develop the skills of staff as well as fostering a person-centered culture within educational institutions.

The utility of the PcCF is apparent within current commentaries on healthcare professionals' education. For example, recent research has identified that existing curricula in undergraduate nursing educational programs in Ireland have a strong focus on person-centered care, but this needs to be enhanced (Ryder et al. 2024). Equally, McAteer and Brown (2024) reported in their research study that participant paramedical students identified that their educational program was focused on person-centered practice; however, findings suggest the need to incorporate meaningful disciplinary application in practice environments and a generalized standardized language for person-centered concepts within healthcare. In this regard, the PcCF provides a useful guide for healthcare educationalists to explicitly embed person-centered care and its philosophy within curricula, while allowing for flexibility for related integrated disciplinary practice development.

The Application of Person-Centered Approaches in Higher Education

The core intention in developing the PcCF was to create a universal curriculum framework for person-centered health and social care practitioner education with relevance and applicability to contexts where learning occurs. The framework considers that person-centered principles are universal, albeit context-dependent, and therefore, it has relevance and can underpin both healthcare education and practice across disciplines. As the PcCF is underpinned and shaped by the McKinsey 7S methodology (Waterman, 1980; Peters & Waterman, 1982), it inherently applies ways of thinking about a complex system to educational contexts. The framework includes key considerations aimed at bringing about the conditions for developing healthcare practitioners to practice in person-centered ways which in some countries is a regulatory requirement (NMC 2018). Whilst the PcCF is an educational framework, its purpose is not education for education's sake but its potential to positively impact learning, self-knowing and practice outcomes (O'Donnell et al., 2020).

The PcCF is operationalized through thematic actions (O'Donnell et al., 2022). The thematic actions provide an implementation strategy for curriculum teams by offering a range of indicators that evidence person-centeredness in the curriculum. A set of thematic actions has been identified for each of the 7S elements. These provide pragmatic exemplars of how the 7S elements contribute to a holistic and effective curricular system. Thematic actions can apply to learning in academic and clinical settings. Fundamental to the effective functioning of the system is a reliance on shared values. In relation to person-centeredness in education, the curricular team's shared values should be mutually agreed upon to provide a frame of reference about ways of being and working. Importantly, team members hold themselves and others to account in implementing the PcCF. Consequently, shared values foster and sustain the healthy learning cultures that enable effective learning incubating the development of healthcare professionals with the knowledge, skills and commitment to advancing person-centered practice. The thematic actions are not offered as an exhaustive list of approaches but provide a basis to generate thought and discussion among curriculum teams that espouse person-centeredness. However, in addition to the thematic actions, it is acknowledged that learning facilitators will have other toolkits and strategies to draw upon that are specific to their discipline, curriculum, learning context and the S or Ss that they influence.

The pursuit of person-centeredness in healthcare education is a shared responsibility between all those who support and engage with learning associated with any aspect of the curriculum. It involves a commitment to enlivening shared values that are consistently manifest through ways of being and working. The PcCF recognizes that a curriculum is a dynamic and living phenomenon rather than a course document, an outcome to be achieved or a destination to be reached. Without an appreciation of the value of person-centered practice and a commitment to it, the curricular framework will remain aspirational and intangible. To truly embed person-centeredness, academic and practice learning teams, in collaboration with learners, people who use healthcare services and other stakeholders, depending on the context, are encouraged to consider and robustly evaluate how their values, knowledge and practices contribute to healthful learning cultures. By establishing an understanding of current successes and areas for further development at both individual and collective levels, the program team can continue to capitalize on person-centeredness in the curriculum to optimize its transformative impact in healthcare practice. However, there is a need to remain vigilant about the fact that a change in one or more of the 7Ss over time may impact the stability and effectiveness of the entire system. For this reason, it is considered prudent to factor in cycles of monitoring and enhancement activity to anticipate, identify and be responsive to changes in system dynamics.

One example of how a team has embraced person-centeredness in Higher Education is the work of the School of Nursing and Paramedic Science at Ulster University in Northern Ireland. The team has developed expertise in person-centeredness over almost two decades. Like many other Higher Education Institutions, the staff team supports an extensive portfolio of healthcare programs, including professionally regulated provision, across multiple campuses and modes of delivery, including fully online options. In addition, over 8,000 internationally educated nurses, nursing associates and midwives are assessed at the Nursing and Midwifery Council's Competence Test Centre at Ulster University. Against this backdrop, multiple curricula and approaches to learning and assessment have been developed, delivered and evaluated in partnership with a diverse range of stakeholders who work collaboratively to drive and embed person-centeredness in healthcare curricula. This approach enables the team to cultivate inclusive, authentic learning experiences that are healthful and responsive to the needs of individuals, communities and the health service. The work of the team extends locally, nationally and internationally. Central to this work is the belief that a curriculum philosophy should be explicit and of meaning to all who are engaged in supporting teaching and learning. The philosophy guides approaches and decision-making so that ways of working together are co-constructed, pragmatic and relational. In the context of a person-centered curriculum, the philosophy creates the vision of a transformative learning journey through a program of education that privileges personhood and values the contribution of all who are engaged in teaching and learning. This conceptual learning framework maps to recommendations within the OECD (2019) for students, where creating new value, reconciling tensions and dilemmas and taking responsibility are central transformative competencies to be embedded in curricula learning outcomes.

A person-centered curricular philosophy has collaboration at its core. The primary aim is to educate healthcare professionals with the prerequisites to practice in person-centered ways and to act as a role model and ambassador for person-centeredness. At Ulster University, this is achieved by leading innovation in curriculum design, developing educators (in academia and clinical settings) to facilitate and lead person-centered curricula and undertaking curriculum evaluation including pedagogic research to impact curriculum renewal. Agency is demonstrated by fostering inclusive, authentic learning experiences that are healthful and responsive to the needs of individuals, communities and the health service. This demands leadership to drive the translation of person-centeredness in healthcare curricula through a program of collaborative person-centered pedagogic research focused on improving healthcare education and practice across the healthcare education sector.

From its inception, the approach at Ulster University was to strategically influence the whole curriculum system to align a vision about the value of education in terms of its impact on learning and practice cultures. This began by identifying and embedding shared values through a culture change project that highlighted the need for values clarification and shared decision-making regarding the preferred curriculum philosophy. Agreement was gained in consultation with stakeholders to embed the curriculum in a person-centered ethos given its primacy in healthcare policy and practice. Team members were supported to undertake doctoral research in pedagogically aligned studies. For example, a regionally commended participatory action research project demonstrated how caring attributes of undergraduate student nurses could be developed and sustained over time when students learned in a program grounded in person-centered principles (Cook et al., 2018). Another study, within Ulster University, developed an instrument to measure students' perceptions of their person-centered practice (O'Donnell et al., 2021). The instrument was then used in a subsequent mixed methods study and the findings demonstrated that, on completion of their studies, and having experienced a person-centered curriculum, students' perceptions of their person-centered practice had improved (O'Donnell et al., 2022).

Concurrently, a priority focus was to facilitate meetings and workshops locally, regionally and internationally to develop a network of people with similar aspirations and were committed to the advancement of person-centered practice through Higher Education curricula. Those with expertise in facilitation worked with peers to cascade knowledge and skills which built capacity among educators in theory and practice contexts and the space and skills to re-imagine approaches to facilitating learning rather than the transactional banking of knowledge. Stakeholder engagement events became a routine and integral aspect of curriculum planning and development activities with investment in the co-development of the team and our partners. Mutuality was nurtured across the curricular community as a shared understanding of pedagogy and its relevance to supporting healthful learning cultures emerged. A summary of various approaches used to promote person-centeredness through pedagogic practice is shown in Table 16.4.

In recognition of outstanding impact, value and reach which has been verified as sector-leading in Higher Education, the team at Ulster's School of Nursing and Paramedic Science was awarded an Advance Higher Education Collaborative Award for Teaching Excellence in 2023.

TABLE 16.4 Approaches to promoting person-centeredness in healthcare curricula (drawn from developmental work by Brown et al., 2023)

Role modeling principles of mutuality and reciprocity
Including students, patients and carers, as key members of program approval teams and in course committee meetings
Co-designing and delivering curricula with students, service users, academic and practice partners
Supporting academic and practice learning facilitators to develop their knowledge of person-centeredness
Developing and sequencing modules across a curriculum to align with the curricular philosophy and curriculum framework
Creating psychologically safe environments where everyone can engage in collaborative, authentic and professional interactions to support learning and innovation
Designing authentic assessment aligned with person-centered approaches to practice
Translating a regional person-centered learning framework into a digital platform to support practice learning

Conclusion

This chapter has considered how community-centered care can be implemented in the third-level institutional setting. Using the principles of person-centered care and applying the McKinsey 7S framework has offered a unique way to conceptualize the development of health and social care curricula that traverse academic and clinical settings. Utilizing an organizational approach enables the intersectionality of reconfiguring structure, strategy, style, skill, staff and system which are founded on the shared values of personhood. This is reflected in a collaborative and creative journey for students, academics, healthcare staff, regulators and service users toward the goal of enabling flourishing, healthful lives within educational programs. While the impact has been demonstrated in Ulster University's implementation of person-centered curricula experiences, the PcCF offers flexible guidance for other third-level institutions to review, assess and transform their educational agendas and foci. Most importantly, such curricula can provide person-centered experiences within educational communities that translate to health and social care cultures, thus enriching not only the individual personhood of educational stakeholders but also the personhood of service user communities within the broader healthcare system.

References

Australian Commission on Safety and Quality in Healthcare (2022). *Person-Centred Care.* Retrieved from https://www.safetyandquality.gov.au/our-work/partnering-consumers/person-centred-care.

Brown, D., O'Donnell, D., Cook, N., Dunleavy, S., McCance, T. & McGarvey, H. (2023) *The Person-centred Collaborative Operational Group.* Ulster University submission for Advance HE Collaborative Award for Teaching Excellence [Unpublished].

Bryan, L. (2008). *The 7S Framework.* Retrieved from https://www.mckinsey.com/capabilities/strategy-and-corporate-finance/our-insights/enduring-ideas-the-7-s-framework.

Chavis, D. M. & Lee, K. (2015). What is community anyway? *Stanford Social Innovation Review.* Retrieved from https://doi.org/10.48558/EJJ2-JJ82

Channon, D. F. & Caldart, A. A. (2015). McKinsey 7S Model. In *Wiley Encyclopedia of Management* (Cooper, C.L., McGee, J. & Sammut Bonnici, T. eds). 12, 1.

Clarke, M., Kenny, A. & Loxley, A. (2015). *Creating a Supportive Working Environment for Academics in Higher Education: Country Report Ireland.* The Teachers' Union of Ireland and The Irish Federation of University Teachers, John Wiley & Sons, New Jersey: Dublin.

Cook, N. F., Brown, D., O'Donnell, D., McCance, T., Dickson, C. A. W., Tønnessen, S., Dunleavy, S., Lorber, M., Falkenberg, H. K., Byrne, B. & McCormack, B. (2022). The Person-centred curriculum framework: A universal curriculum framework for person-centred healthcare practitioner education? *International Journal of Practice Development, 12*(5). Retrieved from https://www.fons.org/library/journal/volume12-suppl/article4.

Demir, E. & Kocaoglu, B. (2019). The use of McKinsey's 7S framework as a strategic planning and economic assessment tool in the process of digital transformation, *Press Academia Procedia, 9*(1), 114–119.

Dickson, C., van Lieshout, F., Kmetec, S., McCormack, B., Skovdahl, K., Phelan, A., Cook, N. F., Cardiff, S., Brown, D., Lorber, M. & Magowan, R. (2020). Developing philosophical and pedagogical principles for a pan-European person-centred curriculum framework. *International Practice Development Journal, 10*(2), 1–20. https://doi.org/10.19043/ipdj.10Suppl2.004.

Dunleavy, S., Falkenberg, H. K., Cardiff, S. & Kmtec, S. (2024). Chapter 7- Staff. In: *Developing Person-Centred Cultures in Healthcare Education and Practice: An Essential Guide,* (McCormack, B. ed.). 157–192. Wiley Blackwell, London. pp. 157–192.

Gechkova, T. & Kaleeva, T. (2020). The McKinsey 7S model in the airport system protection. *Knowledge-International Journal, 42*(5), 843–848.

Greenway, K, Butt, G. & Walthall, H. (2019). What is a theory-practice gap? An exploration of the concept, *Nurse Education in Practice, 34,* 1–6.

Health Foundation (2016). *Person-Centred Care Made Simple What Everyone Should Know About Person-Centred Care.* Health Foundation, London.

Health Service Executive (2013). *Person-Centred Care and Support.* Retrieved from https://www.hse.ie/eng/about/who/qid/resourcespublications/qaandiworkbook1.pdf

Khalaf, B. K., & Mohammed Zin, Z. B. (2018). Traditional and inquiry-based learning pedagogy: A systematic critical review. *International Journal of Instruction, 11*(4), 545–564.

Knowles, M. S. (1970). *The Modern Practice of Adult Education: From Pedagogy to Andragogy.* Cambridge, New York.

Liu, H. (2020). Research on library data management reform: discussion on Mckinsey 7s system thinking model. *6th International Conference on Information Management (ICIM),* London, UK, 2020, pp. 295–298. https://doi.org/10.1109/ICIM49319.2020.244714

Mamun, M. Z., Syah, T. Y., Pusaka, S., & Darmansyah, H. S. (2020). Implementation of McKinsey 7S management strategy concepts for startup business: Fruit combining. *Russian Journal of Agricultural and Socio-Economic Sciences, 97,* 133–141.

McArdle, C. & Luiking, M. L. (2022). Implementing a pan-European Person-centred Curriculum Framework: The need for a strategic whole systems approach: Commentary. *International Journal of Practice Development, 12*(5). Retrieved from https://www.fons.org/Resources/Documents/Journal/Vol12Suppl2/IDPJ_12_Suppl_05.pdf

McAteer, L. & Brown, D. (2024). Exploring undergraduate paramedic students' understanding and experiences of person-centred care while on practice placement. *Paramedicine, 21*(5), 186–199. https://doi.org/10.1177/27536386241251499

McCormack, B. (2022). Developing a pan-European Person-centred Curriculum Framework: A whole systems approach, *International Journal of Practice Development, 12*(5). Retrieved from https://www.fons.org/Resources/Documents/Journal/Vol12Suppl2/IDPJ_12_Suppl_01.pdf

McCormack, B. (2024). *Developing Person-Centred Cultures in Healthcare Education and Practice: An Essential Guide.* Wiley Blackwell, London.

McCormack, B., Magowan, R., McCance, T., O'Donnell, D., Tønnessen, S., Štiglic, G., van Lieshout, F., Lorber, M., Kmetec, G., Phelan, A., Dickson, C., Dunleavy, S., Falkenberg, H. E., Cardiff, S., Cook, N., Byrne, G., & Brown, D. (2024). Introduction. In *Developing Person-Centred Cultures in Healthcare Education and Practice: An Essential Guide.* (McCormack, B. ed). pp. 1–28. Wiley Blackwell, London.

McCormack, B., Mcgowan, R., O'Donnell, D., Phelan, A., Štiglic, G. & van Lieshout, F. (2022). Developing a person-centred curriculum framework: A whole-systems methodology. *International Journal of Practice Development, 12*(5). Retrieved from https://www.fons.org/library/journal/volume12-suppl/article2

McKinsey & Company (2008). *Enduring Ideas: The 7-S Framework.* Retrieved from https://www.mckinsey.com/capabilities/strategy-and-corporate-finance/our-insights/enduring-ideas-the-7-s-framework

Monaghan, T. (2015). A critical analysis of the literature theoretical perspectives on the theory-practice gap amongst qualified nurses within the United Kingdom. N*urse Education Today, 35*(8), e1–e7. https://doi.org/10.1016/j.nedt.2015.03.006

Nouraey, P. & Al-Badi, A., Riasati, M. & Maata, R. L. (2020). Educational program and curriculum evaluation models: A mini systematic review of the recent trends. *Universal Journal of Educational Research, 8*, 4048–4055. https://doi.org/10.13189/ujer.2020.080930.

Nursing & Midwifery Council (2018). *Standards of Proficiency for Registered Nurses.* NMC, London.

Odeh, G. (2021). Implementing Mckinsey 7S model of organizational diagnosis and planned change, best Western Italy case analysis. *Journal of International Business and Management.* Retrieved from https://www.researchgate.net/profile/Ghadeer-Odeh-2/publication/355859980_Implementing_Mckinsey_7S_Model_of_Organizational_Diagnosis_and_Planned_Change_Best_Western_Italy_Case_Analysis/links/6188656261f09877206f112b/Implementing-Mckinsey-7S-Model-of-Organizational-Diagnosis-and-Planned-Change-Best-Western-Italy-Case-Analysis.pdf

O'Donnell, D., Dickson, C. A. W., Phelan, A., Brown, D., Byrne, G., Cardiff, S., Cook, N. F., Dunleavy, S., Kmetec, S. & McCormack, B. (2022). A mixed methods approach to the development of a Person-centred Curriculum Framework: surfacing person-centred principles and practices. *International Journal of Practice Development,* 1*2*(5). Retrieved from https://www.fons.org/Resources/Documents/Journal/Vol12Suppl2/IDPJ_12_Suppl_03.pdf.

O'Donnell, D., McCormack, B., McCance, T. & McIlfatrick, S. (2020). A meta-synthesis of person-centredness in nursing curricula. *International Practice Development Journal, 10*(Suppl 2), Article 2, 1–22. https://doi.org/10.19043/ipdj.10Suppl2.002.

O'Donnell, D., Slater, P., McCance, T., McCormack, B. & McIlfatrick, S. (2021). The development and validation of the Person-centred Practice Inventory-Student instrument: A modified Delphi study. *Nurse Education Today, 100.* https://doi.org/10.1016/j.nedt.2021.104826.

Organisation for Economic Cooperation & Development (OECD) (2019). *OECD Future of Education and Skills 2030 Conceptual Learning Framework: Transformative Competencies for 2030.* OECD, Paris.

Peters, T. J. & Waterman, R. H. (1982). *In Search of Excellence.* Harper & Row, New York.

Phelan, A., McCormack, B., Dewing, J., Brown, D., Cardiff, S., Cook, N. F., Dickson, C., Kmetec, S., Lorber, M., Magowan, R., McCance, T., Skovdahl, K., Štiglic, G. & van Lieshout, F. (2020). Review of developments in person-centred healthcare. *International Practice Development, 10*(3), https://doi.org/10.19043/ipdj.10Suppl2.003

Putra, R. P., Syah, T. Y., Pusaka, S. & Indradewa, R. (2019). Human resources implementation using the Mckinsey 7s method for business startup: duck nugget frozen food. *Journal of Multi-disciplinary Academics, 3*(3). Retrieved from https://www.kemalapublisher.com/index.php/JoMA/article/view/366

Putri, A. D., Ghazali, A. & Ahluwalia, L. (2021). Analysis of company capability using the 7S McKinsey framework to support corporate succession (Case study: part x Indonesia). *Manajemen Bisnis, 11*(1), 44–53.

Ryder, M., Browne, F., Curtin, M., Furlong, E., Connolly, M., Larkin, J., Geraghty, S., Prendergast, M., Meegan, M., Zampiero, N. & Brenner, M. (2024). *A Report of the Review of Undergraduate Nursing and Midwifery Curriculum leading to Registration in Ireland.* Retrieved from https://researchrepository.ucd.ie/entities/publication/125cffb2-c3dc-4b29-b93e-98e3e998469f/details

Scerri, A., Innes, A. & Scerri, C. (2020). Dementia care in acute hospitals-A qualitative study on nurse managers' perceived challenges and solutions. *Journal of Nursing Management, 28*(2), 399–406.

Torralba, K. D., Jose, D. & Byrne, J. (2020). Psychological safety, the hidden curriculum, and ambiguity in medicine. *Clinical Rheumatology, 39*, 667–671.

van der Walt, J. L. (2019). The term "self-directed learning"—Back to knowles, or another way to forge ahead? *Journal of Research on Christian Education, 28*(1), 1–20.

Waterman, J., Peters, T. & Phillips, J. (1980). Structure is not organization. *Business Horizons, 23*(3), 14–26.

Waterman, R. (1980). Structure is not organisation. *Business Horizons, 23*(3), 14–26.

Waterman, R. (1982). The seven elements of strategic fit. *Journal of Business Strategy, 3*, 68–72.

INDEX

Note: **Bold** page numbers refer to tables and *italic* page numbers refer to figures.

For Product Safety Concerns and Information please contact our EU representative GPSR@taylorandfrancis.com
Taylor & Francis Verlag GmbH, Kaufingerstraße 24, 80331 München, Germany

www.ingramcontent.com/pod-product-compliance
Lightning Source LLC
Chambersburg PA
CBHW072130170526
45158CB00004BA/1317

* 9 7 8 1 0 3 2 6 6 2 6 2 6 *